ETHNOBOTANY OF INDIA

Volume 3

North-East India and the Andaman and Nicobar Islands

ETHNOBOTANY OF INDIA

Volume 3

North-East India and the Andaman
and Nicobar Islands

Edited by
T. Pullaiah, PhD
K. V. Krishnamurthy, PhD
Bir Bahadur, PhD

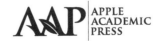

Apple Academic Press Inc.
3333 Mistwell Crescent
Oakville, ON L6L 0A2 Canada

Apple Academic Press Inc.
9 Spinnaker Way
Waretown, NJ 08758 USA

© 2018 by Apple Academic Press, Inc.

First issued in paperback 2021

Exclusive worldwide distribution by CRC Press, a member of Taylor & Francis Group
No claim to original U.S. Government works

Need to add somewhere, preferably on the copyright page.

Cover photo 1 by Wouter Hagens. Used with permission via public domain. https://commons.wikimedia.org/wiki/File:Houttuynia_cordata_A.jpg
Cover photo 2 by Karsten Heinrich. Used with permission via the Creative Commons Attribution license. https://commons.wikimedia.org/wiki/Category:Mahonia_napaulensis#/media/File:Mahonia_napaulensis_Nepal.JPG
Cover photo 3 by Kristian Peters. Used with permission under the terms of the GNU Free Documentation License. https://commons.wikimedia.org/wiki/Mentha_arvensis#/media/File:Mentha_arvensis.jpeg
Cover photo 4 by JeremiahsCPs. Used with permission by via public domain. https://commons.wikimedia.org/wiki/File:Nepenthes_khasiana.jpg

ISBN 13: 978-1-77-463121-8 (pbk)
ISBN 13: 978-1-77-188477-8 (hbk)

Ethnobotany of India, 5-volume set

International Standard Book Number-13: 978-1-77188-600-0 (Hardcover)
International Standard Book Number-13: 978-1-315-18662-7 (eBook)

Library and Archives Canada Cataloguing in Publication

Ethnobotany of India / edited by T. Pullaiah, PhD, K. V. Krishnamurthy, PhD, Bir Bahadur, PhD.
Includes bibliographical references and indexes.
Contents: Volume 3. North-East India and Andaman and Nicobar Islands.
Issued in print and electronic formats.
ISBN 978-1-77188-477-8 (v. 3 : hardcover).--ISBN 978-1-315-36583-1 (v. 3 : pdf)
1. Ethnobotany--India. I. Pullaiah, T., author, editor II. Krishnamurthy,
K. V., author, editor III. Bahadur, Bir, author, editor

GN635.I4E85 2016	581.6'30954	C2016-902513-6	C2016-902514-4

Library of Congress Cataloging-in-Publication Data

Names: Pullaiah, T., editor. | Krishnamurthy, K. V., editor. | Bahadur, Bir, editor.
Title: Ethnobotany of India. Volume 3, North-east India and Andaman and Nicobar Islands / editors: T. Pullaiah, K. V. Krishnamurthy, Bir Bahadur.
Other titles: North-east India and Andaman and Nicobar Islands Description: Waretown, NJ : Apple Academic Press, [2016] | Includes bibliographical references and index.
Identifiers: LCCN 2016022113 (print) | LCCN 2016024704 (ebook) | ISBN 9781771884778 (hardcover : alk. paper) | ISBN 9781315365831 ()
Subjects: LCSH: Ethnobotany--India, Northeastern. | Ethnobotany--India--Andaman and Nicobar Islands.
Classification: LCC GN476.73 .E857 2016 (print) | LCC GN476.73 (ebook) | DDC 581.6/309541--dc23
LC record available at https://lccn.loc.gov/2016022113

CONTENTS

List of Contributors .... *vii*

List of Abbreviations .... *ix*

Preface .... *xi*

Acknowledgements ....*xv*

Ethnobotany of India 5-volume Series .... *xvi*

About the Editors .... *xvii*

1. **Introduction** 1

   T. Pullaiah, K. V. Krishnamurthy, and Bir Bahadur

2. **Ethnic Diversity of North-East India** 15

   Shuvasish Choudhury, Bir Bahadur, K. V. Krishnamurthy,
   and S. John Adams

3. **Ethnoagriculture in North-East India: Pros, Cons,
   and Eco-Sustainable Model** 35

   Prabhat Kumar Rai

4. **Ethnic Food Plants and Ethnic Food Preparation
   of North-East India** 55

   Robindra Teron

5. **Ethnomedicinal Plants of North-East India** 93

   Suvashish Choudhury, Bir Bahadur, and T. Pullaiah

6. **Ethnobotany of Other Useful Plants in North-East India:
   An Indo-Burma Hot Spot Region** 163

   Prabhat Kumar Rai

7. **Ethnoveterinary Practices in Northeast India and Andamans** 177

   Bipul Saikia

8. **Ethnobotany of Andaman and Nicobar Islands** 207

   T. Pullaiah, Bir Bahadur and K. V. Krishnamurthy, S. John Adams,
   and Robindra Teron

9. **Documentation and Exchange of Ethnobotanical Knowledge**........... 249

C. L. Ringmichon and Bindu Gopalakrishnan

10. **Quantitative Ethnobotany: Its Importance in Bioprospecting and Conservation of Phytoresources**.. 269

Chowdhury Habibur Rahaman

11. **Ethnobotany of Turmeric and Its Medicinal Importance**.................. 293

Sujatha Samala and Ciddi Veeresham

12. **Traditional Use of Herbal Plants for the Treatment of Diabetes in India** 317

G. Revathi, S. Elavarasi, K. Saravanan, and Bir Bahadur

13. **Ethnobotany of Oral and Dental Problems in India**........................... 353

K. V. Krishnamurthy, Bir Bahadur, S. John Adams, and Gautam Srivastava

Index *375*

LIST OF CONTRIBUTORS

S. John Adams
Department of Pharmacognosy, R&D, The Himalaya Drug Company, Makali, Bangalore, India,
E-mail: s.johnadams13@gmail.com

Bir Bahadur
Department of Botany, Kakatiya University, Warangal–506009, India,
E-mail: birbahadur5april@gmail.com

Shuvasish Choudhury
Central Instrumentation Laboratory, Assam University, Silchar – 788011, India,
E-mail: shuvasish@gmail.com

S. Elavarasi
P.G. & Research Department of Zoology, Holy Cross College (Autonomous), Tiruchirappalli,
Tamilnadu, India

Bindu Gopalakrishnan
Department of Botany, Mithibai College, Vile Parle (W), Mumbai-56,
E-mail: bindu_phd@rediffmail.com

K. V. Krishnamurthy
Consultant, R&D, Sami Labs Ltd, Peenya Industrial Area, Bangalore–560058, India,
E-mail: kvkbdu@yahoo.co.in

T. Pullaiah
Department of Botany, Sri Krishnadevaraya University, Anantapur–515001, India,
E-mail: pullaiah.thammineni@gmail.com

Chowdhury Habibur Rahaman
Department of Botany, Visva-Bharati University, Santiniketan – 731235, West Bengal, India,
E-mail: habibur_cr@rediffmail.com, habibur_cr@yahoo.co.in

Prabhat Kumar Rai
Department of Environmental Science, School of Earth Science and Natural Resource Management,
Mizoram University, Aizawl–796004, Mizoram, India, E-mail: prabhatrai24@gmail.com

G. Revathi
P.G. & Research Department of Zoology, Nehru Memorial College (Autonomous),
Puthanampatti–621007, Tiruchirappalli, Tamilnadu, India

C. L. Ringmichon
K.V. Pendharkar College, Dept. of Botany, Dombivli (E), Thane Dist., Mumbai, Maharashtra,
E-mail: ringmi2005@rediffmail.com

Bipul Saikia
Department of Botany, Chaiduar College, Gohpur – 784168, Sonitpur, Assam,
E-mail: bipul_sai@yahoo.com

Sujatha Samala
University College of Pharmaceutical Sciences, Kakatiya University, Warangal, Telangana–506009,
India

K. Saravanan
P.G. & Research Department of Zoology, Nehru Memorial College (Autonomous),
Puthanampatti–621007, Tiruchirappalli, Tamilnadu, India,
E-mail: kaliyaperumalsaravanan72@gmail.com

Gautam Srivastava
Government Dental College and Hospital, Vijayawada, Andhra Pradesh, India

Robindra Teron
Department of Life Science and Bioinformatics, Assam University, Diphu Campus, Karbi Anglong,
Diphu, Assam – 782462, E-mail: robin.teron@gmail.com

Ciddi Veeresham
University College of Pharmaceutical Sciences, Kakatiya University, Warangal, Telangana–506009,
India, E-mail: ciddiveeresham@yahoo.co.in

LIST OF ABBREVIATIONS

BP	British Pharmacopoeia
BUN	blood urea nitrogen
CAI	cultural agreement index
CBD	convention on biological diversity
CI	cultural importance index
CII	cultural importance index
CPI	conservation priority index
CR	citation richness
DA	degree of attention
DM	diabetes mellitus
EI	ethnobotanicity index
EVP	ethnoveterinary practices
FAO	Food and Agricultural Organization
FL	fidelity level
HIV	human immunodeficiency virus
ICAR	Indian Council of Agricultural Research
IJTK	Indian Journal of Traditional Knowledge
IP	Indian Pharmacopoeia
IUCN	International Union for Conservation of Nature
IVI	importance value index
LCPI	local conservation priority index
NBPGR	National Bureau of Plant Genetic Resources
NE	north eastern
NER	north eastern region
NIDDM	non insulin dependent diabetes mellitus
NTFP	non-timber forest produce
PRA	participatory rural appraisal
QUAV	quality use agreement value
QUV	quality use value
RD	relative density
RFC	relative frequency of citation

RI	relative importance index
RRA	rapid rural appraisal
SOC	soil organic carbon
SQI	soil quality index
STZ	streptozotocin
TBGRI	Tropical Botanic Garden and Research Institute
TKDL	Traditional Knowledge Digital Library
USP	United States Pharmacopoeia
UV	use value
WHO	World Health Organization
WII	Wildlife Institute of India

PREFACE

Humans are dependent on plants for their food, medicines, clothes, fuel, and several other needs. Although the bond between plants and humans is very intense in several 'primitive' cultures throughout the world, one should not come to the sudden and wrong conclusion that post-industrial modern societies have broken this intimate bond and interrelationship between plants and people. Rather than plants being dominant as in the 'primitive' societies, man has become more and more dominant over plants after industrial revolution, leading to over-exploitation of the latter, and resulting in a maladapted ecological relationship between the two. Hence a study of the relationships between plants and people- ethnobotany and, thus, between plant sciences and social sciences, is central to correctly place humanity in the earth's environment. Because ethnobotany rightly bridges both of these perspectives, it is always held as a synthetic scientific discipline that bridges science and humanity.

Most people tend to think that ethnobotany, a word introduced by Hershberger in 1896, is a study of plants used by 'primitive' cultures in 'exotic' locations of the world, far removed from the mainstream people. People also think wrongly that ethnobotany deals only with non-industrialized, non-urbanized and 'non-cultured' societies of the world. Ethnobotany, in fact, studies plant-human interrelationships among all peoples and among all. However, since indigenous non-westernized societies form the vast majority of people now as well as in the past, a study of their interrelationships with people becomes important. Tens of thousands of human cultures have existed in the past and a number of them persist even today. They contain the knowledge system and wisdom about the adaptations with nature, particularly with plants, for their successful sustenance. Thus, ethnobotanical information is vital for the successful continuance of human life on this planet.

Ethnobotany is of instant use in two very important respects: (i) providing vital ecological knowledge, and (ii) source for economically useful plants. The first will help us to find solutions to the increasing environmental degradation and the consequent threat to our biodiversity. In indigenous societies biodiversity is related to cultural diversity and hence any threat to biodiversity would lead to erosion in cultural diversity. Indigenous cultures are not only repositories of past experiences and knowledge but also form the frameworks for future adaptations. Ethnic knowledge on economically useful plants has resulted in detailed studies on bioprospection for newer sources of food, nutraceuticals, medicines and other novel materials of human use. Bioprospecting has resulted in intense research on reverse pharmacology and pharmacognosy. This has given rise to attendant problems relating to intellectual property rights, patenting and the sharing of the benefits with the traditional societies who owned the knowledge. This has also resulted in efforts to seriously document all types of traditional knowledge of the different cultures of the world and to formalize the methods and terms of sharing this traditional knowledge. It has also made us to know not only *what* plants people in different cultures use and *how* they use them, but also *why* they use them. In addition it helps us to know the biological, sociological and cultural roles of plants important in human adaptations to particular environmental conditions that prevailed in the past, and may prevail in future.

This series of the five edited volumes on ethnobotany of different regions of India tries to bring together all the available ethnobotanical knowledge in one place. India is one of the most important regions of the old world which has some of the very ancient and culturally rich diverse knowledge systems in the world. Competent authors have been selected to summarize information on the various aspects of ethnobotany of India, such as ethnoecology, traditional agriculture, cognitive ethnobotany, material sources, traditional pharmacognosy, ethnoconservation strategies, bioprospection of ethnodirected knowledge, and documentation and protection of ethnobotanical knowledge.

The first volume is on *Eastern Ghats and Adjacent Deccan Region of Peninsular India,* while the second one is on *Western Ghats and Western Peninsular India.* This third volume is on *North-East India and Andaman and Nicobar Islands,* one of the Hot Spots of Biodiversity. Published information is summarized on different aspects. We have added three general chapters on ethnobotany of turmeric, dental care and antidiabetic plants.

Our intention is that the information contained in this volume may lead in future to discovery many new drugs, nutraceuticals, novel molecules and other useful products for the benefit of mankind.

Since it is a voluminous subject we might have not covered the entire gamut but we have tried to put together as much information as possible. Readers are requested to give their suggestions for improvement of the remaining volumes in this series.

ACKNOWLEDGMENTS

We wish to express our grateful thanks to all the authors who have contributed their chapters. We thank them for their cooperation and erudition. We also thank several colleagues for their help in many ways and for their suggestions from time to time during the evolution of this volume.

We wish to express our appreciation and help rendered by Ms. Sandra Jones Sickels and her staff at Apple Academic Press. Above all, their professionalism that made these books a reality is greatly appreciated.

We thank Mr. John Adams, Senior Research Fellow of Prof. K. V. Krishnamurthy, for his help in many ways.

We wish to express our grateful thanks to our respective family members for their cooperation.

We hope that this book will help our fellow teachers and researchers who enter the world of the fascinating subject of Ethnobotany in India with confidence.

—Editors

Ethnobotany of India 5-volume Series

Editors: T. Pullaiah, PhD, K. V. Krishnamurthy, PhD, and Bir Bahadur, PhD

Volume 1: Eastern Ghats and Deccan

Volume 2: Western Ghats and West Coast of Peninsular India

Volume 3: North-East India and the Andaman and Nicobar Islands

Volume 4: Western and Central Himalaya

Volume 5: The Indo-Gangetic Region and Central India

ABOUT THE EDITORS

T. Pullaiah, PhD

Former Professor, Department of Botany, Sri Krishnadevaraya University, Andhra Pradesh, India

T. Pullaiah, PhD, is a former Professor at the Department of Botany at Sri Krishnadevaraya University in Andhra Pradesh, India, where he has taught for more than 35 years. He has held several positions at the university, including Dean, Faculty of Biosciences; Head of the Department of Botany; Head of the Department of Biotechnology; and Member, Academic Senate. He was President of the Indian Botanical Society (2014), President of the Indian Association for Angiosperm Taxonomy (2013), and Fellow of the Andhra Pradesh Akademi of Sciences. He was awarded the Panchanan Maheswari Gold Medal, the Dr. G. Panigrahi Memorial Lecture Award of the Indian Botanical Society, the Prof. Y. D. Tyagi Gold Medal of the Indian Association for Angiosperm Taxonomy, and a Best Teacher Award from the Government of Andhra Pradesh. He has authored 45 books, edited 15 books, and published over 300 research papers, including reviews and book chapters. His books include *Flora of Eastern Ghats* (4 volumes), *Flora of Andhra Pradesh* (5 volumes), *Flora of Telangana* (3 volumes), *Encyclopedia of World Medicinal Plants* (5 volumes), and *Encyclopedia of Herbal Antioxidants* (3 volumes). He was also a member of the Species Survival Commission of the International Union for Conservation of Nature (IUCN). Professor Pullaiah received his PhD from Andhra University, India; attended Moscow State University, Russia; and worked as postdoctoral Fellow during 1976–78.

K. V. Krishnamurthy, PhD

Former Professor, Department of Plant Sciences, Bharathidasan University, Tiruchirapalli, India

K. V. Krishnamurthy, PhD, is a former Professor and Head of Department, Plant Sciences at Bharathidasan University in Tiruchirappalli, India, and is at present a consultant at Sami Labs Ltd., Bangalore. He obtained his PhD degree from Madras University, India, and has taught many undergraduate, postgraduate, MPhil, and PhD students. He has over 48 years of teaching and research experience, and his major research areas include plant morphology and morphogenesis, biodiversity, floristic and reproductive ecology, and cytochemistry. He has published more than 170 research papers and 21 books, operated 16 major research projects funded by various agencies, and guided 32 PhD and more than 50 MPhil scholars. His important books include *Methods in Cell Wall Cytochemistry* (CRC Press, USA), Textbook of Biodiversity (Science Publishers, USA), and *From Flower to Fruit* (Tata McGraw-Hill, New Delhi). One of his important research projects pertains to a detailed study of the Shervaroy Hills, which form a major hill region in the southern Eastern Ghats, and seven of his PhD scholars have done research work on various aspects of Eastern Ghats. He has won several awards and honors that include the Hira Lal Chakravarthy Award (1984) from the Indian Science Congress; Fulbright Visiting Professorship at the University of Colorado, USA (1993); Best Environmental Scientist Award of Tamil Nadu state (1998); the V. V. Sivarajan Award of the Indian Association for Angiosperm Taxonomy (1998); and the Prof. V. Puri Award from the Indian Botanical Society (2006). He is a fellow of the Linnaean Society, London; National Academy of Sciences, India; and Indian Association of Angiosperm Taxonomy.

Bir Bahadur, PhD
Former Professor, Department of Botany, Kakatiya University, Warangal, Telangana, India

Bir Bahadur, PhD, was Chairman and Head of the Department and Dean of the Faculty of Science at Kakatiya University in Warangal, India, and has also taught at Osmania University in Hyderabad, India. During his long academic career, he was honored with the Best Teacher Award by Andhra Pradesh State Government for mentoring thousands of graduates and postgraduate students, including 30 PhDs, most of whom went onto occupy high positions at various universities and research organizations in India and abroad. Dr. Bahadur has been the recipient of many awards and honors, including the Vishwambhar Puri Medal from the Indian Botanical Society for his research contributions in various aspects of plant Sciences. He has published over 200 research papers and reviews and has authored or edited dozen books, including *Plant Biology and Biotechnology* and *Jatropha, Challenges for New Energy Crop*, both published in two volumes each by Springer Publishers. Dr. Bahadur is listed as an Eminent Botanist of India, the Bharath Jyoti Award, New Delhi, for his sustained academic and research career at New Delhi and elsewhere. Long active in his field, he has a member of over dozen professional bodies in India and abroad, including Fellow of the Linnean Society (London); Chartered Biologist Fellow of the Institute of Biology (London); Member of the New York Academy of Sciences; and a Royal Society Bursar. He was also honored with an Honorary Fellowship of Birmingham University (UK). Presently, he is an Independent Director of Sri Biotech Laboratories India LTD, Hyderabad, India.

CHAPTER 1

INTRODUCTION

T. PULLAIAH,[1] K. V. KRISHNAMURTHY,[2] and BIR BAHADUR[3]

[1]*Department of Botany, Sri Krishnadevaraya University, Anantapur–515001, India, E-mail: pullaiah.thammineni@gmail.com*

[2]*Consultant, R&D, Sami Labs ltd, Peenya Industrial Area, Bangalore–560058, India, E-mail: kvkbdu@yahoo.co.in*

[3]*Department of Botany, Kakatiya University, Warangal–506009, India, E-mail: birbahadur5april@gmail.com*

CONTENTS

Abstract 1
1.1 Study Region 2
1.2 Vegetation and Flora 4
1.3 Ethnic Diversity 5
1.4 Utilization Aspects of Ethnobotanical Knowledge 6
1.5 General Reviews on Ethnobotany of India 10
Keywords 12
References 13

ABSTRACT

This introductory chapter summarizes the various aspects discussed in the subsequent 12 chapters of this volume dedicated to the Ethnobotany of North-East India and Andaman and Nicobar Islands. The first section deals with a description of the location, physiography, geological features, vegetation/forest types and flora. The second section summarizes the ethnic diversity of this region, its origin and its cultural, social and linguistic aspects. The third section gives an introduction to the various utilitarian aspects of the study region focusing on attention of ethnoagriculture, ethnofood plants/food system, ethnomedicinal plants, plants of ethnoveterinary importance, plants which are otherwise useful, ethnobotany of Andaman and Nicobar Islands and documentation and exchanges of ethnobotanical knowledge. The last section of this chapter deals with introductions respectively to the quantitative aspects of ethnobotany and ethnobotany of turmeric, antidiabettic plants and plants involved in oral and dental problems. This introduction to all these 12 chapters also emphasizes the type of future attention that needs to be focused on the various topics covered in these chapters.

1.1 STUDY REGION

The Indian subcontinent consists of Himalayan Mountains girdling the northern border, the more or flat Indogangetic plains in the middle, the uplands and plateaus of peninsular India and the narrow coasted plains along the seaboards. Each of these regions is structurally and lithographically contrasted and geomorphically distinct with different geoevolutionary histories (Valdiya, 2010). The Himalayan Mountain with its northwest, north and northeast parts isolated the Indian sub-continent from the rest of Eurasia. It is a 2,400 Km long and 300 to 400 Km wide mountain. It comprises the Kirthar and the Sulaiman mountain chains in the west, the main Himalaya in the center, and Patkai-Naga-Kachin-Arakan Yoma arcuate chains (of about 1,300 km long) of hills in the east. It embodies four physiographically contrasted terranes: the Siwalik, the Himachal (Lesser Himalaya), the Himadri (Greater Himalaya) and the Tethys Himalayas. The Siwalik part abruptly rises above the flat Indogangetic plains and is of 250 to 800 m height and forms the southern front of the Himalayas. North of the Siwalik is the outer Lesser Himalaya which consists of the Pir Panjal–Dhauladhar–Mussoorie–Nanital–Mahabharat Ranges; it is generally more than 2,000 m high. North of these in the central sector (Kumaun and Nepal) is the 600–2,000 m high middle lesser Himalayas. The Himadri or Greater Himalayas is Perennially snow-capped and extremely rugged (3,000 to more than 8,000 m in height). The most important Himalayan peaks are Nanga Parbat, Nun-Kun, Kedarnath, Badrinath, Nanda Devi, Doulagiri, Sagarmath or Everest, Kanchajangha and Namcha barwa. The Tethyys Himalaya lies beyond the Himadri. It is a cold desert bereft of vegetation on the whole. The Himalayan region ends up against the zone of collision of India with Asia. This is a 50–60 Km wide zone and is of 3,600 to 5,000 above mean sea level. North of this is the uplifted Tibet plateau.

As already stated the northeast Himalayas consists of Patkai-Naga-Kachin-Arakan Yoma arcuate chains of hills or the Indo-Myanmarese Range and the Arunachal Himalayan Ranges truncated by the Lohit-Mishmi Ranges. The Lohit terrane extends south-southeast into Myanmar, embracing the Malaysian province. Some peaks of the Patkai and Naga ranges are more than 4,000 m high; mount Victoria in Chin hills is 3,201 m high, while Mount Padaung in the Arakan Yoma is 1,3201 m high. The spectacular feature of the north-east Himalayas is the syntaxial knee-bend that extends southwards up to the Bay of Bengal and continues further south for another 1,700 km under water embracing in its sweep the island arc of Andaman and Nicobar. The Mishmi bends southwards in northern Myanmar, forming the 1,700 km long China, Myanmar border ranges. These ranges comprise the Kachin mountains in the north, the Shan Massif in the Middle and the Tenasserim Range in the south. The last one continues into the Malaysian Peninsula. The average elevation of these border ranges is 4,000 m.

An important geological feature of the North-East Indian is the extension of the Satpura range of hills. The Meghalaya massif of North-East India is an extension of the Satpura range; this range about against the Patkai-Arakan Yoma along the Indo-Myanmar border. The Meghalaya massif is also known as the Shillong plateau and consists of the Garo hills (900 m), the Khasi-Jaintia hills (1,500 m) and the Mikir hills (700 m). The Meghalaya massif is composed of pre Cambrian gneisses and metasedimentary rocks overlain by Cretaceous to tertiary sedimentary rock formations. The general elevation varies from 600 to 1,800 m and its highest peak (1,961 m) is the Shillong peak. This Massif deflects the Brahmaputra river westwards to skirt around the upland, before joining the Ganges river in Bangladesh. The Mikir hills are detached from the Meghalaya Masssif and occurs a midst the alluvial sediments of Brahmaputra (Valdiya, 2010). The Renga peak of 900 m high is located in Mikir hills. The states in North East India are Arunachal Pradesh, Assam, Manipur, Meghalaya, Mizoram, Nagaland, Tripura and Sikkim (Figure 2.1 of Chapter 2).

There is a 850 km long chain of islands between the Bay of Bengal and the Andaman Sea. This forms the central part of the 5,000 km long Myanmar-Indonesia mobile Belt. The Andaman, Nicobar and Mentawai groups (Figure 8.1 of Chapter 8). It is made up of upper Cretaceous-Tertiary flysch-Naga-Arakan Orogenic belt and active volcanoes. The island Arc is divided by the Ten Degree Channel of 150 km into the Andaman group and the Nicobar group of islands. The Maximum elevation of Andaman Islands is 732 m (Saddle peak) and of Nicobar Islands is 670 m (Thuiller Point). There are two volcanic islands also, namely Narcondam and Barren Islands.

1.2 VEGETATION AND FLORA

The Eastern Himalayas are far more evenly humid than the Western Himalayas because of the close vicinity of the former to the Bay of Bengal. This region catches the bulk of the monsoon. The highest humidity and heavy rains are conducive to vegetation growth and as a result its timber-line is up to 4,570 m as compared to 3,600 m only in the W. Himalayas. E. Himalayas is also far richer in species diversity and, in fact, is one of the richest botanical provinces of the world. Most of the states of this region have more than 60% of their area under forest cover. Four district vegetation regions are recognized on the basis of altitude and vegetation types: sub-tropical, temperate, sub-alpine and alpine; about 51 forest types are found in this region. Phytogeographically it is a distinct region, with a very rich flora including more than 4,000 species (Jain, 1982) and perhaps up to 7,000–8,000 species (Haridasan, personal communication), although many areas are still unexplored for their plant wealth. Some interesting aspects of the flora are as follows: (i) presence of more than 80 species of *Rhododendron*; (ii) rich representation of Zingiberaceae, particularly the genus *Hedychium*; (iii) rich in wild and cultivated bananas and in species of *Impatiens* (more than 200 species); the National Bureau of Plant Genetic Resources (NBPGR), India has highlighted this region as being rich in wild relatives of a few other crop plants; (iv) presence of taxa with disjunct distribution, such as *Celastrus stylosa, Malaxis acuminata,* and *Stellaria reticulata;* presence of primitive angiosperms like species of *Tetracentron, Euptelia,* and *Magnolia;* (v) presence of several floristic elements of other countries such as Tibet, Nepal, Myanmar, China, Malaysia, etc.; a list of such species is given in Jain (1982); (vi) very rich region in endemics; it is likely to contain more than 25% of Indian Endemics; (vii) presence of several species are of economic importance and these have been brought to our attention by the tribals of this region; (viii) rich in threatened plants taxa; more than 800 endangered plant species are known from this region; a partial list is provided in Jain (1982); (ix) one of the biodiversity hot spots of the world as well as a priority Global Ecosystem as per WWF; (x) the region has five National Parks and two Wild Life Sanctuaries.

The terrain of most of the islands in Andaman and Nicobar groups is hilly with undulating mountain ranges enclosing narrow valleys. The vegetation consists of the littoral swamps containing *Areca* and *Pandanus* and mangrove forests on the seashore and evergreen and mixed evergreen forests on the interior. The total forest area is around 200 km^2 (Dagar and Singh, 1999) in a total area of 8250 km^2. There is also man-made vegetation in the form of plantations. There are more than 2,650 species of vascular plants under 150 families (personal communication from Dr. D. Narasimhan). There are around 300 endemic plants many of which come under threatened categories (Dagar and Singh 1999; Sinha, 1999).

1.3 ETHNIC DIVERSITY

The North-East India is very rich in ethnic diversity. It is often described as the cultural mosaic of India with Diverse tribal communities and linguistic and ethnic identities. There are about 130 ethnic tribes with about 300 subtribes in this region, out of the about 427 to 450 tribes of the country (Chatterjee et al., 2006; Mao et al., 2009). The most important tribes are listed state-wise in Dutta and Dutta (2005). It is generally believed that humans had spread to different parts of India by the middle of Paleolithic period, including N. East India (Misra, 2001).

This region has about 220 languages coming broadly under Indo-European, Sino-Tibetan, Tai-Kadai and Austroasiatic that share some common structural features and Assamese, an Indo-Aryan language and its pidgin/creoles like Nagamese (in Nagaland) and Nefamese (in Arunachal Pradesh). The Austro-Asiatic Family is represented by Khasi, Jaintia and war of Meghalaya. The Tai-Kadai languages include Ahom, Tai Phake, Khamti, etc. The Sino-Tibetan languages are represented by Bodo, Rabha, Karbi, Mishing, Tiwa, Deuri, Garo, Ao, Tangkhul, Angami, Sema, Lotha, Konyak, Mizo, Hmar, Chakma, Hrusso, Tanee, Nisi, Adi, Abor, Nocte, Apatani, Misimi, etc. Manipuri and Naga languages such as Thadour, Paite, Sylheti, Tripuri, Bengali, etc. Indo-Tibetan languages include Limbu, Bhuta and Lepcha (Moral, 1997). Although the earlier religions of most ethnic communities were basic religions of animism and totemism now most of them follow Christianity followed by Hinduism, Buddhism, Islam, etc.

The Andaman and Nicobar Islands (also known as Bay Islands) are inhabited by six indigenous tribal populations: Great Andamanese, Onges, Jarawas, Sentineles, Nicobarese and Shom Pen. The studies by Thangaraj and his group (see Thangaraj et al., 2005) suggested that the Andamanese "Negritos" have closer affinities with Asian rather than with African populations, while the Nicobarese have originated in mainland S.E. Asian tribals and arrived from the east during the past 18,000 years. The Onge and the great Andamanese have evolved in the Andaman Islands independently from other south and S.E. Asian population. These lineages have likely been isolated since the initial penetration of the northern coastal areas of Indian Ocean by anatomically modern humans about 50,000 to 70,000 years ago. The very rich ethnic diversity of North-East India and Andaman & Nicobar Islands has resulted in very rich ethnobotanical knowledge exploiting the abundantly available floral elements. Choudhury et al. provide a detailed account on the ethnic diversity, culture and practices of people of N.E. Indian in Chapter 2 of this volume. The details on the ethnic diversity of Andaman and Nicobar Islands are given by Pullaiah et al. in Chapter 8.

1.4   UTILIZATION ASPECTS OF ETHNOBOTANICAL KNOWLEDGE

Traditional knowledge of primitive tribal and ethnic communities, both in the Old World and New World, have great relevance in three important spheres of human life: Utilitarian, cultural and social. These three spheres are not isolated from one another but are mutually interrelated and interdependent. Of these three Utilitarian sphere of traditional knowledge encompasses the ways and means of utilizing such knowledge on plants (and animals) relating to hunting-gathering, agriculture and associated crop biodiversity, food plants, medicinal plants, plants of ethnoveterinary importance and other requirements of humans as well as the identification of such source plants through bioprospecting.

Ever since the origin of modern humans in E. Africa around 200,000 years ago and his subsequent spread to different parts of the world initiated around 75,000 years ago, man has been exploiting various natural resources from the environment around him for all his different requirements until about 12,000 years ago from the present man has been a nomadic and hunter-gatherer and forager 12,000 years back, agriculture evolved and a settled life ensued for many human populations. Many useful plants that were identified during the hunter-gatherer stage were slowly beginning to be domesticated and brought into cultivation. Different forms of agriculture evolved depending on the landscape around human settlements and these included Jhum cultivation in hilly tracts and cultivation in plains using river water, ground water or rain-water. In India agriculture may be said to have been initiated around 6,000 to 8,000 years ago depending on the place. In North East region of India agriculture and farming have been the biggest occupation of the tribal people. This region water cultivation and these are continued till today by the diverse ethnic communities of this region. The major agricultural crops of this region are rice, tea, many fruit trees, dwarf cotton, bananas, curcumas, ginger, etc. It is recorded that Bodo community introduced rice and tea in this region. Rai has given a detailed account in Chapter 3 on ethno-agriculture of this region of India and how this agricultural activity is ecosustainable.

It is a very well-known fact that unlike the modern food systems (food resources and methods of preparation) those of the traditional communities of the world (including those in India) cover the full spectrum of life. They also use locally available food resources that are prepared according to local requirements and environmental conditions. However, in last few centuries a great disconnection has been caused between traditional ethnic communities and the food they used to prepare and take and the modern communities and their food. The main reasons for this are increased globalization, liberalization and homogenization of food and food resources. There was also the large-scale introduction of high-yield crops (which incidentally required high-put agricultural technologies, monoculture and use of chemical pesticides and fertilizers) that have almost replaced traditional crop varieties and land races of the local people. These crops have also largely degraded the ethnic agricultural ecosystems, partly the Jhum ecosystems of N. E. India. Moreover, modern food systems have introduced diet related chronic diseases as well as malnutrition, thus distorting greatly the local food safety and security. Thus, there is an urgent need to protect the food heritage and the health of the culturally-determined food systems of the local ethnic communities from being lost totally. Traditional foods are also of nutraceutical and therapeutic value. We have to document the local food resources after a detailed inventory and also the local food preparation techniques. In Chapter 4 of this volume, Robindra Teron has dealt in detail with ethnic food plants and food preparation of N. E. India. He has highlighted the intricate link between food systems and the ethnic linguistic, cultural and biological diversity. He has also highlighted the role of women in traditional food systems. He has raised serious concerns about the loss of wild food resources.

Ever since the emphasis made by botanists in many parts of the world about the utilitarian or economic approach to the study of ethnobotany from around the middle of the 20th century, people in different parts of the world have concentrated their attention on the traditional knowledge held by diverse ethnic communities. This ethnodirected approach to bioprospecting has resulted in the discovery and identification of several medicinally useful ethnic plant resources, particularly newer sources of nutraceuticals, pharmaceuticals and molecules of medicinal importance. North-East India has a rich niche ethnic diversity as well as floristic diversity, a combination of which has resulted in the very rich traditional knowledge on plants. Suvashish Chaudhury et al. have given a detailed account on the medicinal plants used by the diverse ethnic communities of N. E. India. Their account will form the basis for very intensive bioprospection studies in the coming years.

Plant species form the main source for a vast array of products used by mankind throughout the world. While some plants have been directly exploited from the wild with very little or some further processing many others need to be processed substantially. Some plant sources need to be brought under domestication and cultivation. One of the best means of knowing these plant resources is to go for ethnic knowledge as the traditional communities have been in constant association with nature over vast periods of history such knowledge on plant resources from these traditional communities has not been adequately translated into more wider and popular use. Besides foods and medicines as mentioned above, plants have been good sources of other human requirements such as ornamentals, timbers, fibers, dyes, fuel and a host of other materials. North-East India and its tribal knowledge have been a very good source of the above materials. Prabhat Kumar Rai has given a very useful account on the ethnobotany of other useful plants of N. E. India.

Many ancient ethnic communities are hunter-gatherers and/or nomadic pastorals. The latter have been chiefly instrumental in identifying useful wild animals and birds, in domesticating them as well as in maintaining the domesticated ones, besides the wild native stocks for any future breeding programs. Pastoralists were also mainly dependent on these domesticated animals not only as a source of food but also for providing milk, manure and fuel or to serve as draft animals, during these processes, they because aware of the various problems in successfully maintain these animals, particularly about the various ailments/diseases that these animals face. Hence, they identified potential ethnoveterinary, as well as fodder plants taxa that are found around them respectively for curing the ailments/diseases and for feeding them. The N.E. Indian and Andaman tribal communities did the same things mentioned above as they also depended on animal husbandry and poultry for their sustenance, if not fully, partially at least of this volume Bipul Saikia deals with the prevalent ethnoveterinary practices in North-East India and Andamans.

The Andaman and Nicobar Islands constitute an archipelago of over 572 islands (550 in Andamans and 22 in Nicobar) with a total area of about 8250 Km^2 (6400 in Andamans and 1850 in Nicobar). These islands are blessed with unique tropical rainforests with floral elements of India, Myanmar, Malaysia, Indonesia and Australia. There are also wild relatives and land races of cultivated taxa which are believed to have originated (primary or secondary) there. This is the homeland of six tribal groups, inhabiting for thousands of years in the verdant rain forests. Because of their intimate association with the flora around them as hunter-gatherers they have developed a very rich traditional knowledge on the plants of importance in food, medicine and other requirements. An inventory of such plants would be of great value in bioprospection and use in human welfare. Pullaiah et al. have given details on the ethnobotany of Andaman and Nicobar Islands in Chapter 8.

Ethnobotanical research has historically played a very vital role in understanding the relationship between people and the plants around them. Today it is a rapidly growing field of research attracting the attention of diverse stakeholders. However, ethnobotanists have been rather slow in adopting and applying tools of bioinformatics revolution and also in integrating the already obtained research data into a meaningful entity. Many of them still follow traditional approaches to gathering and disseminating ethnobotanical information. Electronic storage and retrieval databases have been started to be organized in increasing numbers (Berlin and Berlin, 2005; Bisby, 2000; Thomas, 2003). Documentation, retrieval and exchange of ethnobotanical information from the organized databases will not only help preserving and protecting traditional knowledge but also will help in bioprospection and commerce. Ringmichon and Bindu Gopalakrishnan have provided detailed information on the documentation and exchanges of ethnobotanical knowledge of North-East India in Chapter 9 of this volume. They have provided very useful information derived from the various kinds of databases and published literature, on the ethnobotany of the various tribes of this regions; they have covered on medicinal plants, food plants, beverages and other uses of plants associated with rituals/ceremonies.

1.5 GENERAL REVIEWS ON ETHNOBOTANY OF INDIA

This volume also contains a few review chapters on the ethnobotany of India, in which details pertaining to North-East India and Andaman are also included. The first of these chapters is on Quantitative approaches to Ethnobotany by Dr. Chowdhury Habibur Rahman. Initially when ethnobotany became a separate subject under the discipline of Botany, it was more descriptive based on data collected from different tribal communities of the world. Subsequently the subject of ethnobotany was broadly divided into cultural, social and utilitarian ethnobotany. The third branch gained more and more importance because the traditional knowledge on food medicinal ethno-veterinary and other uses of plants was subjected to intensive research by those involved in bioprospection and discovery of newer molecules of importance. Simultaneously documentation of ethnic traditional knowledge using information, technology and bio informatics tools as well as detailed quantitative approach to the study of ethnobotany also developed in order to make meaningful and correct exploitation of traditional knowledge. The advances in the field of Quantitative ethnobotany, drawing information from Indian examples are discussed in Chapter 10 of this volume by Dr. Rahman.

Turmeric, botanically known as *Curcuma longa* L. (Family: Zingiberaceae), is esteemed by the Indo-European race of people (Aryans) for its golden-yellow colored dye that resembles sunlight; this race which worshiped the sun attributed special protective properties to turmeric. Turmeric has been used for several centuries in India, both in folk medical systems as well as a coloring agent for various media such as silk, cotton, wood, paper, food stuffs and cosmetics. Turmeric, a native of south and southeast Asia, is believed to have had its origin and initial domestication in Western Ghats of India. The genus *Curcuma* along with *C. longa* has more than 100 species as well as a number of varieties about 40 of which are found in India. *Curcuma* not only has morphological diversity but also a very rich chemical diversity; the most important chemicals of turmeric are the curcuminoids. In view of its very high contemporary relevance turmeric has been a subject of interest to botanists, phytochemists and medical people for a very long time. In Chapter 11 Samala and Veeresham have given a good account of the ethnobotany of turmeric and its medicinal importance.

According to WHO over 400 million people in the world suffer from Diabetes mellitus, commonly abbreviated as Diabetes. This is one of the most common metabolic diseases of humans and is often controlled by several factors. It may be due to defect in insulin secretion, insulin gene or both. These lead to chronic hyperglycemia with attendant disturbances in carbohydrate (and protein and lipid) metabolism. Diabetes also leads to a number of complications like retinopathy, neuropathy, nephropathy, cardiovascular diseases, eye problems and ulcers. In recent years Diabetes cases have been on rapid rise, essentially due to changing life styles and food habits/systems (Youssef and McCullough, 2002). Revathi et al. have given a detailed account on the traditional use of herbal plants for the treatment of diabetes in India. However, we feel that in the list of antidiabetic plants prepared from ethnic knowledge sources, only very few plants have been analyzed phytochemically and clinically in order to verify their claimed efficacy and a great deal of research must be done in the near future.

A critical review of the ethnobotany of oral and dental *hygiene* has indicated that there is a serious lack of a baseline catalog containing details of the Plants used of the ethnomedical treatments of oral and dental problems/diseases (Colvard et al., 2006). Most publications, particularly from India which has a rich data on ethnomedical aspects of oral problems, has been essentially give a list of plants for different problems without attendant data on phytochemistry or the therapeutic basis for prevention/ cure of these problems (Soejarto, 2005). There is also a lack of clinical documentation of the ethnomedicinal treatments for oral diseases experience by people in their own cultural and ecological environments (Elkin and Elisabetsky, 2005). There is, thus, an immediate need for ethnobotanists, ethnomedical experts and modern allopathic dental doctors to come together and take up a detailed multidisciplinary study of the plants listed by Krishnamurthy et al. in Chapter 13 of this volume.

KEYWORDS

- **Andaman and Nicobar Islands**
- **diabetes**
- **ethnic diversity**
- **ethno documentation**
- **food plants**
- **medicinal plants**
- **northeast India**
- **oral and dental hygiene**
- **quantitative enthobotany**
- **turmeric**
- **veterinary plants**

REFERENCES

1. Berlin, E. A., & Berlin B. (2005). Some field methods in medical ethnobiology. *Field Methods 17*, 235–268.
2. Bisby, F. A. (2000). The Quiet Revolution: Biodiversity Information and the internet. *Science289*, 2309–2312.
3. Chatterjee, D., Saikia, A., Dutta, P., Ghosh, D., Pangging, G., & Goswami, A. K. (2006). Biodiversity significances of North East India. WWF-India, New Delhi.
4. Colvard, M. D., Cordell, G. A., Villalobas, R. et al. (2006). Survey of Medical ethnobotanicals for dental and oral medicine conditions and pathologies. *J. Ethnopharmacol. 107*, 134–142.
5. Dagar, J. C., & Singh, N. T. (1999). Plant Resources of the Andaman and Nicobar Islands. Vol. 1. Bishen Singh Mahendra Pal Singh, Dehra Dun, India.
6. Dutta, B. K., & Dutta, P. K. (2005). Potential of ethnobotanical studies in North East India: An Overview. *Indian J. Trad. Knowl. 4*, 7–14.
7. Elkin, N. L., & Elisabetsky, E. (2005). Seeking a transdisciplinary and culturally germane science: the future of ethnopharmacology. *J. Ethnopharmacol. 100*, 23–26.
8. Jain, S. K. (1982). Botany of Eastern Himalayas. pp. 201–217. In: Paliwal, G. S. (Ed.). The Vegetations Wealth of the Himalayas. Puja Publication, Delhi.
9. Mao, A. A., Hyniewto, T. M., & Sanjappa, M. 2009. Plant Wealth of Northeast India with reference to ethnobotany. *Indian J. Trad. Knowl. 8*, 93–103.
10. Misra, V. N. (2001). Prehistoric human colonization of India. *J. Biosci. 26*, 491–531.
11. Moral, D. (1997). North-East India as a linguistic are. *Mon-Khmer Studies 27*, 43–53.
12. Sinha, B. K. (1999). Flora of great Nicobar Islands. Botanical Survey of India, Calcutta, India.
13. Soejarto, D. D. Fong, H. H., Tan, G. T. et al. (2005). Ethnobotany/ethnopharmacology and mass bioprospecting: issues on intellectual property and benefit-sharing. *J. Ethnopharmacol. 100*, 15–22.
14. Thangaraj, K., Chaubey, G. Kivisild, T., Reddy, A. G., Sigh, V. K., Rasalkar, A. A., & Singh, L. (2005). Reconstructing the origin of Andaman Islanders *Curr. Sci. 308*, 996.
15. Thomas, M. B. (2003). Emerging synergies between information technology and applied ethnobotanical research. *Ethnobotany Research & Application 1*, 65–73.
16. Valdiya. (2010). The Making of India. Macmillan, New Delhi, India.
17. Youssef, W., & McCullough, A. J. (2002). Diabetes mellitus obesity, and Hepatic steatosis. Semin. *Gastrointest Dis 13*, 17–30.

CHAPTER 2

ETHNIC DIVERSITY OF NORTH-EAST INDIA

SHUVASISH CHOUDHURY,[1] BIR BAHADUR,[2]
K. V. KRISHNAMURTHY,[3] and S. JOHN ADAMS[4]

[1]Central Instrumentation Laboratory, Assam University,
Silchar – 788011, India, E-mail: shuvasish@gmail.com

[2]Department of Botany, Kakatiya University, Warangal–506009,
India, E-mail: birbahadur5april@gmail.com

[3]Consultant, R&D, Sami Labs Ltd, Peenya Industrial Area, Bangalore,
India, E-mail: kvkbdu@yahoo.co.in

[4]Department of Pharmacognosy, R&D, The
Himalaya Drug Company, Makali, Bangalore, India,
E-mail: s.johnadams13@gmail.com

CONTENTS

Abstract 16
2.1 Introduction 16
2.2 Ethnic Diversity 18
2.3 Tribes of Arunachal Pradesh 24
2.4 Tribes of Nagaland 25
2.5 Tribes of Manipur 26
2.6 Tribes of Tripura 27
2.7 Tribes of Mizoram 27

2.8   Tribes of Meghalaya 28

2.9   Tribes of Assam... 29

2.10 Tribes of Sikkim.. 29

2.11 Conclusion 31

Keywords 31

References.. 32

ABSTRACT

The North Eastern (NE) region of India houses considerable ethnic multiplicity, which largely differ in their traditions, customs and language. Majority of these tribes are forest dwellers and live in communities under the rule of despotic chiefs. These tribes are classified according to their origin, language, race, religion and their geographical location. These tribal communities are distinct from each other and considerable variations are found even among closely related tribal groups of the region. In this chapter, we focus on the different ethnic communities of NE India, their distribution, their cultural activities, religion and languages.

2.1   INTRODUCTION

India is a multicultural country and perhaps nowhere in the world people in a small geographic area are distributed as a large number ethnic, caste, religious and linguistic groups as in India (Bhasin et al., 1994). People of different groups live side by side for hundreds or even thousands of years but yet retained their support entities through endogamy. These diverse groups of people started migrating to India from different directions in an unbroken sweep over at least 5,000 years from the present and have con-tributed very significantly to the present day rich human gene pool of the sub-continent (Gadgil et al., 1998; Allchin and Allchin, 1982; Sankalia, 1974; Misra, 1992; Kashyap et al., 2003). The diverse ecological regimes of India seems to have nurtured this diversity (Gadgil and Guha, 1992). The major waves of historical migration into Indian sub-continent include Austro-Asiatic languages speakers soon after 65,000 BP, probably from the Middle East, Indo-European language speakers, in several waves, after 4,000 years BP and Sino-Tibetan language speakers, in several waves, after 6,000 years BP (Gadgil et al., 1998). The *ethnic racial groups* of India include the Caucasoid, Negrito (or Negroid), Australoid and Mongoloid who differ from one another in certain morphological features, but one should remember that there are no strict lines of demarcation between these four racial groups. The first and last racial groups are mainly concentrated in the north and northeastern parts of India, the third confined mostly to central, western and southern India while the second is essentially restricted to Andaman Islands (Cavalli-Sforza et al., 1994). The linguistic groups of India include the Dravidian (Dravida), Austro-Asiatic (Nishada), Tibeto-Burman or Sino-Tibetan (Kirata) and Indo-European (Indo-Aryan). They together speak about 187 languages and 544 dialects. The first group is spread essentially over southern part of India, the fourth essentially over northern part of India, the third essentially over northeast India, while the second is restricted to certain tribes such as Korkus, Mundas, Santals, Khasis and Nicobarese (Kashyap et al., 2003). The *People of India* project recognized 4635 distinct communities in India, although the actual number of endogamous groups may be of the order of 50 to 60 thousand (Cavalli-Sforza et al., 1994; Singh, 1998). The religious groups of India include, Hindus, Muslims, Christians, Sikhs, Buddhists, Jains, Parsi and Jews.

The northeast region of India is a very important region known for its cultural heritage, rich floristic and faunal diversity, diverse ethnicity and unique biogeography. It is located in the North eastern corner of India comprising of eight states/ territories of Assam, Meghalaya, Nagaland, Manipur, Mizoram, Arunachal Pradesh, Tripura and Sikkim. It comprises 8% of the total land size of India. According to the census of 2001, the total population of North East India is approximately 40 million (2011 census), representing 3.1% of India's total population. This region borders on China and Bhutan in the North, Myanmar in the east, Bangladesh and West Bengal on the West and the Bay of Bengal of the South. It is connected to the mainland of India with a 22 km long "Chicken Neck corridor (Bijukumar, 2013) or Siliguri corridor. Although this region shows ecological and cultural contrasts between the hilly terrains and the plains, there are significant features of continuity (Kumar et al., 2004).

Interdependence and interaction (Dutta and Dutta, 2005). With more than 150 tribes speaking as many language, the northeast region of India is a "Melting pot of variegated Cultural Mosaic" of races, languages, religions and "ethnic tapestry of many hues and shades" (Dutta and Dutta 2005). This chapter deals with ethnic diversity of northeast India and the rich cultural diversity associated with it.

2.2   ETHNIC DIVERSITY

The tribal segment of Indian population reflects an interesting profile of India's ethnic richness and diversity. There are about 427 tribal communities all over India, of which about 145 major tribal communities and a total sub-tribes of 300 (Kala, 2005) are found in northeast India. It has been estimated that of the approximately 40 million people inhabiting this region, around 10 million are tribal or 25% (Ali and Das, 2003).

The first settlers of North East India were Austro-Asiatic speaking people and later people of Tibeto-Burmese and Indo-Aryan origins settled there. It is the home for major tribal communities like Abor, Garo, Khasi, Kuki, Naga, Apatani, Adi, Hmar, Mizo, Reang, Chorei, Tripuri, etc. Studies have indicated that due to immense biological and crop diversity and availability of fertile land, the primary tribal settlers were mostly farmers although they were preceded in some parts by hunter-gatherers/foragers. The major tribal groups are of Mongoloid origin, who came to the region at different times, possibly earlier than Caucasoid (Das et al., 1987; Kumar et al., 2004). The tribes that belong to the Mongoloid racial stock usually belong to the Tibeto-Chinese or Tibeto-Burmese linguistic family, while the Caucasoid are related to Indo-European linguistic stock (Kumar et al., 2004). Both Mongoloid and Caucasoid represent definite degree of differences in cultural and biological traits. Some workers have suggested that the Australoids came to North East India before the Mongoloids and the physical feature of different tribes of this region suggests the presence of Australoid element in some of the tribes (Das, 1970; Ali and Das, 2003). The diversity of tribal communities varies considerably. In Assam, Tripura and Manipur, the tribal communities represents 12.82%, 30.95% and 34.41% respectively of the total population, while ~90% of the total population in other states are represented by tribal communities.

The most important tribal communities in the various states of northeast India are shown in Table 2.1. It is evidenced from this table that among all the major tribes of North East India, the largest groups comprise the Bodos, Khasi, Garo, Naga, Mizo, Karbis and Mishing. The Bodo tribes are widely distributed from areas bordering North Bengal to the western Nagaon and Darrang districts of Assam, while Khasi and Garo have well defined homeland in the state of Meghalaya. Mizo are characteristically found in the state of Mizoram, while a small population is also residing in some parts of Southern Assam (Cachar district) and regions of Manipur. Karbi tribe belongs to the Karbi-Anglong district of Assam but also spread over some parts of Dima-Hasao district in Assam and parts of western Nagaland and north-eastern Meghalaya. In Nagaland, the major tribal communities include the Ao, Sema, Konyak and Angami. Bulk of the Naga population belonging to Tangkhul, Kabui and Thado are found in the state of Manipur. Hmar tribal population is widely distributed in states of Manipur and Mizoram, while a major population is also found in three districts of Southern Assam. In Arunachal Pradesh, the major tribes include the Nishi, Apatani, Adi, Mishing, Wancho and Galong. These tribes represent extreme heterogeneity in terms of population distribution and socio-cultural structure and pattern (Ali and Das, 2003). Each of the tribe has distinct sub-divisions and their customs and societal structure varies considerably. For examples, among the sub-divisions of Khasis like Wars, Khynriams, Pnars and Bhois follow distinctive the socio-cultural traits, which varies considerably with each other (Ali and Das, 2003). The geographical distribution has a strong impact on social, cultural and economic aspects of each of the tribes. The Dimasa-Kacharis residing in Dima-Hasao district of Assam have mostly retained their traditional practices, while those living in Cachar district have a strong influence of Bengali culture and customs. Most of the tribes which are in vicinity of non-tribal groups are mostly influenced by the non-tribal customs and in due course of time they have acquired such customs and culture in their day to day life (Ali and Das, 2003). The diversity of the cultural heritage gives the tribal communities of North East India their specific identity. The North Eastern region of India, which is represented by bulk of the tribal population of the country have cultural and traditional similarities with inhabitants of China, Tibet and Myanmar. After the post-independence era, these tribal communities of North East India have faced identity crisis and as a result there is a strong divergence of these communities towards modern life. Further, loss of traditional cultural among the tribal youths has also resulted in loss of traditional knowledge and heritage. This situation appears to be extremely alarming and needs special attention to conserve the precious traditional knowledge.

The culture of North-East Indian Tribal communities is reflected in their food, dance, music, drama, festivals (including harvest, pottery), arts and crafts, songs, dressing, jewelry and ornaments, tattooing, and social ceremonies and rituals, which vary in different communities. The most important festivals celebrated are Nyokam, Ngada, Kashad Suk Nongkrum, Mimkuut, Khaskain, Wangala, etc. Their arts and crafts include weaving (cotton, silk, and wool) with different motifs printed (manual) using vegetable dyes, crafts and furniture made out of canes, bamboo and wood, basket weaving (using canes and wild twinners and climbers) etc. The major dance forms include Ponung, RekhamPada, Ajima Rao, and Chambilmpa when string and wind blowing instruments.

TABLE 2.1 Major Ethnic Tribes of Northeast India

Sl. No	Ethnic Tribes	State
1.	Abor	AR
2.	Adi (Ashhing, Bogun, Bokar, Bori, Botang, Gallong, Karka, Komar, Lodung, Milang, Miniyong, Padam, Pailibo, Pangi, Ramo, Shimong, Tangam)	AR, NA
3.	Aimol	MA
4.	Aka	AR
5.	Anal	MA
6.	Angami	MA, NA
7.	Ao	NA
8.	Apatani	AR
9.	Bangni	AR
10.	Barmans	AS
11.	Bhil	TR
12.	Bhoi	AS, ME
13.	Bhutia	TR, SI
14.	Boro	AS, ME

TABLE 2.1   (Continued)

Sl. No	Ethnic Tribes	State
15.	Borokachari	AS
16.	Chaimal	TR
17.	Chakma	AS, MI, ME, TR
18.	Chethe	MA
19.	Chiru	MA
20.	Deori	AS, AR
21.	Dimasa	AS, ME, MI, NA
22.	Galong	NA, AR
23.	Gangte	AS, ME, MI, NA, TR
24.	Garo	AS, ME, MI, NA, TR
25.	Hajong	AS, ME, MI
26.	Halam	TR, MI
27.	Hmar	AS, MA, ME, MI
28.	Idu/Chulikata Mishmi	AR
29.	Jaintia	AS, ME, MI, NA, TR
30.	Jamatia	TR
31.	Kabui	MA
32.	Kacha Naga	MA
33.	Karbi (mikir)	ME, NA, MI
34.	Kaur	TR
35.	Khamba	AR
36.	Khampti	AR
37.	Khanmiang	AR
38.	Khanti	AR
39.	Khasi	AS, ME, MI, Na, TR
40.	Khowa	AR, ME, NA
41.	Koch	ME
42.	Koineng	MA

TABLE 2.1   (Continued)

Sl. No	Ethnic Tribes	State
43.	Koirao	MA
44.	Kom	MA
45.	Kuki (Baiate, Belalhut, Chhalya, Chongloi, Doungel, Fun, Gamalhou, Gangte, Guite, Hanpit, Hao, Haolai, Hengna, Henneug, Hongsungh, Hranghwal, Jangtei, Khareng, Khawanthlang, Khawchung, Khelma, Khephong, Kholhou, Khothalong, Kiggen, Kip, Kuki, Laifaung, Lengthang, Lentei, Lhangum, Lhoujen, Lhouvum, Misao, Mizelnamte, Paitu, Rangchan, Rangkhole, Raokohl, Riang, Sairhem, Selnam, Singsom, Sithale, Sukto, Thado, Thangiuya, Thangngen, Tongbe)	NA, MI, TR, ME
46.	Lakher	AS, ME, MI
47.	Lalung	AS
48.	Lamgang	MA
49.	Lepcha	TR, SI
50.	Limboo (Tsongs)	SI
51.	Lushai	TR, MA
52.	Lyngngam	AS, ME
53.	Mag	TR
54.	Man (Tai speaking)	AS, ME, MI
55.	Mao	MA
56.	Maram	MA
57.	Maring	MA
58.	Mech	AS
59.	Memba	AR
60.	Meyor	AR
61.	Miji	AR
62.	Mikir	AS, MI, ME
63.	Miri (hill)	AR, AS
64.	Miri (Mishing)	AR
65.	Mishmi	AR
66.	Mizo (Lushai)	AS, MA, MI, NA, ME
67.	Momba	NA, AS

TABLE 2.1 (Continued)

Sl. No	Ethnic Tribes	State
68.	Monpa	AR
69.	Monsang	MA
70.	Moyon	MA
71.	Munda	TR
72.	Naga (Chakhesang, Chang, Chini, Khiemnungan, Konyak, Lotha, Makwani, Sangtam, Sema, Tikhir, Yimchungnee, Zeliang)	ME, MI, AR
73.	Nishang	AR
74.	Nishi	AR
75.	Noatia	TR
76.	Nocte	AR
77.	Nyshi	AP
78.	Orang	TR
79.	Paite	MA
80.	Pawi	AS, ME, MI
81.	Pnar	AS, ME
82.	Purum	MA
83.	Rabha	AS, ME
84.	Ralte	MA
85.	Rengma	NA, AS
86.	Rlang	TR
87.	Santhal	TR
88.	Sema	MA
89.	Sherdukpen	AR
90.	Sherpa	SI
91.	Simte	MA
92.	Singpho	AR
93.	Suhte	MA
94.	Sulung	AR
95.	Synteng	AS, ME, NA, MI
96.	Tagin	AR
97.	Tamang	SI

TABLE 2.1   (Continued)

Sl. No	Ethnic Tribes	State
98.	Tangkhul	MA
99.	Tangsa	AR
100.	TawangMonpa	AR
101.	Thandou	MA
102.	Tippera	TR
103.	Tripuri	TR
104.	Uchai	TR
105.	Wancho	AR
106.	War	AS, ME, MI
107.	Yobin (lisu)	AR
108.	Zakhring	AR
109.	Zou	MA

Key: AR – Arunachal Pradesh; AS – Assam; MA – Manipur; Me – Meghalaya; MI – Mizoram; NA – Nagaland; SI – Sikkim; TR – Tripura.

2.3   TRIBES OF ARUNACHAL PRADESH

The tribal of Arunachal Pradesh constitutes 64.20% of the total state population. There are 35 ethnic groups in the state, which are widely distributed in 13 districts. Almost 86% of the tribal population thrives in rural areas with farming and animal rearing as their principal occupation. Among the tribes, the female population exceeds the male population in the state. The tribal population of Arunachal Pradesh is of Asiatic origin and have facial proximity with people of Tibet and Myanmar. In the western part of Arunachal Pradesh, the major tribe include Nishi, Sulung, Sherdukpen, Aka, Monpa, Apatani and Miri. Adis are one of the largest groups in the states after Apatani, which occupies the central region of the state. The Wancho, Nocte and Tangsa are mainly distributed in Tirap district, while Mishmis are mostly concentrated in northeastern hills. These groups differ among themselves in their culture, tradition, customs and religious beliefs. There are almost 50 different languages and dialects. Majority of the languages spoken by these tribes belong to the Tibeto-Burmese branch of Sino-Tibetan language family. Beside their own language, the tribes are well conversant in English, Hindi and Assamese. Mompa tribe has six subgroups, which include the Sherdukpens, Akas, Khowas and Mijis that are inhabitants of Kameng district. In the east Kameng district, Sulungs, Mijis and Akas are the pre-dominant tribes. Among Adis and Tangsas, there are about 15 sub-groups, while Mishmis are divided into 3 sub-groups. The Mishmi tribes are distributed mainly in the Dibang valley and Lohit district of Arunachal Pradesh. In addition to the Mishmis, the Lohit district is also inhabited by other tribes including Zhakrings, Meyors, Khantis and Khamiyangs (Ali and Das, 2003). The main religious practices among the Arunachal tribes is based on worshiping the deities of nature and spirits. Ritual sacrifice of animals like Mithun is commonly observed among all the major tribes of Arunachal Pradesh. Religious beliefs based on Hinduism and Buddhism can also be observed among several tribes of the state.

2.4   TRIBES OF NAGALAND

Nagaland has around 30 ethnic communities. The Naga tribe of North East India is one of the most diverse tribal communities of India. In the 1991 census of India, there are 35 different Naga tribes that are enlisted among the schedule tribes in India, out of which 17 in Nagaland, 15 in Manipur and 3 in Arunachal Pradesh. Each of the tribal inhabited regions of Nagaland has its own definite population and usually governed by despotic chiefs. The current geographical regions of Nagaland comprises of some former Naga districts of Assam and Tuensang frontier divisions. It is divided into eight main districts viz., Mokokchung, Tuensang, Mon, Wokha, PhekZunheboto, Kohima and Dimapur. The most predominant Naga tribes include the Angami, Ao, Chakesang, Chang, Chirr, Konyak, Lotha, Khiamngam, Makware, Phom, Rengma, Sangtam, Sema, Yimchunger and Zeliang (Ali and Das, 2003). Each of these tribes have their own legend, which articulates about the original course of their migration. The Khaimungan, Pochury, Sangtam and Chang regard themselves as original descendants of Naga Hills, while Angami, Chakhesang, Lotha, Rengma and Sema have originated from same racial stock but got separated and congregated their own identity. However, conflicting views regarding their origin and ancestry exists. It is assumed that larger tribes like the Ao and Angami kept on shifting from one place to another and gradually encroached into territories of smaller tribes, but later due to economic and social compulsion they started settling into specific territories and maintained principles of patrilineal descent. Smaller group of Naga tribes like Kahha came from Phom, which in their local dialect means cloud. Pochury, which is the smallest group among all Naga tribes have originally descended from the Chakhesang tribe and widely distributed in about 24 villages of Nagaland. People of Pochury tribe are engaged in spinning, carpentry, stone craving and leather works. The Rengma are divided into two distinct territorial groups' viz., Nteyne and Nzong, which occupies the subdivisions constituting Nidzurku Hills to Wokha Hills. Both Nteyne and Nzong groups of Rengma tribe have different dialect. It is also believed that a major section of Rengmas have gradually migrated to the Mikir Hills in Assam. The Yimchunger is a relatively small group of Naga tribe that is divided into three sub-tribes viz., Tikir, Makware and Chirr. They speak different dialect and live in a well-defined territory under the headship of tribal chiefs. The Sangtams of Nagaland are divided mainly into two distinct territorial groups in Chare and Kiphire sub-divisions of Nagaland. Sema is widely scattered in almost in all major parts of Nagaland and also distributed in some parts of Assam. The Zemi, Liangmei and the Rongmai belongs to single ethno-cultural entity and collectively known as the Zeliang in Nagaland. Among the Naga, there is no concept of caste or class. Each clan is exogamous, which occupies a definite territorial boundary. The clans have their independent political and economic rights and distinguishes itself from the other in terms of the custom, language and ethnicity.

2.5 TRIBES OF MANIPUR

The state of Manipur is distinctly divided into two geographical regions. This includes the fertile plains and hilly tracts. Manipuri belonging to the Methai community are the primary inhabitants, however, tribal groups belonging to Naga and Kuki-Chin-Mizo are also the native of Manipur. As per the 2001 census, Manipur comprises of 34.2% tribal population, under about 30 tribes the total tribal population of Manipur, Thadou is considered as the largest with a total population of 1.80 lakhs, representing 24.6% of the total tribal population. Other major tribes of Manipur include Tangkhul (19.7%), Kabui (11.1%), Paite (6.6%), Hmar (5.8%), Kacha Naga (5.7%) and Vaiphui (5.2%). Other major tribal groups of Manipur are Maring (3.1%), Anal (2.9%), Zou (2.8%), Lushai (2.0%), Kom (2.0%) and Simte (1.5%). About 95% of the tribal population resides in rural areas, who predominantly practices agriculture. Agriculture is the main occupation of males, while the womenfolk are engaged in weaving and looming.

2.6 TRIBES OF TRIPURA

Tripura is one of the smallest states of India with a total population of 3,199,203. According to the 2001 Census report, the tribal communities comprise 31.1% of the total population. They come under 40 different ethnic communities The Tripuri are the main tribal group of the state and accounts for 54.7% of the total tribal population. Other tribal groups of Tripura include Reang (16.6%), Jamatia (7.5%), Chakma (6.5%), Halam (4.8%), Mag (3.1%), Munda (1.2%), Any Kuki Tribe (1.2%) and Garoo (1.1%). Tripura is a meeting point of both tribal and non-tribal culture, generating a unique combination of unusual cultures. Currently, Tripura is largely dominated by Bengali population, which constitutes the major portion of the population. The state is divided as North and South Tripura including hilly terrains and fertile land. These zones are home for tribal communities. The principal occupation of tribes of Tripura is agriculture, mainly in the form of Jhum cultivation. They live in elevated houses made of bamboo, known as the thong. Music and Dance are integral part of tribal culture of Tripura and each community is known for their specific forms of Dance and Music. Handicrafts and handloom practiced by the tribes of the state are famous and earned international recognition.

2.7 TRIBES OF MIZORAM

The Mizos belong to the mixed racial stock of Huns. They migrated from Chamdo region of Tibet to the Upper Burma and subsequently kept moving southwards and occupied what is now known as Patkai Hills and

Hukwang Valley. The Mizo as an ethnic group assimilates many tribes, sub-tribes and clans. The transformation of diverse clans into a single common ethnicity was driven by common basic interest and also facilitated by adoption of Christianity, Roman Script and West Education. According to the Census of 2001, out of the total population of 888,573, the tribal communities comprises 94.5% of it. There are around 65 ethnic communities of which Lushai or Any Mizo Tribe is the largest group comprising of 77% of total tribal population. Other major tribal groups includes the Chakma (8.5%), Pawi (5.0%), Lakher (4.3%), Any Kuki Tribe (2.5%), Hmar (2.2%), Khasi (0.2%) and Any Naga Tribe (0.1%). Beside these, other smaller groups include Syntheng, Dimasa, Garo, Mikir, Man and Hajong. The broad groups of Mizo are classified into 15 different communities, which include Ngente, Khiangte, Chwangthu, Renthlei, Zowngte, Khwlhring, etc. These groups though have distinct identity, still they are no longer considered separate. Religious beliefs of all Mizos are strictly based in Christianity. Literacy rate is significantly high among the Mizos.

2.8   TRIBES OF MEGHALAYA

Meghalaya constitutes 85.9% tribal population mainly comprising of Khasis (56.4%) and Garos (34.6%). Out of the total population of 2,318,822, the tribal population comprises 1, 992,862 persons. The state has registered 31.3% decadal growth in Tribal population in the period 1991–2001. There are around 25 tribal communities of which Khasis constitute almost half of the total tribal population, followed by the Garos and both together comprise 91% of the total tribal population. In Meghalaya smaller tribal groups include the Hajong (1.6%), Raba (1.4%), Koch (1.1%), Synteng (0.9%), Mikir (0.6%), AnyKuki Tribe (0.5%), Lushai (0.2%), Naga (0.2%), Boro-Kacharis (0.1%) and Hmar (0.1%). The tribal population is pre-dominantly rural (97.2%), while only a small part of the population resides in urban areas. The state was carved out from Assam in 1973 and divided into seven administrative districts. Khasis are the group, who follows matrilineal social structure. They are Mon-Khmer speaking people mostly residing in East and West Khasi Hills and the Jaintia Hills. Garos are predominantly concentrated in the Garo Hills and preferred to be called the Mande or Achik (Ali and Das, 2003). The social structure of these tribes are predominantly matrilineal, which follows the matriarchal law of inheritance (Ali and Das, 2003). Females have the custody of property and holds key position in the family, which is passed onto the youngest daughter from mother. The Khasis and Jantias speak the language that belongs to the Mon-Khmer family of Austric connection, while the Garo language has proximity with Bodos belonging to Tibeto-Burmese family of languages (Ali and Das, 2003).

2.9 TRIBES OF ASSAM

The state of Assam comprises of 12.4% of tribal population, registering 15.1% decadal growth in population in 1991–2001. There are around 80 tribes that are distributed in different parts of the state. In addition to recorded major tribal population, good numbers of other tribal communities belonging to Naga, Mizo, Kuki, Chorei, Reang and Tripuri are also existent in Assam. Topographically, Assam is distinguished into three distinct zones viz., the Brahmaputra Valley in the North, Karbi-Anglong or Dima-Hasao comprising the central regions and Barak Valley in the south. About 95.3% of the tribal population of Assam are rural and practice agriculture and handicraft as their primary occupation. Bodos represent almost half of the total tribal population, followed by other tribes. The district-wise breakup of tribal population of Assam shows that more that 68% of the population in Dima-Hasao are tribal, which is followed by Karbi-Anglong with ~55% tribal population. In Dhemaji and Kokrajhar districts the tribal population is 47.3% and 33.7%, respectively. The majority of the tribal communities in districts like Kamrup, Cachar, Karimganj, Hailakandhi and Dibrugarh are urban, while a small portion of them are located in rural areas.

2.10 TRIBES OF SIKKIM

Sikkim is one of the most beautiful States of North east India with an area of 7300 sq. km. The state is interlaced with jungle-clad ridges and deep ravines created by the Mountain Rivers, emerald valleys and dense forests. The original Lepcha inhabitants call Sikkim Myel Lyang – "the land of hidden paradise". To the Bhutias, it is Beyul Demojong – the hidden valley of rice and the Limbus call it Sukhim, which means 'the new house'. The landscape of this tiny State is dominated by the world's highest mountain peaks like Kangchendzonga, the third highest mountain on earth. It has played a major unifying role among these three major ethnic communities of Sikkim. This mountain has been worshipped by the Lepchas from very early times. It is equally revered by the Bhutias and Nepalese. Pang Lhabsol is an annual festival celebrated. The population of Sikkim is about 5.5 lakhs, mainly consisting of the Nepalese, the Lepchas and the Bhutias. Of these, the Nepalese are the largest in number followed by the Bhutia and Lepcha communities. A small number of people from other parts of the country have also settled in Sikkim. Despite such an ethnic diversity, a remarkable feature of Sikkimese society is the tolerance and acceptance of different cultures and their harmonious co-existence. The Lepchas are the earliest settlers of Sikkim. Lepchas belong to one of the Naga tribes or are associated with the Jimdars and Mech in their eastward migration from Nepal. Some scholars have found a similarity between the Lepachas and the tribes in Arunachal Pradesh. Yet some others contend they are related to the Khasis in Meghalaya. The Lepchas themselves are convinced that their home has always been the legendary kingdom of Mayel in the vicinity of Mt. Kangchendzonga. The Lepchas have their own language and script. The Lepcha dances, songs and folk tales reflect a wonderful synthesis between men and nature. The Bhutias are mainly descendants of the early settlers in Sikkim from Tibet and Bhutan who accompanied the ancestors of the first Chogyal, Phuntsok Namgyal. Tibetan Buddhism played a special role in shaping the Bhutia society. Every household ritual, marriage, birth, death ceremonies and agricultural rites are conducted by the monks from the Gompas. Like the Lepchas and the Nepalese, the Bhutias are fond of their "chang", the local brew. This preparation from fermented millet is served in bamboo containers. It has become an indispensable part of every Sikkimese ceremony, whether religious or secular. The Bhutias are famous for their weaving, woodcarving and the Thanka painting. Important festivals observed by the Bhutia community include Losoong, Pang Lhabsol, Kagyat dance and Saga Dawa. The Nepalese community of Sikkim is itself a conglomeration of diverse ethnic groups, some speaking their own vernacular. These ethnic groups can be roughly divided between the Magars,

Murmis, Tamangs, Gurungs, Rais, Limbus, Damis, Kamis, Bahuns and the Chhetris. Most Nepalese are Hindus or Buddhists. Some of them have also adopted Christianity. The Rais, Limbus, Magars, Murmis, Tamangs and Gurungs have somewhat similar physical characteristics inasmuch as they are all Mongoloid. But each group has its own distinctive culture. The major festivals of the Hindu Nepalese in Sikkim are Dasain, Teohar, Makar Sankranti and Baisakhi.

2.11   CONCLUSION

Studies have shown that each of the tribal communities of North-East India differ in terms of their culture and tradition, which provides them a distinct identity. North-East India is a very important region of India with very rich cultural heritage. The region is very rich in ethnic diversity with varied origins. Several languages and dialects are spoken. As a part of their various culture and social behavior they have utilized the diverse flora (and fauna) for their day-to-day requirements and thus have contributed to a very rich traditional knowledge. With the increase in urbanization and eagerness to adopt modern ways of life, the traditions and culture are becoming extinct day-by-day. It is important to note that the impact of development in terms of improving the living standard has affected traditional culture significantly. Most of the ethnic population, particularly in state of Assam have preferred to adopt urban way of life. It is, therefore, imperative to emphasize that the conservation and preservation of ethnic culture and traditions *vis-à-vis* socio-economic development of the tribes requires important and pointing attention.

KEYWORDS

- **Arunachal Pradesh**
- **Assam**
- **culture**
- **ethnic languages**

- Manipur
- Meghalaya
- Mizoram
- Nagaland
- origin of tribes
- Sikkim
- society
- Tripura

REFERENCES

1. Ali, A. N. M. I., & Das, I. (2003). Tribal Situation in North East India. *Stud. Tribes Tribals, 1(2)*, 141–148.
2. Allchin, B., & Allchin, R. (1982). The Rise of Civilization in India and Pakistan. Cambridge University Press, Cambridge.
3. Bhasin, M. K., Walter, H., & Dankor-Hopfe (1994). An investigation of biological variability in Ecological Ethno-economic and Linguistic Groups. Kamla-Raj Enterprises, Delhi, India
4. Bijukumar, U. (2013). Social exclusion and ethnicity in northeast India. *NEHU Jour. 9*, 19–35.
5. Cavalli-Sforza, I., Menozzi, P., & Piazza, A. (1994). The History and Geography of Human Genes. Princeton University Press, Princeton, New Jersey.
6. Das, B. M. (1970). Anthropometry of the Tribal groups of Assam, India. Florida: Field Research Project
7. Das, B. M., Walter, H., Gilbert, K., Lindenberg, P., Malhotra, K. C., Mukherjee, B. N., Deka, R., & Chakraborty R. (1987). Genetic variation of five blood polymorphisms in ten populations of Assam India. *Int. J. Anthrop, 2*, 325–340
8. Dutta, B. K., & Dutta, P. K. 2005. Potential of ethnobotanical studies in North East India: An overview. *Indian J. Tradit. Knowl. 4*, 7–14.
9. Gadgil, M., & Guha, R. (1992). The Fissured Land: AN Ecological History of India. Oxford Univ. Press, New Delhi, India.
10. Gadgil, M. Joshi, N. V., Prasad, U. V., Manoharan, S., & Patil, S. (1998). Peopling of India. pp. 100–129. In: Balasubramanian, D., & Appaji Rao, N. (Eds.). The Indian Human Hertiage. Universties Press, Hyderabad, India
11. Kala, C. P. (2005). Ethnomedicinal botany of the Apatani in the Eastern Himalayan region of India. *J. Ethnobiol. Ethnomed. 1*, 11.
12. Kashyap, V. K., Sarkar, N., Sahoo, S., Sarkar, B. N & Trivedi, R. (2003). Genetic variation at fifteen microsatellite loci in human populations of India. *Curr. Sci. 85*, 464–473.

13. Kumar, V., Basu, D.,& Reddy, B. M. (2004). Genetic Heterogeneity in Northeastern India: Reflection of Tribe–Caste Continuum in the Genetic Structure. *Amer. J. Human Biol. 16*, 334–345.

14. Misra, S. (1992). The age of the Achenlian in India: New evidence. *Curr. Anthropol, 33*, 325–328.

15. Sankalia, H. D. (1974). Prehistory and protohistory of India and Pakistan. Deccan College, Poona, India.

16. Singh, K. S. (1998). People of India. Anthropological Survey of India and Oxford University Press, Delhi, India.

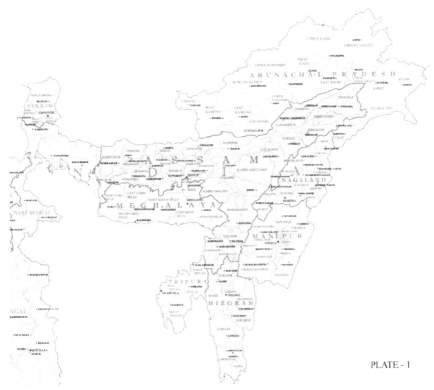

PLATE 1: Map of North East India (Source: National Atlas and Thematic Mapping Organization, Govt. of India).

CHAPTER 3

ETHNOAGRICULTURE IN NORTH-EAST INDIA: PROS, CONS, AND ECO-SUSTAINABLE MODEL

PRABHAT KUMAR RAI

Department of Environmental Science, Mizoram University, Aizawl – 796004, Mizoram, India, E-mail: prabhatrai24@gmail.com

CONTENTS

Abstract 35
3.1   Introduction 36
3.2   Shifting Cultivation 36
3.3   Ethnoagriculture in Other Parts of the World 41
3.4   Case of Apatanis in Arunachal Pradesh 42
3.5   Alternate of Shifting Cultivation 43
3.6   Agroforestry: Prospects and Potential for Sustainable
       Development of NE India 44
Acknowledgement 49
Keywords 50
References 50

ABSTRACT

Ethnoagricuture is intimately and inextricably linked with the society and livelihood of North East India. It is strongly interwoven with tradition, culture and festivals of North East India. Shifting cultivation is linked with ethnicity of North East India. Its pros and cons to the environment are discussed in this chapter. Further, case study on ethnoecology of Apatanis of Arunachal Pradesh is mentioned. Finally, agroforestry implications in ethno-agriculture is discussed and explained through an eco-sustainable model developed by the author.

3.1   INTRODUCTION

Ethnoagricuture is inextricably linked with ethnoecology as well as traditional knowledge like shifting cultivation in North East India. The large and varied body of knowledge that farmers possess and employ is an important, yet often overlooked, element in the analysis of traditional agriculture (Brosius et al., 1986). Shifting cultivation and deforestation are major constraints in developing sustainable food-production systems in the north-eastern hill region, due to their detrimental effects on soil and water resources (Borthakur et al., 1985; Singh et al., 1994). At the same time the region has some excellent indigenous resource-based land use systems. Most of them are tree based, having unique fertility restoration capacity by preventing soil loss, improving soil organic matter status and replenishing the nutrients through effective recycling mechanism (Chauhan and Dhyani, 1989; Dhyani and Chauhan, 1994).

3.2   SHIFTING CULTIVATION

Different anthropogenic and socio-economic factors have perturbed the pristine ecology of NE India, leading to the degradation of environment and natural resources. Shifting cultivation is a form of ethnoagriculture in North East India. Particularly, the practice of unregulated shifting cultivation (*jhooming*) exacerbates the gloomy situation. Shifting agriculture, or slash and burn agriculture is locally called "*jhooming.*" Figure 3.1 demonstrates a patch of forest which underwent shifting cultivation. Practiced since time immemorial (originating during Neolithic times), it is still the major form of agriculture in the NE Himalaya. Practiced by about half a million tribal families, it affects about 2.7 million ha, and about 0.45 million ha remain under shifting cultivation per year. This accounts

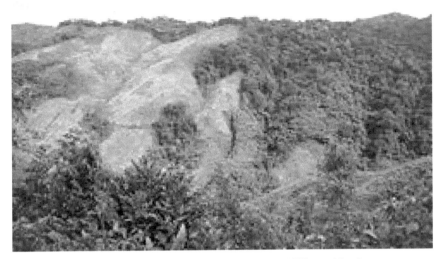

FIGURE 3.1   Figure showing patch of forest underwent shifting cultivation.

for 85% of the land cultivated each year. Normally, shifting cultivation involves: (i) forest cutting during December-January; (ii) burning of the slashed forest after removing tree trunks and large branches during mid-February to mid-March; (iii) cultivation of crops in April-May (cereals, vegetables, and oil-yielding crops) in various mixes; (iv) shifting to another forest site; and (v) returning to the original site (in earlier times after 20–30 yr.) but currently, owing to the population pressure, after 5 years or even less (Singh and Singh, 1987).

In the NE India, shifting cultivation is a major land use that is practiced by almost all the tribal groups (Ramakrishnan, 1993; Ramakrishnan et al., 1996). There is wide recognition across the globe, and disciplines, that regions of ecological relevance like NE India exhibit a symbiotic relationship between their habitat and the culture within (Ramakrishnan et al., 1996, Ramakrishnan, 2001). Moreover, *jhoom* practice among various tribes of Mizoram is closely linked with socio-cultural life of the people. Various festivals are organized on the onset of *Jhooming* as well as at the time of harvesting of crops. Shifting cultivation could be said to have evolved as a response to special physiographic characters of the land, and the economy and socio-cultural traditions of the cultivators practicing it (Ramakrishnan, 1993, 2001). Earlier, shifting cultivation was supposed to be a sustainable use of forest ecosystems while cultivators had plenty of forest areas available (Ramakrishnan, 2001). However, today this form of cultivation accounts for about 61% of total tropical forest destruction, thus posing socio-economic constraints. Further, it leads to biological invasions hampering the native forest resources (Gupta and Mukherjee, 1994; Raman, 2001). Moreover, under the strain of increasing population pressure, the fallow period became drastically reduced and the system degenerated, resulting in serious soil erosion and decline in the soil's fertility and productivity (Ramakrishnan, 2001). The tribal cultivators of NE India replaced traditional jhooming with non-traditional jhooming as their source of livelihood (Arunachalam et al., 2002).

The net decrease in forest cover due to shifting cultivation in NE India was estimated to be 387 km^2 between 1989 and 1991, 448 km^2 between 1991 and 1993 and 175 km^2 between 1993 and 1995 (Satapathy and Bujarbaruah, 2006). During this period, the rate of forest loss has declined in NE states such as Arunachal Pradesh and Meghalaya, increased in Nagaland and Manipur and fluctuated in other states (Satapathy and Bujarbaruah, 2006).

In 1957, the Food and Agricultural Organization (FAO) officially condemned shifting cultivation as a waste of land and human resources, and as major cause of soil erosion and deforestation. Traditional shifting cultivation were able to maintain subsistence crop yields at a low but sustained level for centuries; if fallow length was respected. In the tropics, where rain and sunshine are abundant throughout the year, secondary forest develops wherever cultivated land has been forsaken for a long period. Notwithstanding, the practice causes a severe loss of biological diversity. Moreover, in area of high demographic growth and increasing land short-ages (like Aizawl, the capital city of Mizoram, NE India), intensification of slash and burn system can be highly detrimental. Intensified land use under shifting cultivation not only increase invasive weed biomass but also changes weed species composition difficult to control (Rai, 2009). The creation of secondary forests composed of a few dominant coloniz-ing plant species, bamboo thickets, and thatch grasslands has adversely affected plant diversity (Gupta, 2000). Plant diversity is also affected by the almost total cessation of the natural regeneration of shade loving species of Orchidaceae and Dipterocarpaceae following changes in the light regimes on the forest floor due to wide openings in the canopies created by large-scale jhoom clearings (Gupta, 2000).

In nutshell, general impact of unregulated shifting cultivation in tropics altered the landscapes that were once large tracts of evergreen dense primary forests, into fragmented mosaics of small habitat islands of degraded primary forests, secondary forests and low quality bamboo forests (Rai, 2009). The frequent periodic clearing of forests as in non traditional jhooming creates an ecosystem where secondary plant species are totally different from the parent forest (Rai, 2009). These changes in habitat also affect forest resources (Arunachalam et al., 2002), animals, birds, and microorganisms (Raman, 2001). After slash and burn agriculture (jhoom) at lower elevations in North-East (NE) India, the secondary succession passes from a herbaceous weedy community to bamboo forest (Rai, 2009). During the intervening fallow period, the vegetation grows back through the 'succession' (Raman, 2001; Rai, 2009). In NE India, where shifting cultivation is a common practice, a typical fallow period theoretically lasts about 10 years.

Some ecologists have suggested that jhoom may increase biodiversity because it creates new habitats, while others see it as a largely destructive practice (Raman, 2001). Several workers (Singh and Singh, 1987; Raman, 2001) addressed this debate by measuring the change and recovery of plant and bird communities after shifting cultivation. One group of researchers (Raman, 2001) from Wildlife Institute of India (WII) concluded that jhoom cultivation leads to the invasion of widespread bird species at the expense of forest species that are often rare or restricted in range. They recommended that to avoid substantial changes in natural communities, jhoom cycles would need to be at least 25 years (for birds) to 50 years (for vegetation) as the current 8–10 years cycles are clearly inadequate to conserve forest bird and plant communities.

Due to excessive non-traditional jhooming, forest area and vegetation cover have shrunk by about 22.9% and 12.4%, respectively in last 40 years in Tripura, a NE state (Gupta, 2000). According to Gupta (2000), open, less diverse, moist and dry mixed deciduous secondary forests have replaced the dense primary forests of NE India due to the shifting cultivation with reduced fallow period. Repeated jhooming on short fallow rotation coupled with grazing and other human disturbances (encroachment, over-exploitation for timber, fuel wood, fodder, and construction materials, etc.) have arrested secondary succession at the serial community stages, favoring weed infestation, loss of accumulation of woody biomass, and reduction of floral diversity. It has also resulted in the creation of *Imperata cylindrica* grasslands, and degraded bamboo forests (Gupta, 2000; Rai, 2009).

As far as soil physico-chemical parameters change pertaining to aforesaid practice is concerned before the forest is cleared for jhooming, a closed nutrient cycle exists in the soil- forest system. Within this system, most nutrients are stored in the biomass and topsoil, and a constant cycle of nutrient transfer from one compartment of system to another operates through the physical and biological processes of rain-wash (i.e., foliage leaching), litter fall, root decomposition, and plant uptake. However, clearing and burning the vegetation leads to a disruption of this closed nutrient cycle. During the burning operation the soil temperature increases and afterwards, more radiation falling on the bare soil-surface results in the higher soil and air temperature. This change in the temperature regime causes changes in biological activity in the soil. The addition of ash to the soil through burning causes important changes in soil chemical properties and organic matter content (Stromgaard, 1991). In general, exchangeable bases and available phosphorus increase slightly after burning; pH values also increase, but usually temporarily. Burning is also expected to increase organic matter content, mainly because of the unburnt vegetation left behind (Yadava and Devi, 2004, 2005; Devi and Yadava, 2007). Yadava and Devi (2004) reported higher values of C, N, P, and microbial biomass than the native forest site in the immediate slash and burnt site of Manipur, NE India. The rate of ammonification and N-mineralization were also recorded to be higher in the slash and burnt site as compared to the protected forest site (Yadava and Devi, 2005; Devi and Yadava, 2007). These changes in the soil after clearing and burning result in sharp increase of available nutrient but in following years it declines significantly. The main reasons for the decline in crop yields are soil fertility depletion, increased weed infestation, deterioration of soil physical properties, and increased insect and disease attacks. Ramakrishnan (1992) studied the effect of jhoom on soil fertility at high elevations of Meghalaya, NE India, using 15, 10 and 5 years jhoom cycles and found that longer fallows gave greater improvement in humus and nutrients.

Bhadauria and Ramakrishnan (1996) investigated the role of earthworms in the Nitrogen cycle in a shifting agriculture system under a 5- and a 15-year jhum system fallow period intervening between two croppings on the same site. Earthworms participated in the N cycle through worm cast egestion, mucus production, and dead tissue decomposition. Soil N was initially depleted by volatilization during slash and burn operations, and subsequently during cultivation processes. These losses were more pronounced under the 15-year Jhum system. The total soil N made available for uptake by the plant through the activity of earthworms in this agro-ecosystem was higher than the total input of N to the soil through the addition of slashed vegetation, inorganic and organic manure, and recycled crop residue and weeds.

Nevertheless, in view of current demographic, economic, and land use patterns in NE states, it will be too ambitious attempt to revert to traditional shifting cultivation. Also, such traditional practices are further linked with their culture and sentiments. Moreover, most of the human population depends on shifting-agriculture in the NE region. Only we have to find out alternate ways and an ecologically relevant hypothetical growth model.

3.3   ETHNOAGRICULTURE IN OTHER PARTS OF THE WORLD

Ethnoagriculture record of Mexico has been overviewed by Butzer (1990). Growth of sedentary agricultural settlement was seen over the 2000 years prior to "Classic" Teotihuacan (demographic growth rate only 0.09% annually when 14C dates are calibrated to absolute years). Yet locally the ecological impact was enormous, with strong pollen peaks of maize (to over 30%) (Butzer, 1990). Around Lake Texcoco, a much more modest peak of maize and disturbance plants was delayed until the Teotihuacan phase (ca. A.D. 300–750) (Rai, 2012). Population centers were, then, prone to shift over time, with long intervening periods of agricultural recession. That pattern is reflected in the overall population history. For the early 1500s, extrapolating for the 20% or so of the arable lands not surveyed, a population of 800,000 to 1.2 million is suggested (Sanders, 1981; Butzer, 1990). This compares with 230,000 during the earlier maximum of the

Teotihuacan era, which was followed by a protracted decline, to a low of only 130,000 between about A.D. 950–1150, a time of considerable settlement retraction in many areas and disintensification in some. The remarkable growth of the Late Aztec period is linked by Sanders to agricultural expansion and intensification. In Classic times, floodwater and canal irrigation had been limited to a small part of the basin, primarily around Teotihuacan. During the 150 years of Aztec rule, irrigated agriculture expanded greatly along the alluvial lowlands, up into the piedmont zone, while chinampa cultivation was developed in the Xochimilco-Chalco area, and hill slope terracing brought higher ground into cultivation (Butzer, 1990). In other words, the elaborate system of intensified agriculture that characterized the basin in 1519 was of comparatively recent origin. Although Sanders prefers to see intensification and agricultural expansion as a response to growing population pressure, the three centuries or more of demographic decline after A.D. 750 shows that growth was not linear and that the systemic interactions were more complex. The several cycles of settlement nucleation evidently corresponded to times of administrative centralization and population growth that were repeatedly terminated by periods of decentralization, with settlement dispersal and population decline. This suggests that systematic integration or dissipation, with increasing or decreasing energy (tribute) demands, must be considered as major factors in the equation (Butzer, 1990).

3.4   CASE OF APATANIS IN ARUNACHAL PRADESH

One other well-known example that can be cited as an example of TEK is wet rice cultivation of the *Apatanis*, which is a unique and highly integrated land use system in the State Arunachal Pradesh of NE India (Ramakrishnan et al., 2002). The estimated diversity of rice found in the entire region is about 9650 (Mao et al., 2009; Chaliha and Kant, 2011). The state of Arunachal Pradesh itself yielded around 616 germplasm collections of rice from 1987 to 2002 (Hore, 2005; Chaliha and Kant, 2011).

The Apatanis of Ziro valley in lower Subansiri district of Arunachal Pradesh are one such tribe which grow a wide variety of paddy in very small land holdings (Chaliha and Kant, 2011). This tribe, known to be relatively advanced among other tribal societies, grows paddy varieties of unique grain characteristic, nutrition requirement, duration, productivity and resistance to disease and insect pests, in highly evolved wet paddy cultivation coupled with pisciculture (Chaliha and Kant, 2011). Wetland rice cultivation in Ziro valley is practiced in broad and well-leveled terraces with strong bunds in which the hill streams are trapped, channelized and diverted into primary, secondary and tertiary networks to provide water in the terraces. Water from one terrace reaches another through bamboo or wooden pipes. Fish pits in the plots ensure water remains for pisciculture even when the field is drained off especially in the flowering and the grain maturity stage (Chaliha and Kant, 2011).

The paddy varieties of Apatanis have been reported by different researchers and their accounts vary greatly (Dabral, 2002; Pulamte, 2008; Dollo et al., 2009; Nimachow et al., 2010; Chaliha and Kant, 2011) on account both of limited tools at their disposal as also the geographical areas actually explored.

Further, the inventory of medicinal plants used by the *Apatani* by Kala (2005) opened new avenues to scrutinize such a rich natural resource for further analysis in order to develop the potential of herbal medicine.

3.5   ALTERNATE OF SHIFTING CULTIVATION

Shifting cultivation, which is the prime concern of policy makers in the context of natural resource management, cannot sustain for the long term because increasing population in the absence of an abundant supply of land is bound to shorten the cycle of shifting cultivation, bringing about continuous deterioration in soil fertility and ecological changes. Studies conducted in the Philippines, Gambia, Malawi, Zambia, and in India (Ganguly, 1968; Saha, 1970) reveal that land carrying capacity under shifting cultivation is very low-about six persons per sq. km. Therefore, conservation of biodiversity will largely depend on creating conditions to revert to traditional long fallow shifting cultivation, finding suitable alternatives to such farming practices, or a combination of both. In view of earlier mentioned demographic, economic, and land use patterns in NE states, it may be too ambitious attempt to ban traditional shifting cultivation. The efforts of the government to control forest resources could not be enforced against strong local needs of subsistence and income generation.

Therefore, the best solutions may lie in finding suitable alternatives that make an appropriate balance between socio-economic considerations and natural resource management.

In order to remove the ecological and economic constraints imposed due to non traditional shifting cultivation, TEK and scientific approach can be practiced in an integrated way in NE India through the broad implementation and extension of agroforestry practices on *jhoom* lands.

Agroforestry is a collective name for land use systems and technologies where woody perennials (trees, shrubs, palms, bamboos, etc.) are deliberately used on the same land management units as agricultural crops and/ or animals, in some form of spatial arrangement or temporal sequence. Community forestry, farm forestry, social forestry in nutshell describes the "tree growing by the people, for the people" and in general, all these terminologies encompass agroforestry concepts and technologies. In agroforestry systems, there are both ecological and economic interactions between the different components. The mixture of crops grown in agroforestry is so evolved that the root systems of different plants reach out to varying depths. In this way, different crops are able to use the nutrients of different layers of the soil in the field. In contrast, all plants under monoculture system (common in conventional shifting cultivation) draw up from the same strata. Secondly, the varieties of plants in *jhoom* system are arranged in a multi-storied pattern so that the leaf area of all vegetation in the field together is extraordinarily large. This helps in harvesting the solar energy much more efficiently than in a mono crop area. The multi-storied pattern also provides a better cover for the land against soil erosion. Further, aforesaid monoculture pattern may be more prone to pest attack when compared to multiple cropping pattern followed in agroforestry.

3.6 AGROFORESTRY: PROSPECTS AND POTENTIAL FOR SUSTAINABLE DEVELOPMENT OF NE INDIA

Various approaches have been suggested as alternatives and/or improvements to shifting cultivation (FAO, 1985), and most of them emphasize the importance of retaining or incorporating the woody vegetation into the fallow phase and even in the cultivation phase, as the key to the maintenance of soil productivity (Nair, 1993). However, suitable eco-friendly methods are to be applied for true and all round agricultural development in the hills. Depending on the ways in which the woody species are incorporated, the alternate land-use system can be agroforestry (Nair, 1993).

Agroforestry is a collective name for land use systems and technologies where woody perennials (trees, shrubs, palms, bamboos, etc.) are deliberately used on the same land management units as agricultural crops and/ or animals, in some form of spatial arrangement or temporal sequence. In agroforestry systems there are both ecological and economic interactions between the different components (Nair, 1993). Community forestry, farm forestry and social forestry in nutshell describe the "tree growing by the people, for the people." In general, these terminologies all encompass agroforestry concepts and technologies (Nair, 1993). The mixture of crops grown in agroforestry is so evolved that the root systems of different plants reach out to varying depths. In this way different crops are able to use the nutrients of different layers of the soil in the field. In contrast, all plants under monoculture system (common in conventional shifting cultivation) draw up from the same strata. Secondly, the varieties of plants in jhoom system are arranged in a multi-storied pattern so that the leaf area of all vegetation in the field together is extraordinarily large. This helps in harvesting the solar energy much more efficiently than in a mono crop area. The multistoried pattern also provides a better cover for the land against soil erosion. Further, aforesaid monoculture pattern may be more prone to pest attack when compared to multiple cropping pattern followed in agroforestry. There are wide scope of sloppy land development and management in the hilly region with application of agronomical, mechanical soil and water conservation measures and intervention of agroforestry systems. The soil conservation measures and agroforestry systems are to be generally planned and taken up in the areas retrieved from *jhooming* to provide protective cover to the barren lands. These will help in prevention of soil erosion, improving water regime particularly of the catchments areas and general restoration of the balance of the ecology of nature (Sonowal et al., 2006). Tiwari and Jha (1995) surveyed 22 watersheds in Mizoram. These have been placed in three class, i.e., low priority, high priority or very high priority as per the requirement of swift soil conservation measures. Effective planning, development, and utilization of all natural resources in hills towards sustainable production are possible on the basis of watershed programs, aimed to check soil erosion, improve soil fertility and productivity (Satapathy and

Bujarbaruah, 2006). Further, TEK, as discussed earlier in the text may also encourage agroforestry approaches in an effective and systematic way. For instance, TEK was integrated into institution building in the sustainable management of the traditional slash and burn agroecosystem in the State of Nagaland in NE India. Traditional tribal societies of Nagaland in NE India organize nutrient-use efficient crop species on the upper slopes and less efficient species along the lower slopes, corresponding to the soil fertility gradient of a steep slope. By shortening the shifting agricultural cycle the farmer tends to place emphasis on tuber and vegetable crops rather than cereals with longer cycles. Operating a mixed cropping system, where species are sown simultaneously following the first rain during the monsoon, the farmer harvests crops one after the other as they mature over a period of a few months. After the harvest, the biomass is recycled into the agricultural plot. Weed biomass taken from the plots are put back into the system; about 20 per cent of weed biomass serves an important nutrient conservation role on the hill slope, which would otherwise be lost through leaching processes. Socially selected species of traditional agricultural systems and those from natural systems often have an ecologically significant keystone value; these keystone species often play a major role in the nutrient enrichment of soil. Traditional eco-technologies, such as systems for water harvesting during the period of the monsoon, have been shown to be of value in altering biological processes in soil and thus improving soil fertility (Ramakrishnan, 1992).

There should be an inextricable link between plants and animals in agroecosystems. Animal husbandry with fish or prawn aquaculture may be an integral component of agroforestry in NE India. Livestock management, for example, pig and bee culture may also be practiced in agroforestry systems. Animal husbandry is an important component of the local economy and the status of a tribal family is often also assessed on the basis of the number of animals of its own (Satapathy and Bujarbaruah, 2006). By pollinating the diverse group of plants Bees perform vital and often unappreciated roles. At least 30% of our agricultural crops require the movement of pollen between flowers mediated by bees. We are dependent upon these "forgotten pollinators" for most of what we eat. Furthermore, in agroforestry, selective breeding of livestock for meat extraction may prevent frequent hunting of wildlife leading to their extinction. Concomitantly, animal husbandry in agroforestry systems may boost the socioeconomic status of peoples, for example, breeding of pig is particularly popular in Mizoram and it provides a sound contribution to economy.

Similarly, Agroforestry may be Teak based, Subabul based, Fruits mixed with Subabul, Medicinal plants mixed with Subabul, Bamboo based agroforestry, Hedgerow cropping, Coffee based agroforestry, Sole Banana based cropping, and Medicinal plant based, which further ameliorate the socio-economic sector. Medicinal plant cultivation has many more advantages, as this practice brings economic benefit to the community while also addressing conservation concerns (Chettri and Sharma, 2007). Jha and Lalnunmawia (2003) studied the ecological and economic aspect of Bamboo and Ginger based agroforestry system. Lalramnghinghlova and Jha (1996) mentioned prominent multipurpose trees in farming system of Mizoram. Such sort of studies in context of agroforestry systems need focused attention and further work in this direction. Home gardens are very common and age old practice of agroforestry in every village of NE India, which may be encouraged further. A home garden is an assemblage of plants which may include trees, shrubs, bamboos, and herbaceous plants in or adjacent to a home or home compound. Banana, papaya, mango, peach, plum, jack fruit, pine apple and some other domesticated wild fruit and vegetables are commonly cultivated in home gardens. Fodder and fuel trees are also planted in home garden for home consumption throughout the year. Besides, a number of the home gardens of rare and endangered orchids (epiphytic and ground/terrestrial), medicinal plants (both as vegetables and medicinal) and wild fruit plants (both lianas and trees) are grown in the garden. Live fence of different species (both thorny and non-thorny) are planted around the orchard for providing protection from the livestock and for additional production and risk diversification. The species widely planted for the purpose are: *Erythrina indica*, *Gliricidia* sp, *Thysanolaena maxima*, *Emblica officinalis*, etc. Large cardamom (*Amomum subulatum*) is the most important native cash crop of Sikkim in agroforestry systems of NE India and traditional agroforestry systems also encompasses different economic crops (Rai et al., 1994, 1997, 2002). Therefore, agroecosystems as well as natural ecosystems harbor immense genetic potential (Lalramnghinghlova, 1999a,b,c,d, 2000, 2001, 2002a,b).

Agroforestry systems promote an increase in the soil organic carbon stocks and fractions, thus improving soil quality (Ramesh et al., 2015). Certain plants, for example, *Alnus nepalensis* in particular, can, therefore, be recommended as an alternative soil management strategy for food production, and for the maintenance of soil quality and agricultural sustainability through increased Soil Organic Carbon (SOC) sequestration in the highly fragile agro-ecosystems of northeast India (Ramesh et al., 2015).

In this context, agroforestry systems, land use systems in which woody plants are grown in association with agricultural crops, pasture or livestock, have been widely promoted as a sustainable food production system, and would be particularly attractive for under-developed regions, where the use of external inputs is not feasible (Nair et al., 1999). It is also considered to be a viable option for better soil use, favoring environmental functions and increasing carbon sequestration (Takimoto et al., 2009). These agroecosystems can improve nutrient cycling and enhance soil structure (Maia et al., 2006), reducing water erosion and increasing SOC stocks depending upon the quantity and quality of litter reaching soil surface and rate of litter decomposition and nutrient release (Aguiar et al., 2010).

Soil hydro-physical behavior was studied under a 20-year old agroforestry plantation consisting of five multipurpose tree species (*Pinus kesiya* Royle ex Gordon, *Alnus nepalensis* D. Don, *Parkia roxburghii* G. Don, *Michelia oblonga* Wall. and *Gmelina arboria* Roxb.) maintained under normal recommended practices at Indian Council of Agricultural Research (ICAR) Complex, Umiam, Meghalaya, India (Saha et al., 2007). Of the tree species, *Pinus kesiya, Michelia oblonga* and *Alnus nepalensis* were found to be rated best for bio-amelioration of soils as these tree covers had more root and shoot biomass and more litter fall compared to other species (Saha et al., 2007).

Ethnopedology is the documentation and understanding of local approaches to soil perception, classification, appraisal, use and management (WinklerPrins and Sandor, 2003; Nath et al., 2015). It is widely recognized that farmers' hold important knowledge of folk soil classification for agricultural land for its uses, yet little has been studied for traditional agroforestry systems (Nath et al., 2015). Nath et al. (2015) explored the ethnopedology of bamboo (*Bambusa* sp.) based agroforestry system in North East India, and establishes the relationship of soil quality index (SQI) with bamboo productivity.

Author of this chapter made a self-explainable eco-sustainable model (Figure 3.2) for the integrated management of natural and human resources on the basis of abovementioned discussions. Further, integrated

work and cooperation among social workers, scientists, ecologists, wildlife workers, academicians from Mizoram University and North-Eastern
Hill University, NGO's and policy makers is recommended for sustainable
development of natural resources of NE India (Rai, 2012).

ACKNOWLEDGEMENT

The author is thankful to Professor Amar Nath Rai, Former Director,
NAAC, Vice chancellor Mizoram and North Eastern Hill University, India.

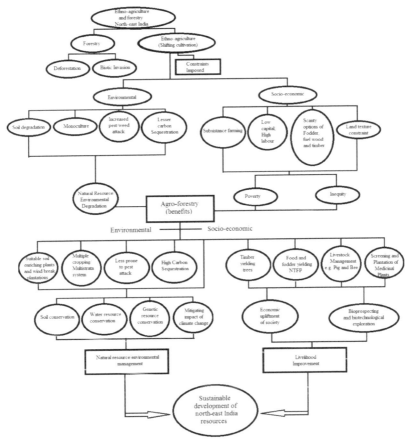

FIGURE 3.2   Alternate to ethno-agriculture in the form of shifting cultivation for eco-
sustainable development of North East India (Redrawn and modified after Rai, 2012, 2015).

KEYWORDS

- **agroforestry**
- **apatanis**
- **eco-sustainable model**
- **ethnoagriculture**
- **ethnoecology**
- **shifting cultivation**

REFERENCES

1. Aguiar, A. C. F., Bicudo, S. J., Costa Sobrinho, J. R. S., Martins, A. L. S., Coelho, K. P., & Moura, for example, (2010). Nutrient recycling and physical indicators of an alley cropping system in a sandy loam soil in the Pre-Amazon region of Brazil. *Nutr. Cycl. Agroecozyst.* 86, 189–198.
2. Arunachalam. A., Khan, M. L., & Arunachalam, K. (2002). Balancing traditional jhum cultivation with modern agroforestry in eastern Himalaya – a biodiversity hotspot. *Curr. Sci. 33,* 117–118.
3. Bhadauria, T., & Ramakrisnan, P. S. (1996). Role of earthworms in nitrogen cycling during the cropping phaseof shifting agriculture (Jhum) in north-east India. *Biol. Fertil. Soils. 22,* 350–354.
4. Borthakur, D. N., Singh, A., & Prasad, R. N. (1985). Shifting cultivation in north-east India and strategy for land and water resources management. *Beitrage zur Tropischen Landwirtschaft und Veterinarmedizin. 23,* 147–158.
5. Brosius, J. P., Lovelace, G. W., & Marten, G. G. (1986). Ethnoecology: An approach to understanding Traditional Agricultural Knowledge. In: Traditional Agriculture in South East Asia: A Human ecology perspective. Aarten, G. G. (ed.). Boulder and London, Westview Press. pp. 24–220.
6. Butzer, K. W. (1990). Ethnoagriculture and cultural ecology in Mexico: Hostorical Visatas and modern implications. In: Conference of Latin Americanist Geographers. BENCHMARK (1991/1992), University of Texas Press. *17/18,* 139–152. Accessed: 04-06-2015 00:07 UTC.
7. Chaliha, S., & Kant. P. (2011). Adapting to Climate Change: Conserving rice biodiversity of the Apatani tribe in North East India. Institute of Green Economy IGREC Working Paper IGREC-24: 2011.
8. Chauhan, D. S., & Dhyani, S. K. (1989). Traditional agroforestry practices in N. E. Himalayan region of India. *Indian J. Dryland. Agric. Res. Dev. 4(2),* 73–81.
9. Chettri, N., & Sharma, E. (2007). Firewood value assessment: A comparison on local preference and wood constituent properties of species from a trekking corridor, West Sikkim, India. *Curr. Sci., 92*(12), 1744–1747.

10. Dabral, P. P. (2002). Indigenous techniques of soil and water conservation in North Eastern region of India. Paper presented at 12th ISCO Conference, Beijing, China, 26–31 May 2002

11. Dollo, M., Samal, P. K., Sundriyal, R. C., & Kumar, K. (2009). Environmentally sustainable traditional natural resource management and conservation in Ziro Valley, Arunachal Himalayas, India. *J. American Sci., 5(5)*, 41–52

12. Devi, A. S., & Yadava, P. S. (2007). Wood and leaf litter decomposition of *Dipterocarpus tuberculatus* Roxb. in a tropical deciduous forest of Manipur, North East India. *Curr. Sci. 93(2)*, 243–246.

13. Dhyani, S. K., & Chauhan, D. S. (1994). Agroforestry practices of north-eastern hill region of India. In: *Agroforestry Traditions and Innovations*. Narain, P., Dadhwal, K. S., & Singh, R. K. (eds.). Central Soil and Water Conservation Research and Training Institute, Dehradun. pp. 19–23.

14. FAO. (1985). Changes in shifting cultivation in Africa: Seven case studies. *FAO Forestry Paper* 50/1. FAO, Rome, Italy.

15. Ganguly, J. B. (1968). Economic problems of Jhumias of Tripura. Bookland Private. Calcutta.

16. Gupta, A. K. (2000). Shifting Cultivation and conservation of biological diversity in Tripura, Northeast India. *Hum. Ecol. 28(4)*, 605–629.

17. Gupta, A. K., & Mukherjee, S. K. (1994). Status of wildlife in Tripura—problems in its management. *Environ. 2*, 34–49.

18. Hore, D. K. (2005). Rice diversity collection, conservation and management in northeastern India. *Genetic Resources and Crop Evolution. 52*, 1129–1140.

19. Jha, L. K., & Lalnunmawia, F. (2003). Agroforestry with bamboo and ginger to rehabilitate degraded areas in North East India. *J. Bamboo and Rattan, 2*(2), 103–109.

20. Kala, C. P. (2005). Ethnomedicinal botany of the Apatani in the Eastern Himalayan region of India. *J. Ethnobiol. Ethnomedicine*. doi: 10.1186/1746–4269, 1–11.

21. Lalramnghinghlova, H. (1999a). Ethnobotany: A Review. *J. Econ. Taxon. Bot. 23 (1)*, 1–27.

22. Lalramnghinghlova, H. (1999b). Prospects of Ethnomedicinal plants of Mizoram in the new millennium. In: *Proc. Symp. On Science & Technology for Mizoram in 21st Century.* 17–18 June, Aizawl. pp. 119–126.

23. Lalramnghinghlova, H. (1999c). Status paper on bamboo in Mizoram. *Arunachal Forest News. 17(1&2)*, 34–37.

24. Lalramnghinghlova, H. (1999d). Ethnobotanical and agroecological studies on genetic resources of food plants in Mizoram state. *J. Econ. Taxon. Bot. 23(2)*, 637–644.

25. Lalramnghinghlova, H. (2000). Ethnomedicinal plants development in Mizoram. In: *Proc. Int. Workshop on Agroforestry and Forest Products, Aizawl.* November, 28–30. pp. 395–404.

26. Lalramnghinghlova, H. (2001). Ethnobotanical interpretations and future prospects of ethnobotany in the North-East India. *Science Vision. 1*, 24–31.

27. Lalramnghinghlova, H. (2002a). Bioresources of Mizoram: An overview. *J. North Eastern Council.* pp. 56–64.

28. Lalramnghinghlova, H. (2002b). Ethnobotanical study on the edible plants of Mizoram. *Ethnobotany 14*, 23–33.

29. Lalramnghinghlova, H., & Jha, L. K. (1996). Prominent agroforestry systems and important multipurpose trees in farming systems in Mizoram. *Indian Forester, 122*(7), 23–33.

30. Maia, S. M. F., Xavier, F. A. S., Oliveira, T. S., Mendonca, E. S., & Araujo, Filho, J. A., (2006). Impactos de sistemas agroflorestais econvencional sobre a qualidade do solo no semi-a'rido cearense. *R Arvore. 30*, 837–848.

31. Mao, A., Hynniewta, T. M., Sanjappa, M (2009). Plant wealth of North east India with reference to ethnobotany. *Indian J. Trad. Knowl. 8(1)*, 96–103.

32. Nair, P. K. N., Buresh. R. J., Mugendi, D. N., & Latt, C. R. (1999). Nutrient cycling in tropical agroforestry systems: myths and science. In: *Agroforestry in sustainable agricultural systems.* Buck, L. E., Lassoie, J. P., & Fernandes. E. C. M. (eds.). CRC Press LLC, Boca Raton. pp. 1–31.

33. Nair, P. K. R. (1993). An Introduction to Agroforestry. Kluwer Academic, Netherlands.

34. Nath, A. J., Lal. R. &Das, A. K. (2015). Ethnopedology and soil quality of bamboo (*Bambusa* sp.) based agroforestry system. *Sci. Tot. Environ. 521–522*, 372–379.

35. Nimachow, G., Rawat, J. S., Dai, O., & Loder, T. (2010). A sustainable mountain paddy fish farming of the Apatani tribes of Arunachal Pradesh, India. *Aquaculture Asia Magazine, 15(2)*, 25–28.

36. Pulamte, L. (2008). Linkage between indigenous agriculture and sustainable development – Evidences from two Hill communities in Northeast India. National Institute of Science, Technology and Development Studies (CSIR).

37. Rai, P. K. (2009). Comparative Assessment of soil properties after Bamboo flowering and death in a Tropical forest of Indo-Burma Hot spot. *Ambio 38(2)*, 118–120.

38. Rai, P. K. (2012). Assessment of multifaceted environmental issues and model development of an indo-Burma hot spot region. *Environmental Monitoring and Assessment, 184*, 113–131.

39. Rai, P. K. (2015). Environmental issues and sustainable development of North East India. Lambert Publisher, Germany.

40. Rai, S. C., Sharma, E., & Sundriyal, R. C. (1994). Conservationin the Sikkim Himalaya: Traditional knowledge and land use of the Mamlay watershed. *Environmental Conservation, 15*, 30–35.

41. Rai, M., Chandel, K. P. S., & Gupta, P. N. (1997). Occurrence, distribution, and diversity in the genus *Citrus* in the Indian Gene Centre. *Proceedings of International Citriculture Congress, 1996, 2*, 1228–1234.

42. Rai, Y. K., Chettri, N., & Sharma, E. (2002). Fuelwood value index of woody tree species from forests of Mamlay Watershed, South Sikkim, India. *Forests, Trees and Livelihoods, 12*, 209–219.

43. Ramakrishnan. P. S. (1992). Shifting Cultivation Agriculture and Sustainable Development: An Interdisciplinary Study from North Eastern India. Man and Biosphere Series. Volume 10, United Nations Educational Scientific and Cultural Organization (UNESCO), Paris.

44. Ramakrishnan. P. S. (1993). Shifting agriculture and Sustainable development: An Interdisciplinary Study from North-East India. Oxford University Press, Delhi.

45. Ramakrishnan. P. S. (2001). Ecology and sustainable development, National Book Trust, New Delhi.

46. Ramakrishnan, P. S., Rai, R. K., Katwal, R. P. S., & Mehndirtta, M. (Eds.) (2002). Traditional ecological knowledge for managing biosphere reserves in South and Central Asia UNESCO and Oxford and IBH, New Delhi.

47. Ramakrishnan, P. S., Das, A. K., & Saxena, K. G. (1996). Conserving biodiversity for sustainable development. Indian National Science Academy, New Delhi.

48. Raman, T. R. S. (2001). Effect of slash-and-burn shifting cultivation on rainforest birds in Mizoram, northeast India. *Conserv. Biol. 15*, 685–698.

49. Ramesh, T., Manjaiah, K. M., Mohopatra, K. P., Rajesekar, K., & Ngachan, S. V. (2015). Assessment of soil organic carbon stocks and fractions under different agroforestry systems in subtropical hill agroecosystems of north-east India. *Agroforest. Syst.* DOI 10.1007/s10457-015-9804-z.

50. Saha, R., Tomar, J. M. S., & Ghosh, P. K. (2007). Evaluation and selection of multipurpose tree for improving soil hydro-physical behavior under hilly eco-system of north east India. *Agroforest. Syst. 69*, 239–247.

51. Saha, S. B. (1970). Socio-economic survey of the Noatia tribes. Unpublished report of the Tribal Welfare Department. Government of Tripura, Agartala, Tripura, India.

52. Sanders, W. T. (1981). Ecological adaptation in the Basin of Mexico: 23,000 B.C. to the present. In:. J. A. Sabloff (ed.). Archaeology: Supplement to the Handbook of Middle American Indians. University of Texas Press. Austin, Texas. pp. 147–197.

53. Satapathy, K. K., & Bujarbaruah, K. M. (2006). Slash and burn agriculture: Its practice, effect and problem of development. In: Bhatt, B. P., & Bujarbaruah, K. M. (eds.). Agroforestry in north east India: Opportunities and challenges. ICAR Research Complex for NEH Region, Umiam, Meghalaya. pp. 1–14.

54. Singh, B. P., Dhyani, S. K., & Prasad, R. N. (1994). Traditional agroforestry systems and their soil productivity on degraded alfisols/ultisols in hilly terrain. In: Singh, P., Pathak, P. S., & Roy, M. M. (eds.). Agroforestry systems for degraded lands. Oxford and IBH Publishing Co Pvt Ltd, New Delhi. pp. 205 214.

55. Singh, J. S., & Singh, S. P. (1987). Forest Vegetation of the Himalaya. *Bot. Rev. 53*, 81–181.

56. Sonowal, D. K., Bhatt, B. P., Satapathy, K. K., & Baishya, B. (2006). Soil and water conservation techniques for sustainable land use. In: B. P. Bhatt, & K. M. Bujarbaruah (eds.). Agroforestry in north east India:Opportunities and challenges (pp. 33–53). Uniam, Meghalaya: ICAR Research Complex for NEH Region.

57. Stromgaard, P. (1991). Soil nutrient accumulation under traditional African agriculture in the miombo woodland of Zambia. *Tropical Agric (Trinidad). 68*, 74–80.

58. Takimoto, A., Nair, V. D., & Nair, P. K. R. (2009). Contribution of trees to soil carbon sequestration under agroforestry systems in the West African Sahel. *Agrofor Syst. 76*, 11–25.

59. Tiwari, R. P., & Jha, L. K. (1995). Morphometric analysis of watersheds of Mizoram for estimation of burn-off and sediment yield in natural resource management in Mizoram (Vol. 1). A. P. P. Publications, New Delhi.

60. Winkler Prins, A., & Sandor, J. A., (2003). Local soil knowledge: insights, applications, and challenges. *Geoderma. 111*, 165–170.

61. Yadava. P. S., & Devi, A. S. (2004). Impact of Slash and Burning on Microbial Biomass in Semi-Evergreen Tropical Deciduous Forest of Manipur, North-East India. *Korean J. Ecol. 27(4)*, 225–230.

62. Yadava, P. S., & Devi, A. S. (2005). Effect of Slash and Burning on N-mineralisation in the *Dipterocarpus* Forest of Manipur, NE India. *Intern. J. Ecol. Environment. Sci. 31(10)*, 53–60.

CHAPTER 4

ETHNIC FOOD PLANTS AND ETHNIC FOOD PREPARATION OF NORTH-EAST INDIA

ROBINDRA TERON

Department of Life Science and Bioinformatics, Assam University, Diphu Campus, Karbi Anglong, Diphu, Assam – 782462, E-mail: robin.teron@gmail.com

CONTENTS

Abstract 55

4.1   Introduction 56

4.2   Data Acquisition 60

4.3   Ethnic Food Plants and Ethnic Foods of North-East India 61

4.4   Conclusion 86

Acknowledgement 88

Keywords 88

References 89

ABSTRACT

Ethnic food systems, diversity of food plants, culinary methods and socio-cultural implications of ethnic foods in North Eastern Region (NER) of India are reviewed in this chapter. Evaluation of available information implicates great diversity in food plants among ethnic groups of NER.

In NER though many foods have common ingredients, methods of preparation, nomenclature and their cultural values differ. This speaks of the intricate link of food systems with ethnic, linguistic, cultural and biological diversity. One of the significant aspect of this review is the invaluable role of women in the preservation of ethnic food traditions and the associated traditional knowledge. Maintenance of ethnic food systems or food culture poses a real challenge against the onslaught of globalization, climate change and biodiversity loss. *Jhum* (slash and burn agriculture), particularly in Northeast India, poses serious threat to natural habitats of wild foods. Nonetheless, ethnic foods provide multitude of opportunities for preservation of cultural heritage, research and development. The diverse ethnic foods can provide a platform for ecotourism through which the local food systems can be popularized and promoted. All these can help in realization of the value of ethnic food plants and food systems, and present a case for their conservation.

4.1   INTRODUCTION

Food is not only a necessity of life, but also a significant cultural reflection of people's community and background (Wakefield et al., 2007). It is a necessary commodity for sustenance and is deeply associated with the social facets of life. Food has always been linked to environmental conditions with production, storage and distribution, markets all sensitive to weather extremes and climate fluctuation (Ingram et al., 2010). The geographical and economic environment of a region has a significant impact on foods, their availability and usage. Different cultures or ethnic groups have traditional dietary patterns, preparation methods and eating practices associated with them. Food and food systems play a central role in every culture and eating socially has less to do with nutrition than with communication and relationships. The culinary methods and the ways of serving and consuming food, which vary from culture to culture, can have an important influence on social and familial relationships. Food has also played an important role in religion, helping to define the separateness of one creed from another by means of selective use of foods and dietary taboos. Ceremonies, oral traditions such as stories, songs and oral histories and other cultural practices such as reciprocity are important cultural elements in the maintenance and transmission of knowledge and practices of traditional food and agro-ecosystems. The indigenous tribes residing in different regions of the world largely depend on either shifting cultivation systems or forest based food products for their sustainable survival. The people adhere to their indigenous knowledge pertaining to agriculture, food, medicine and natural resource management. The indigenous people are habituated to live and survive with the forest and *jhum* (slash and burn) cultivation culture, which ensures a range of ethnic foods rich in nutrition and compatible to culture and ethnicity of tribes (Singh et al., 2007). Women, on the other hand, have played a magnificent role in almost all cultures. Women folks have been actively involved in accumulating wild food plants and non-vegetarian foods through trial and error (Kar, 2004; Singh and Singh, 2006). They have been gathering knowledge on wild foods through their long years of collection and utilization of wild products. Collection and conservation of many local crops, ethnic vegetables, and wild edible fruits used in ethnic food systems are mainly practiced by the indigenous women folk. These practices have transformed women into users, preservers and managers of agro-biodiversity (FAO, 1996) and plant genetic resources in general. Women are, therefore, regarded to be the source of traditional knowledge which is passed on from generation to generation maintaining culture through food systems.

Fermentation is also one of the oldest forms of food processing technologies in the world. It is a widespread tradition in all cultural societies. Indigenous fermented foods have been prepared and consumed for thousands of years and are strongly linked to culture and tradition. Knowledge about traditional fermentation technologies particularly alcoholic beverage is usually transmitted through female members only as the task is usually accomplished by women folk. These fermented products have been adopted over generations and have gained importance in meeting the technical, social and economic requirements of the people. Traditional foods both fermented and non-fermented are important for food security, subsistence, livelihoods, conservation, cultural and ethnical practices. Indigenous people also have developed sound knowledge system on survival under intense condition of food scarcity by shifting to unconventional resources during the period.

4.1.1 WHY STUDY ETHNIC FOOD SYSTEMS?

Indigenous people comprise about 5.5% of the world's population, yet they are disproportionately represented among the poor and food insecure, in both developed and developing countries (Woodley et al., 2009). Their relationship with traditional lands and territories forms a core part of their identity and spirituality and is deeply rooted in their culture, language and history. Since land and its resources form the basis of Indigenous Peoples' subsistence activities, losing control of these factors undermines their food and livelihood security and can threaten their survival as well. Furthermore, the people's overall health, well-being and cultural continuity are directly related to their ability to eat traditional foods and continue their traditional food practices. These traditional foods and food practices are deeply intertwined with their cultures and value systems, and play an important role in religious ceremonies and spirituality, as well as in songs, dances and myths. While their agroecological and food systems offer some signs of resilience and adaptation, a range of factors are increasingly threatening these systems and Indigenous peoples' well-being.

Food has always played a major role in addressing major significant issues of the processes of ethnic identity, the transmission of ethnic consciousness and the maintenance of ethnic group boundaries. Therefore, there always exist a link between food and ethnicity, a relationship about which many assumptions have been made with little empirical evidence. There is enormous scope in investigations of traditional food systems. Ethnic foods present opportunities for rural development. Good nutritional contents, nutraceuticals, food security, culture, livelihoods, conservation of crop varieties and tourism are some strong features of traditional foods. In the process of maintenance of traditional food systems, indigenous people around the world have contributed towards conservation of many varieties of crops (popularly referred as 'folk varieties') and biodiversity. When staple foods are in short supply, wild plants have been exploited by indigenous peoples around the world as source of energy and sustenance; even unpalatable plants form source of famine food during shortage of staple foods (Minis, 1991; Turner and Davis, 1993; Paul et al., 2011). Study on ethnic foods of indigenous cultures can promote better understanding, transparency and accountability amidst Indigenous Peoples. Such study would enable the people to monitor the impacts of some key trends and development interventions on their lives; it would rather assist public services, development practitioners, governments, NGOs and international agencies to understand, recognize and respect dimensions of Indigenous Peoples' livelihoods that are important for them. It would also provide decision-makers with the key facts regarding the cultural dimensions of Indigenous Peoples' food and agro-ecological systems that are essential for sound and appropriate policy design. And, it would ensure legitimacy and accountability to all stakeholders by identifying good practices, facilitating lesson-learning as well as measuring progress and achievements.

However, despite great opportunities in ethnic food systems, the impact of globalization triggered by technological development is gradually jeopardizing cultural practice which is likely to create discontinuity in the food-culture relationship. Introduction of fast foods through globalization process, accompanied by decrease in the use of traditional foods by local tribes has resulted in many diseases notably heart diseases and anemia, particularly to pregnant and lactating women (Mao and Odyou, 2007). Linguistic and cultural diversity have been threatened by processes of globalization (such as acculturation, market expansion, and biodiversity loss) as well as through scientific education and assimilation policies and programs. The loss of indigenous languages can undermine their ability to maintain their traditional knowledge and food systems. Endogenous institutions play an important role in ensuring the continuity of traditional food systems and agro-ecosystems through the transmission of related traditional knowledge, beliefs and practices across generations; continuation of this traditional system is valued considering the fact that culture is not static but highly dynamic. In this context, it is critical to identify factors that interfere with or provide opportunities for elders to pass on their knowledge to the youths as well as to identify skills, traditional knowledge and practices that are no longer appropriate to the changing environment. Indigenous peoples' access to forest resources is strongly influenced with places, ecological processes and species. Local food system is susceptible to change with fluctuation in local environment and influence of other cultures. Climatic change stands to impact the species and ecosystem that constitute tribal traditional foods that are vital to tribal culture, economy and traditional ways of life. The preservation and maintenance of traditional knowledge and associated subsistence practices that accompany food acquisition are threatened. As traditional foods are affected by climate change through habitat alterations and change in the abundance and distribution of species, there is a resulting erosion of traditional practices and knowledge (Kuhnlein and Recerveur, 1996; Nabhan, 2010; Lynn et al., 2013).

The main goal of this review is to explore the nature of ethnic food systems, diversity of food plants, culinary methods and socio-cultural implications of ethnic foods in North Eastern Region (NER) of India. The indigenous people of NER live in close proximity with nature and they are well adapted to subsist on forest and forest based products. Although ethnic and cultural diversity vis-a-vis dietary diversity in these two regions have been cited by many reports, a detailed and systematic ethnobotanical study of food plants and food preparation is required for documentation and to promote traditional knowledge of the indigenous tribes and the use of plants and plant products as food and means of their survival. Such effort help in organizing scattered information in one report and provide ready reference for researchers interested in the ethnobotany of Northeast India. It helps to understand the diversity, exploitation and utilization of plant resources by ethnic people and human-food-environment nexus in the regions.

The geographical details and the tribal diversity has been given in Chapter 2.

4.2 DATA ACQUISITION

Information for writing this review was gathered using research publications, books and online repositories. Systematic online searches was also made using the following keywords 'ethnic foods,' 'indigenous cultures of Northeast India,' 'wild edible plants of Northeast India,' 'fermented products of Northeast India' and 'food and culture,' 'indigenous tribes of Andaman Islands' and 'cultural diversity in the Andaman Islands'. Research publications and reports of different organizations were also accessed to collect data on ethnic food plants and food products. The information was then organized into two sections. The first section discusses on the ethnic food system of NER in which ethnic food plants, preparation methods and food products of the region is enumerated. In the next section, ethnic food of the aboriginal tribes of Andaman Islands is presented. Challenges and opportunities for ethnic foods of NER as well as the Andaman Islands are also discussed.

4.3 ETHNIC FOOD PLANTS AND ETHNIC FOODS OF NORTH-EAST INDIA

4.3.1 DIVERSITY OF ETHNIC FOOD PLANTS AND ETHNIC FOODS

The NER is a constituent of two biodiversity hotspots, namely Eastern Himalaya and Indo-Burma. A large number of indigenous and immigrant ethnic groups inhabit this region with bewildering physical and cultural features. Different ethnic groups adhere to different dialects and socio-religious customs. These communities have always generated passed-on traditional knowledge from generations to generations, the knowledge which is based on their needs, instinct, observation, trial and error experiences. Agriculture through *jhum* or shifting cultivation remains their main occupation since time immemorial. However, the agricultural products being inadequate, people of the region indispensably use wild resources for sustenance as well as livelihoods. Forest products do not only account for their food requirement but also supplement traditional medicinal practices, construction materials and animal feeds. Apart from that, the products also harbor cultural value amidst the different ethnic groups. There is great body of information on the ethnobotany of indigenous people of NER (Dutta and Dutta, 2005; Agrahar-Murugkar and Subbulakshmi, 2006; Bhutani, 2008; Shankar and Rawat, 2008; Mao et al., 2009).

Jain and Shanpru (1977) surveyed wild edible plants of bazaar of Meghalaya. Arora (1990) has given an account of native food plants of the tribals in northeast India. Wild edible plants of Arunachal Pradesh were dealt by Haridasan et al. (1990). Maikuri (1991) has given nutritional value of some lesser-known wild food plants and their role in tribal nutrition. Wild edible plants constitute the major food component of the rural life in Mizoram. Diversity, endemism and economic potential of wild edible plants of Indian Himalayas was dealt by Samant and Dhar (1997). Lalramnghinglova (1999) reported 116 food plants from Mizoram. Common wild vegetables of Nyishi tribe of Arunachal Pradesh were given by Murten (2000). Samati (2004) reported 55 taxa of kitchen garden plants documented during field visits in Jaintia Hills, eastern district of Meghalaya, with botanical notes about their local names, useful parts, uses, etc.

Famines in Mizoram are mainly caused by bamboo flowering and they are called 'Thingtam' and 'Mautam'. Thingtam famine is caused by the flowering of *Bambusa tulda* Roxb. (Rawthing) and 'Mautam' famine by flowering of *Melocanna baccifera* (Roxb.) Kurz. (Mau-tak). These two bamboo species produce flowers every 48 years periodically in Mizoram. 'Thingtaan' occurred in 1724, 1785, 1833, 1881, 1929, and 1977 and 'Mautam' famine occurred in 1767, 1815, 1863, 1911, and 1959. During such situation wild edible plants play a significant role in the sustenance of rural life in Mizoram. Lalramnghinglova (2002) enumerated 78 wild edible and famine food plants from Mizoram. The wild edibles of Mizoram include vegetables, fruits, spices and condiments. Three species are reported to use their tubers and rhizomes as vegetables (Sahoo et al., 2010). The tubers of *Amomum dealbatum* and *Diocorea alata* are eaten boiled or roasted vegetables. The rhizomes of *Arisaema leschenaulti* are eaten as boiled vegetables. Young shoots and leaves of different plant species are gathered and then eaten raw or cooked as vegetables. There are 20 species used by the tribals in the studied areas. Young leaves of *Acacia* spp, *Eurya japonica, Garcinia lancifolia* are eaten boiled or fried vegetables. Young shoots from *Adiantum caudatum, Cephalostachyum capitatum, Dysoxylum procerum, Rhus acuminata, Bambusa* spp., *Adiantum phillippense, Melocana bambosoides* are used by the tribes (Sahoo et al., 2010). Fruits are another important NTFPs collected by the villagers mainly for self-consumption but sometimes some fruits are also sold in the market. There are 34 fruit plant species commonly used in the studied villages. The commonly sold fruits are *Artocarpus heterophyllus, Emblica officinalis, Mangifera indica, Musa paradiasica, Protium serratum* and *Rhus javanica* (Sahoo et al., 2010).

Sundariyal and Sundariyal (2000, 2001) described potential of wild edible plants in the Sikkim Himalayas. Das and Choudhury (2003) has surveyed non-conventional foods of southern Assam. Gajurel et al. (2006) described indigenous knowledge on wild plants use by the Adi tribes residing along the banks of Sing river towards south western boundary of the Dehang Debang Biosphere reserve. About 150 wild plant species are utilized by these tribes for various purposes; of these about 85 plant species are found to be edible. Among these, most of the species are utilized as vegetables and fruits, while a few are used as medicine and for other needs. Angami et al. (2006) recorded 118 wild edible plant species from Arunachal Pradesh consumed by the ethnic tribes. Use of traditional and underutilized leafy vegetables of Sub-Himalayan Terai region of West Bengal was given by Jana (2007). A census on edible flowers found in the valley districts of Manipur was given by Devi et al. (2009). Various traditional foods consumed by the ethnic Khasi tribe of Meghalaya were sampled, standardized and evaluated by Blah and Joshi (2013) for their nutritional contents. Diversity of food composition and nutritive analysis of edible wild plants in Northeast India was given by Saha et al. (2014). They recorded 289 plant species used by selected tribal communities, among them 75 species for fruit, 65 vegetables, 18 mushrooms, 163 as medicinal plants, 13 as spices and 11 species for making local drinks and beverages. Devi et al. (2014) discussed the ethnobotanical aspects of *Allium* species of Arunachal Pradesh. They reported that bulbs of 9 species of *Allium* are being used by the tribal communities as vegetable and condiment.

A list of selected ethnic food plants and food items among the indigenous tribes of NER is presented in Table 4.1.

It is evident from the information given in Table 4.1 that the ethnic groups employ common plants from ambient environment for the preparation of their foods. But there is no unanimity among the cultural groups in the preparation method and the names given to the dish. One similarity that has been observed is the use of three species of *Musa* for preparing food additive, which is still vibrant among the people of NER. This herbal additive is generally used for seasoning food and to increase flavor. Another notable feature is the cultural value ascribed to foods among the Karbi ethnic group. In summary it reflects optimum use of plant resources by ethnic cultures for food. Some important ethnic food plants of NER have been supplemented in Plate 1 (Figures 4.1–4.8).

TABLE 4.1   Ethnic Food Plants and Foods of NER

Ethnic food	Tribe	Plants	Products
Saya-aan	Karbi	*Oryza sativa* L.	Consumed during religious feast *Cho-Jun*
Hanmoi	Karbi	*Gnetum gnemon* L., *Rhynchotechum ellipticum* (Wallich ex D. Dietrich) A.DC.	Ritual offerings to household deities
Hanthor	Karbi	*Hibiscus* spp., *Acacia* sp.	Sour dishes
Han-up	Karbi	*Dendrocalamus hamiltonii* Nees & Arn. ex Munro	Ritual offering during harvesting festival
Him-et	Karbi	*Oryza sativa* L., *Curcuma longa* L.	Consumed during religious feast *Cho-Jun*
Him-duk	Karbi	*Oryza sativa* L.	Rice flour
Hanserong anempo	Karbi	*Hibiscus sabdariffa* L.	Consumed during religious feast *Cho-Jun*
Anishi	Naga	*Colocasia* species	Fermented food
Akhuni	Naga	*Glycine max* (L.) Merril	Fermented food
Jadoh	Khasi	*Oryza sativa* L. with pork intestines	Religious food
Tungrymbai	Khasi	*Glycine max* (L.) Merril	Fermented soybean food
Lungseiji	Khasi	*Bambusa nutans* Wall. ex Munro	Fermented food
Kolakhar	All tribes of Assam	*Musa balbisiana* Colla *M. acuminata* Colla *Musa x paradisiaca*	Food additive
Bekang	Mizo	*Glycine max* (L.) Merril.	Fermented food
Aagya	Galo	*Glycine max* (L.) Merril.	Fermented food
Kinema	Ethnic tribes of Sikkim	*Glycine max* (L.) Merril.	Fermented food
Hawaizaar	Meitei	*Glycine max* (L.) Merril.	Fermented food
Soibum	Meitei	Bamboo shoot	Fermented dish
Goyang	Sikkim	*Cardamine macrophylla* Willd.	Fermented vegetable
Tuaithur	Hmar, Baite, Hrangkhol	Bamboo shoot	Fermented food
Khalpi	Gorkha of Sikkim	*Cucumis sativus* L.	Fermented vegetable

PLATE 1

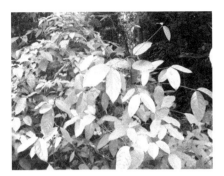

FIGURE 4.1 *Gnetum gnemon* L.

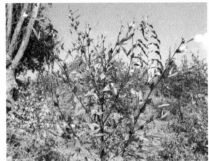

FIGURE 4.2 *Hibiscus sabdariffa* L.

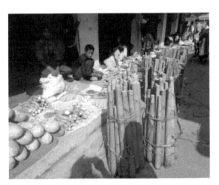

FIGURE 4.3 Bamboo shoots in local market.

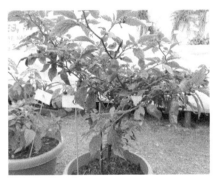

FIGURE 4.4 King chili (*Capsicum chinense* Jacq.).

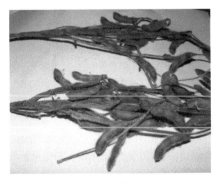

FIGURE 4.5 Pods of *Glycine max* (L.) Merr.

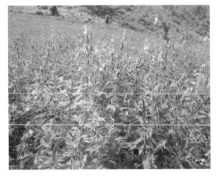

FIGURE 4.6 *Sesamum indicum* L.

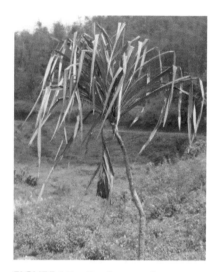
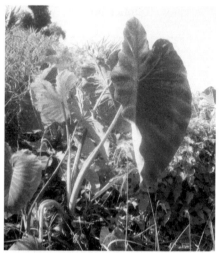

FIGURE 4.7 *Pandanus*, an important staple food in the Andamans.

FIGURE 4.8 *Colocasia esculenta* (L.) Schott.

4.3.2 CULINARY METHODS AND FOOD PRODUCTS

The indigenous people of NER are mostly meat lovers with very few vegetarians. They are also very much fond of boiled foods and the inclusion of chilies in their food. Oil is seldom used for cooking food. Although there are many similarities in the ingredients of food, yet the method of preparation varies among the tribes. The culinary methods of ethnic foods are broadly categorized into different forms:

Boiled: This is the simplest and most common culinary method. Foods are simply cooked with water usually with a pinch of salt; often the dish is flavored with local herbs like garlic, onion, sesame, etc.

Roasted: The food (usually meat) are chopped into fine pieces and screwed in a wooden skewer and placed over fire until the food is ready for consumption.

Smoked: The food materials are spread over a wooden or bamboo mesh and placed above the fireplace till the food is ready to consume. Often raw foods are smoked and stored for future consumption.

Baked: Food is wrapped in plant leaves and shoved in the hot ashes or charcoal. Sometimes food (potatoes, tomato, tubers, yams, meat, fish, etc.)

are shoved under hot ashes and are taken only when the food is ready to be eaten.

Steamed: Food is firstly mixed together with spices and condiments and then shoved in hollow bamboo tubes. The filled bamboo tubes are then placed over fire to cook (Plate 2, Figure 4.9). Food prepared by this method is considered revered.

Stir fried: Vegetables are simply stir fried by adding a pinch of salt and garlic. Very often, powdered black sesame seeds and a few chilies are also added to bring flavor to the dish.

Fermentation: Fermentation is the traditional technology for processing ethnic foods. Fermented foods are source of cultural heterogeneity and usually each type has strong affiliation with ethnic group. Plants like bamboo shoots, soybean and mustard and fish are often fermented to produce foods of strong aroma and taste. Rice and other cereals are fermented to produce beverage, a product that is as diverse as the ethnic tribes of NER.

The diverse ethnic foods of NER come in different taste and aroma. Criteria of food selection differ between cultural societies and thus the preference and palatability. Most ethnic foods have unique aroma that is usually not mistaken by consumer familiar with the region. Some foods emit strong pungent smell that is not liked or tolerable by individuals from other culture. Many foods are prepared from fresh collection while an equal number of plants are fermented to produce desired taste and aroma according to the preference of the people. For larger audience, ethnic foods of NER are discussed under non-fermented and fermented foods. This review however, is limited to plant foods only.

4.3.3 NON-FERMENTED ETHNIC FOODS

Eromba: *Eromba* is an ethnic cuisine of the Meitei people of Manipur. It is prepared from many ingredients but chilli is the major one hence, the item is hot even without addition of spice. Potato, fermented bamboo shoots, taro, chilli and fermented fish are boiled and then smashed to produce a hot item which is taken as side dish (Plate 2, Figure 4.10). Often mint or coriander is added to flavor to the food. *Eromba* is favorite among the Meiteis because of its simple culinary method but great taste. *Eromba* can be prepared with any seasonal vegetables (veg *eromba*) and meat or fish (non-veg *eromba*) as well. Veg types *eromba* are traditionally served in shrines during ritual occasions and household rituals.

Hanmoi: This dish is prepared by the Karbis. It consists of many green herbs including *Gnetum gnemon*, *Rhynchotecum ellipticum*, and *Raphidophora* sp. with the addition of few pieces of dry fish called *Manthu* and a small amount of food additive called *Pholo* (Plate 2, Figure 4.11). *Hanmoi* is used as ritual offerings to local deities and forms integral part of rituals. *Pholo* is prepared out of the ashes of bamboo, sesame, mustard and banana. The ash is placed on a conical bamboo craft called *Pholobisir* and water is poured from above and drained through the plant material which is collected in a container at the bottom. The drained water called *Pholo* is highly alkaline and used in cooking and to certain extent for washing clothes and as hair wash.

Hanserong anempo: It acts as a food additive which is processed and prepared by the Karbi tribe during a religious feast called *Cho-Jun*. The additive is generally prepared from the seeds of the plant *Hibiscus sabdariffa* which is roasted and pounded into fine powder. The powdered substance is then ready to be consumed either in raw form or as food additive.

Hanthor: It is a sour dish and the Karbis generally include this dish in their local diet served at lunch during hot summers. The dish generally consists of plants like *Hibiscus*, *Acacia*, *Polygonum* and *Dillenia* cooked together with either brinjal or lady's finger and by adding a few pieces of dry fish called *Manthu*. Ground powder seeds of *Sesamum* sp. are added if desired, to reduce the sourness of the dish and enhance the taste (Plate 2, Figure 4.12).

Him duk/Sang aduk: This is a very common food of the Karbis which is served in almost all occasions. The food is prepared out of rice grains which are previously soaked and roasted in a cooking pot. The roasted rice grains are then coarsely pounded in a wooden mortar and with pestle by women only. The coarse powder is then taken out and the first handful amount of the *sang aduk* is offered to the local deity; offerings are also made to the deceased ancestors so that they bestow their blessings on the living members before they begin any auspicious or inauspicious occasion or ceremonies. The food is generally taken with pieces of homemade jaggery and red tea.

Him-et: It is another ethnic food of the Karbis which is also prepared during the ritual *Cho-Jun*. On the occasion rice previously soaked is pounded with pestle in wooden mortar usually by women. Then they add fresh rhizomes of turmeric (*Curcuma longa* L.) and pound them together with the rice grains. The mixture is then cooked along with pork fat and consequently salt is added according to individual's taste.

Jadoh: Jadoh is the ethnic food of the people of Meghalaya. The food is generally prepared from rice (*Oryza sativa* L.) cooked together with pork or chicken or fish intestines. It is the most preferred dish in Meghalaya and almost found at every household and every Khasi food stalls. During rituals, Jadoh is cooked with meat of the animals sacrificed (Plate 2, Figure 4.13).

Kolakhar: *Kolakhar* is a type of food additive which is widely used among the rural folk of Assam. The food additive is derived from banana plant (*Musa* sp.) where the rhizomes, trunk and peels are commonly used for the preparation of *Kolakhar*. The plant parts are cut into pieces and dried which is then burnt into ashes and extracted with water. The extracted substance is the *Kolakhar* which is used in the preparation of the dish called *Khar*, a famous ethnic cuisine of Assam. *Kolakhar* is also used widely for washing purposes.

Lungseiji: It is the ethnic food prepared by the Khasi women from tender shoots of *Bambusa nutans*. After cleaning the sheaths, the tender shoots are sliced into thin pieces and cooked by boiling with salt and garlic. This is directly eaten after adding sesame powder or eaten fried.

Nempo: This is powdered seeds of *Sesamum orientale*. The seeds are first fried and then grounded into powder. *Nempo* is the most important food additive of the Karbis and consumed in all occasions. The food is so important that every household is expected to keep *nempo* ready for consumption. Legacy of *nempo* exist in Karbi society as a proverb, *osomar nempo chori, nangning ludet ji* (children should not eat *nempo*, else you will not become wise). The moral of this proverb emphasizes the importance of *nempo*: children are very fond of *nempo*

PLATE 2

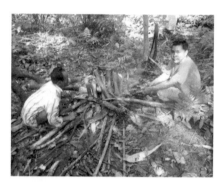

FIGURE 4.9   Rice being cooked in
bamboo tubes.

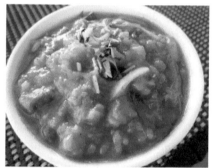

FIGURE 4.10   *Eromba*, ethnic food of
the Meiteis of Manipur.

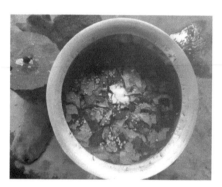

FIGURE 4.11   Leaves of *Gnetum
gnemon* cooked with dry fish for *hanmoi*,
Karbi food for ritual offering.

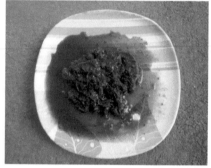

FIGURE 4.12   A sour dish prepared from
hanserong (*Hibiscus sabdariffa*) by the
Karbis.

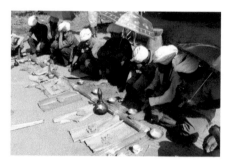

FIGURE 4.13   Jadoh, ethnic food of the
Jaintia tribe being served during ritual
feast.

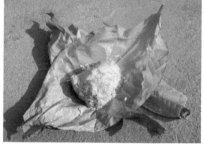

FIGURE 4.14   *Saya a-an*, ethnic food of
the Karbi tribe; rice is cooked with fresh
turmeric.

for its taste and will even exhaust the food, so the proverb is being used as a deterrent.

Saya a-an: This is the ethnic food of the Karbis which is generally cooked and served only during religious feast called *Cho-Jun*. The dish is prepared out of pork blood and pork fat cooked together with broken grain rice (*Oryza sativa* L.). Fresh rhizomes of turmeric (*Curcuma longa* L.) are added so that the food appears yellow (Plate 2, Figure 4.14). This ethnic dish is prepared by women and the dish is served at the end of the occasion when the traditional shamans finishes their propitiations and offerings to *Arnam Kethe*, supreme deity of the Karbis.

Up-vai: It is a dish prepared out of the fresh and tender bamboo shoots by the Karbi tribe. The shoots are usually collected by the women folk and after removing the sheaths, the shoots are cut in thin slices and cooked with the addition of water and salt. For the Karbis, it is taboo to consume *up-vai* before propitiation of community religious festival called Rongker. Often sesame powder and *Ocimun* species are added to enhance the flavor.

4.3.4 FERMENTED ETHNIC FOODS

Based on the intoxicating property, fermented ethnic foods of the NER can be broadly classified into alcoholic and non-alcoholic products. The latter is part of regular diet of the people and usually has strong odor and taste. Alcoholic products or beverages are consumed in daily life and on social occasions. As per tribal culture it is customary to serve beverages during marriages and rituals as offerings to ancestral spirits and deities. A brief description of non-alcoholic and alcoholic ethnic foods is provided in the following subsections.

4.3.4.1 Non-Alcoholic Foods

Aagya: It is the fermented soybean food prepared by the women of Galo tribe of Arunachal Pradesh. Desired quantity of soybeans is boiled and the boiled seeds are wrapped in leaves of *Pyrnium pubinerve* and left for fermentation. The fermented mass is collected as the *Aagya* which is consumed after mixing it with vegetables.

Akhuni: It is the traditional food of the Nagas and it is basically prepared from soybean, *Glyxine max*. The beans are boiled and wrapped in leaves of *Musa, Phrynium* or *Macaranga* (Plate 3, Figure 4.15). It is then kept over the fireplace for the fermentation process for a week. The fermented beans now called *Akhuni* is ready for use and consumed either in the form of *chutney* cooked with tomatoes and chilies or *akhuni* is cooked with meat (Mao and Odyou, 2007).

Anishi: *Anishi* is the traditional fermented food of the Naga tribe prepared from the leaves of *Colocasia* (Plate 3, Figure 4.16). The leaves are properly washed and placed one above the other and wrapped around with banana leaf which is kept aside for few days till the leaves turn yellow in color. The leaves are then ground into paste and cakes are made out of the paste which is dried over the fireplace in the kitchen. The cakes are often cooked with pork which is one of the favorite ethnic dishes of the Nagas (Mao and Odyou, 2007).

Bekang: *Bekang* is the integral food component of all boiled foods in Mizoram. It is prepared by Mizo women out of fermented soybeans. The soybean seeds are crushed and boiled and the boiled seeds are wrapped in leaves of *belphuar* tree. The wrapped seeds are kept near a fireplace and left for fermentation. The fermented mass is then consumed directly after the addition of chilies, ginger and salt.

Hawaizaar: This is a dish made out of fermented soybeans by the women of Meitei community of Manipur. The soybeans are boiled until soft and the beans are wrapped in cotton cloth and tied with banana leaves (Plate 3, Figure 4.17). It is then kept under a bamboo basket and covered with rice husk and pressed with stone and kept above the fireplace for the fermentation process. The fermented soybean is then used in the preparation of the ethnic dish called *Cheigem pomba*.

Kinema: *Kinema* is an important food component of the ethnic communities of Sikkim. It is generally prepared by fermenting whole-soybean seeds. To prepare *Kinema*, soybeans are soaked in water and cooked until the beans are soft and tender. The cooked beans are finely splitted using a wooden mortar and pestle and the paste is wrapped with fern fronds *Glaphylopteriosis erubescens*, *Ficus* leaves or banana leaves. Sometimes fresh firewood ashes are also added during the preparation of *Kinema*. The wrapped bean paste is then kept over the fireplace for the fermentation process. The preparation of *Kinema* varies from place to place and it is restricted to household level.

Soibum: This fermented bamboo shoot is prepared by the women folk of the Meitei community living in Manipur. Women collect the emerging bamboo shoots and after removing the peels, the shoots are cut into pieces and the product is squeezed out and left to dry. The dried bamboo parts are then mixed with salt and bits of turmeric and kept in an earthen pot with an addition of little amount of water. The pot is sealed and left for fermentation (Plate 3, Figure 4.18).

Tuaithur: It is an ethnic fermented bamboo shoot product prepared and consumed by the Hrangkhol, Baite and Hmar of Dima Hasao district, Assam; it is similar to other fermented bamboo shoot products of NER. Bamboo shoots are chopped into pieces with knife. It is thoroughly washed with water, drained and pressed in a conical basket made of bamboo or bottles. The container is made airtight with a lid and fermented under natural anaerobic condition for about a week.

Tungrymbai: *Tungrymbai* is a traditional fermented food product prepared from soybean seeds used in Meghalaya by the indigenous Khasi tribes (Sohliya et al., 2009). Soybean seeds are first soaked in water and cooked until they are soft and tender. The cooked beans are placed in basket lined with leaves of *Phyrnium pubinerve* and covered with jute bags and left to ferment naturally. The fermented mass is collected, cooked by adding salt, ginger and chilies and consumed as a side dish along with rice and vegetables (Plate 3, Figure 4.19).

Up-thor: This is the fermented bamboo shoots processed and prepared by the Karbi tribe. Young and tender shoots of bamboo are collected usually during September to November. The shoots are peeled and either cut in thin slices or pounded in wooden mortar with pestle. The pounded mass or the sliced bamboo shoots are placed in bamboo tubes called *langpong*. The bamboo tubes are sealed tightly and left to ferment naturally. The housekeeper (i.e., woman) checks the bamboo tubes timely and when

PLATE 3

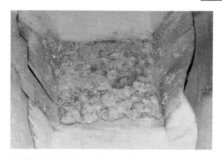

FIGURE 4.15   *Akhuni*, fermented soya bean food of the Angami Naga.

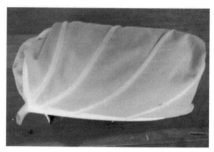

FIGURE 4.16   *Anishi*, ethnic food of the Naga prepared by fermented taro leaves.

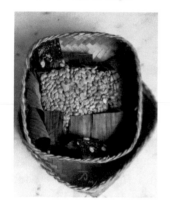

FIGURE 4.17   *Hawaizar*, fermented soya bean based food of the Meitei community of Manipur.

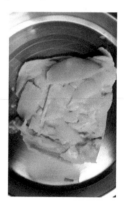

FIGURE 4.18   *Soibum*, fermented bamboo shoots of the Meitei community.

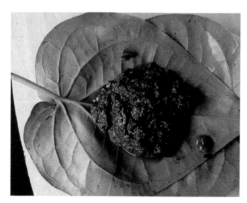

FIGURE 4.19   *Tungrymbai*, a traditional fermented soybean food product of the Khasi tribes.

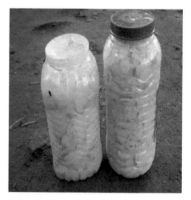

FIGURE 4.20   *Upthor*, bamboo shoots being fermented in plastic containers by the Karbi ethnic tribe.

a particular smell is emitted, it indicates that the shoots are fermented and ready to consume. In the present time due to scarcity of bamboo tubes, bamboo shoots are fermented in plastic, metal or earthen containers (Plate 3, Figure 4.20).

4.3.4.2. Ethnic Beverages (Alcoholic Foods)

Apart from food, people of NER are well known for brewing household beverages. The tribal people of the region have been producing and consuming various kinds of alcoholic drinks since time immemorial. Such methods are unique and are still practiced in its raw form. Each of these beverages prepared by the indigenous tribe holds a special recognition and importance in the social and cultural lives of the tribals in NER. Brewing of alcoholic beverage is regarded as an important household cum societal activity among different tribal communities (Sharma and Mazumdar, 1980). Alcoholic beverage is consumed in day-to-day life both as a refreshing as well as an invigorating drink. Consumption of rice beer is indispensable in almost all the occasions like rituals, festivals, marriages, funerals and social gatherings. But preparation of alcoholic beverage for certain occasions like marriage and rituals is considered sacred and holy where women folk recite incantations for good product. Because during such instances, it is customary to offer rice beer to the deities and ancestral spirits as it is believed to appease them; often guests are honored with rice beer as a mark of respect. The indigenous beverages are consumed in large quantities during auspicious occasions or festivals and hence, the preparation starts months before the occasion. The role of women is indispensable in the brewing of alcoholic beverages either for consumption or for the use in rituals. In all cultures, brewing of alcoholic beverages is the domain of women folk and, therefore, the associated traditional knowledge is transmitted through them. There is no age, gender or status restriction for consumption of indigenous liquor during rituals and ceremonies. Thus, indigenous alcoholic beverages have strong religious importance and are deep rooted with the socio-cultural practices of the various ethnic groups of NER. Beverage is believed to have therapeutic potentials and folks often use it after hard day's work to relive stress and tiring body and muscles.

Preparation of alcoholic beverage is much elaborate than non-fermented foods. All cultures use starter cakes (Plate 4, Figure 4.21) in fermentation of substrates for production of beverages in which rice is the chief ingredient along with many plant parts (Table 4.2). The method of preparation and processing of starter cakes practiced by different cultures is almost similar but there exists prominent variation in the number and types of plants used during the preparation of starter cakes (Figure 4.21a). On evaluation of all reports accessed, sixty four plants distributed in thirty nine botanical families are used in preparation of starter cakes. There is also great variation in the number plants used among the tribes/groups. Highest number of plants (i.e., forty) was used by the Deori ethnic group in the preparation of *mod pitha*, starter cake. These plants are blended to add flavor or aroma and/or to increase the strength of the products. A list of plants employed in the preparation of starter cakes by different ethnic groups of NER is presented in Table 4.2. Depending upon the available regional ingredients and manufacturing procedures, alcoholic beverages are known under a variety of local names, and each type yields unique odor and different taste of the liquor. Rice is the predominant substrate across cultural groups; one publication (Teron, 2006) reported use of other substrates like *Eleusine corocana*, *Musa* and *Citrullus vulgaris* amongst the Karbi ethnic group. Use of millets as substitute of rice for fermentation was also reported among the Khasis (Tanti et al., 2010) and the Adi-Galo tribe of Arunachal Pradesh (Shrivastava et al., 2012).

The methods for beverage production among the tribes differ and follow their own indigenous protocols employing different starter cultures, although most of them use similar substrates for fermentation (Tanti et al., 2010). For its taste and aroma, beer from glutinous rice is considered revered over beer produced from other rice varieties. The principle of alcoholic beverage manufacturing consist of the saccharification of steamed rice starch by fungal enzymes under aerobic solid state fermentation and the molded mass is mixed with water and allowed to undergo submerged alcoholic fermentation by yeasts using traditional starter cakes (Blandino et al., 2003; Sujaya et al., 2004;

PLATE 4

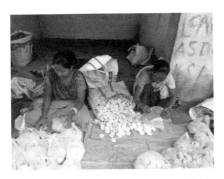

FIGURE 4.21 Starter cakes being sold by women in a local market.

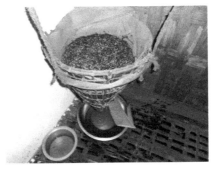

FIGURE 4.22 Extraction of *poro apong*, rice beer of the Mishing community.

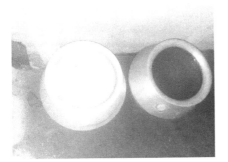

FIGURE 4.23 Fermentation of substrate for production of *atingba*, beverage of the Meitei people.

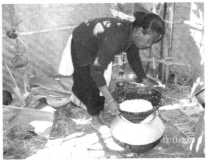

FIGURE 4.24 A Karbi woman extracting *hor*, rice beer.

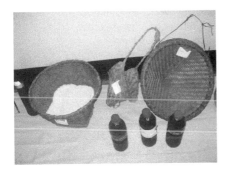

FIGURE 4.25 *Judima*, rice beer (in bottles) of the Dimasa ethnic group prepared from sticky rice variety (in basket).

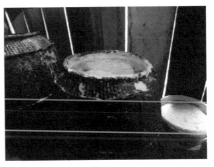

FIGURE 4.26 Production of *zutho*, alcoholic beverage of the Angami tribe.

TABLE 4.2 Plants Used by Ethnic Groups of NER in Preparation of Various Starter Cakes

Starter cake	Ethnic group	Plants (Family)	Reference
Angku	Bodo	*Xanthium strumarium* L., *Scoparia dulcis* L., *Clerodendrum viscosum* Vent.	Das et al., 2012
Thap	Karbi	*Croton joufra* Roxb., *Phlogacanthus thyrsiflorus* Nees., *Solanum viarum* Dunal, *Acacia pennata* (L.) Willd., *Amomum corynostachyum* Walls, *Clerodendrum viscosum* Vent., *Ricinus communis* L., *Cymbopogon citratus* (DC) Stapf, *Ananas comosus* L., *Saccharum officinarum* L., *Solanum indicum* L., *Artocarpus heterophyllus* Lam.	Das et al., 2012; Teron, 2006
Vekur pitha	Ahom	*Oldenlandia corymbosa* L., *Lygodium* sp., *Hydrocotyle sibthorpioides* Lam., *Centella asiatica* (L.) Urb., *Cissampelos pareira* L., *Piper nigrum* L.	Das et al., 2012
E'pob	Mishing	*Centella asiatica* (L.) Urb., *Hydrocotyle sibthorpioides* Lam., *Oldenlandia corymbosa* L., *Saccharum officinarum* L., *Clerodendrum viscosum* Vent., *Cyclosorus extensus* (Blume) H. Ito, *Ipomoea* sp., *Scoparia dulcis* L., *Drymeria cordata* Willd., *Capsicum annuum* L., *Ananas comosus* (L.) Merr., *Lygodium flexuosum* (L.) Sw.	Das et al., 2012; Pegu et al., 2013
Mod pitha	Deori	*Jasminum sambac* (L.) Aiton, *Cinnamomum byolghata*, *Zanthoxylum hamiltonianum* Wall., *Lygodium flexuosum* (L.) Sw., *Acanthus leucostachyus* Wall. ex Nees, *Cyclosorus extensus* (Blume) H. Ito, *Alstonia scholaris* (L.) R. Br., *Alpinia malaccensis* (Burm.f.) Roscoe, *Costus speciosus* (J. Konig) Sm., *Artocarpus heterophyllus* Lamk., *Allium sativum* L., *Ananas comosus* (L.) Merr., *Alpinia malaccensis* Rosc., *Alternanthera sessilis* (L.) R. Br. ex DC., *Capsicum annuum* L., *Cinnamomum bejolghota* (Buch.-Ham) Sw., *Centella asiatica* (L.) Urban., *Coffea bengalensis* Roxb., *Desmodium* sp., *Cyperus* sp., *Desmodium pulchellum* (L.) Benth., *Equisetum* sp., *Lygodium flexuosum* (L.) Sw., *Melastoma malabathricum* L., *Mussaenda roxburghii* Hook. f., *Myxopyrum smilacifolium* (Wall.) Bl., *Naravelia zeylanica* (L.) DC, *Oryza sativa* L., *Psidium guajava* L., *Pothos scandens* L., *Pteridium aquilinum* (L.) Kuhn., *Pycnarrhena pleniflora* Miers., *Rubus* sp., *Saccharum officinarum* L., *Selaginella semicordata* (Wall) Spreng., *Scoparia dulcis* L., *Solanum torvum* Sw., *Thunbergia grandiflora* Roxb., *Zanthoxylum oxyphyllum* Edgw., *Zingiber officinale* Rosc.	Das et al., 2012; Deori et al., 2007

TABLE 4.2 (Continued)

Starter cake	Ethnic group	Plants (Family)	Reference
Siiyeh, Opop	Adi-Galo	*Clerodendron viscosum, Veronia* sp.	Das et al., 2012
Umhu, Humao	Dimasa,	*Acacia pennata* Willd, *Piper betle* L., *Buddleja asiatica* Lour.	Das et al., 2012; Arjun et al., 2014; Terangpi et al., 2013
Bakhor, Surachi, Phap	Rabha	*Ananas comosus* (L.) Merr., *Artocarpus heterophyllus* Lam., *Calotropis gigantea* (L.) W. T. Aiton, *Capsicum frutescens* L., *Clerodendrum viscosum* Vent., *Dennstaedtia scabra* (Wall.) T. Moore, *Ochthochloa coracana* Edgew., *Plumbago indica* L., *Saccharum officinarum* L., *Scoparia dulcis* L.	Deka and Sarma 2010

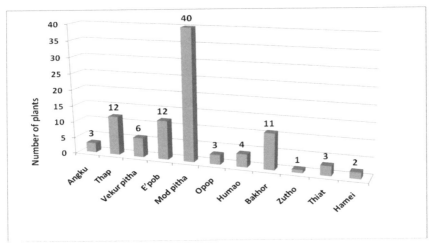

FIGURE 4.21A Plant ingredients used in preparation of starter cakes among cultural groups of NER.

Dung et al., 2007). In western countries barley malt is used as both the source of starch and the saccharifying agent. By contrast, in Asian countries, alcoholic beverages are produced with rice as the major source of starch and the saccharifying agent. The various alcoholic beverage and the methods of brewing the beverages are discussed briefly below:

Apong: *Apong* is an alcoholic beverage prepared by the Mishings of Assam. The starter culture called *e'pob* is prepared with rice flour and leaves of many plants (Table 4.2). Earlier about fifty plants are known to be used, but today, due to erosion of knowledge only 26 plants are used in the preparation of starter cakes (Pegu et al., 2013). The leaves are cleaned and dried on a bamboo mat called *opoh*. Previously soaked rice and the leaves are ground separately and mixed together in a vessel by adding little amount of water to make a dough. From the dough, oval shaped balls are made and sun-dried. For production of *apong*, boiled rice (preferably aromatic variety) is spread on a *kol pat* (banana leaf) and powdered *e'pob* is added to it; the whole mixture is kept in an earthen pot for fermentation. After about 5 days, little water is added to the fermented product and filtered to get the *apong* (Plate 4, Figure 4.22). Two forms of *apong* are produced by the Mishing people (Pegu et al., 2013). The one which is produced by fermentation of cooked rice with locally prepared *e'pob* is called *Nogin Apong*. Another type, *po:ro apong* is produced by fermenting mixture of cooked rice, ash of partially burned paddy husk and straw with *e'pob*. Preparation of *po:ro apong* is tedious and time consuming for which this beverage is usually prepared during festivals and rituals. *Po:ro apong* is usually produced from glutinous or sticky rice varieties, and also use the best quality *e'pob* for fermentation.

Atingba/Yu: It is the alcoholic beverage of the Meitei tribe of Manipur state. The starter culture used for the purpose is *hamei* (Jeyaram et al., 2008) prepared with powdered rice and barks of the plant *yangli* (*Albizia myriophylla*). With the addition of water to the mixture, flat cakes are made out of it and kept over rice husks in bamboo baskets. After a few days, the cakes swell, produces alcoholic flavor and yellowish coloration which are stored for a year (Tamang et al., 2007; Jeyaram et al., 2008, 2009). *Atingba* is produced by fermentation of cooked glutinous rice with powdered *hamei* (5 cakes for 10 kg rice). The substrate is kept in mud pots covered with '*hangla*' (*Alocasia* sp.); it is left for 3–4 days during summer and 6–7 days in winter. This is followed by 2–3 days of submerged fermentation in earthen pots (Plate 4, Figure 4.23). The beverage (i.e., *atingba*) is obtained after filtration (Kar, 2004).

Choko/Jonga-mod: *Choko* or *jonga-mod* is the local rice beer of the Rabhas, one of the large tribal groups of Assam and widely scattered but mostly concentrated in the undivided Goalpara, Kamrup and Darrang districts of Assam (Deka and Sarma, 2010). Several herbs with known medicinal property are used by the Rabhas in the preparation of rice-beer. The starter cake *bakhor*, *surachi* or *phap* is usually prepared by mixing the plant parts (Table 4.2) with rice paste (mainly rice variety *Sali* and *Ahu*) and a considerable amount of old rice beer cakes. To prepare *choko* (rice-beer), firstly cooked rice is placed over a broad bamboo mat and allowed to cool. To this, certain amount of starter cake is added and the mixture is kept in *jonga*, an earthen pitcher. It takes 4–5 days during summer and 7–8 days during winter for the *choko* or rice beer to attain the actual stage of drinking. The rice beer is then again fermented after adding some quantity of water and starter cakes. After 3–4 days, rice beer is again collected through local distillation process using both earthen and metallic pots; the resulting product is strong liquor known as *fotika* (Deka and Sarma, 2010).

Hor: *Hor* is the indigenous alcoholic beverage of the Karbis, the main inhabitants of Karbi Anglong district of Assam state and scattered in almost all the states of NER. The starter cake used in the production of *hor* is called *thap* (Teron, 2006) prepared from rice and many plants, the chief constituent being either leaves of *Croton joufra* or bark of *Acacia pennata* (Table 4.2). The ingredients are pounded into fine powder and some amount of previously prepared *thap* called *thap aphi* is added to the mixture. Round flat cakes are made out of it and they are dried in the sun for a few days and kept near fire place for future use. *Hor* is produced by fermenting cooked rice with *thap*. Cooked rice is mixed with adequate amount of powdered *thap* and the mixture is stored in *pho-le* (cooking utensil) and left for fermentation. After 3–4 days *hor lang* or beer is produced (Plate 4, Figure 4.24). *Hor arak* (alcohol) is distilled from it after addition of aliquot quantity of water (Teron, 2006).

Jou: *Jou* is prepared by the Bodos, one of the largest linguistic groups in Northeast India and among the earliest settlers of Assam (Das and Deka, 2012). The starter cakes known as *angkur* is prepared from rice flour and different plants such as *agarsita* (*Xanthium strumarium*) and *dongphang rakhep* (*Scoparia dulcis*) and either roots or leaves of *lokhu-nath* (*Clerodendrum viscosum*). For preparing the beer, either glutinous or non-glutinous rice is used as substrate. When glutinous rice is used, the product is known as *maibra joubishi* and when non-glutinous rice is the substrate the product is referred as *matha joubishi*. The cooked rice is mixed with powdered *angkur* and the mixture is put inside a container and sealed for one night. After this, a little water is added to it and left in a *baiphu* (earthen pot) covered with banana leaves for at least 3 days. The fermented mass is further mixed with water and strained in order to get the liquid *jou* (Das and Deka, 2012).

Judima: *Judima* is the alcoholic beverage of the Dimasas, one of the earliest indigenous ethnic groups of North-Eastern India (Das et al., 2012; Arjun et al., 2014). They are mostly found in the Dima Hasao district (formerly North Cachar Hills) of Assam and Dimapur in Nagaland State. *Umhu* or *humao* is the starter cake for producing *judima* which is a mixture of rice and bark of *themra* (*Acacia pennata*) (Terangpi et al., 2013). Usually scented variety of rice is boiled, cooled and then mixed with powdered *humao* and kept in a large container for fermentation. After about a week, slightly yellowish *judima* comes out of the substrate which indicates the completion of fermentation; the beer turns red on prolonged storage (Plate 4, Figure 4.25). Often water is added to the fermented mass, mixed properly and the beer is extracted by filtration.

Kiad: Local liquor of the Jaintia tribe (also known as Pnar or Synteng) of Meghalaya, *kiad* is produced by fermentation of rice substrate with the starter cake known as *thiat* (Samati and Begum, 2007; Jaiswal, 2010). *Thiat* is prepared by pounding leaves of *khawiang* (*Amomum aromaticum*) and water-soaked *Kho-so* (local variety of rice); water is added to turn the mixture into dough from which small round cakes are made and processed by exposing to sunlight or held above the fire place. For brewing *kiad*, boiled rice is mixed with 2–3 finely crushed *thiat* and the mixture is left for about 2–3 days. The fermented mash, known as *jyndem*, is distilled and the distillate is known as *kiad* (Samati and Begum, 2007; Jaiswal, 2010).

Opo: *Opo* is the local rice beer produced by the *Adi-Galo* tribe of Arunachal Pradesh who lives in Pasighat sub-division of East Siang district (Das and Deka, 2012). The starter cake *siiyeh* or *opop* is prepared with leaves and barks of the plants *dhapat* (*Clerodendrum viscosum*) and *lohpohi* (*Vernonia* species). For production of *opo*, rice is boiled and spread on a bamboo mat to cool. Then half-burnt rice and powdered *opop* are added and the mixture is put in a plastic container, the walls of which are covered with leaves of a local Zingeberous plant called *oko*. The mouth is also sealed with *oko* leaves and is left undisturbed for about 5 days. The contents are then mixed well and again left in the same manner for a longer duration. The product becomes ready after about 20 days of fermentation and kept for longer durations for production of more beverages. For filtration, a special type of funnel called *perpur* is used where *oko* leaves are used as the filter. To the fermented mass, hot water is poured over slowly in order to obtain *opo* as the filtrate.

Sujen: This beverage is indigenous rice beer of the Deoris who mostly scattered in upper Assam (Deori et al., 2007). The starter cake is called *mod pitha* is prepared from rice flour and various plant parts (Table 4.2). After pounding the mixture into powder in *dheki* (wooden implement) along with the old *mod pithas*, the mixture is made into paste and small round cakes are prepared out of the paste and covered with straws and kept in *Kula* (bamboo container) above the fire place for drying until the *mod pitha* becomes hard. Glutinous rice is fermented with *mod pitha* in an earthen pot for about 4–5 days. It is then diluted and filtered to produce *sujen* which can be stored for up to 1 or 2 months (Deori et al., 2007).

Xaj Pani: *Xajpani* or *kolohpani* is the local beverage prepared by the Ahoms, who are of *Tai* origin scattered all over Assam mostly concentrated in Upper Assam (Das and Deka, 2012). The starter cake known as *vekur pitha*, which literally means fungus-infested balls, consists of rice and parts of several plants (Table 4.2). The mixture is pounded into coarse powder and small round cakes are made from the paste. The cakes are processed by drying in sunlight or placed over fireplace. *Xaj pani* is produced by fermenting rice (either glutinous or non-glutinous) with powdered *vekur pitha* in a *koloh* (earthen pot). This is kept in a closed room for 3 to 5 days. After this, a considerable amount of water is added to the fermented mass and left for about 10 minutes. Filtration is done by straining the mass using a cloth (Das and Deka, 2012).

Zutho and *Litchumsu*: *Zutho* and *Litchumsu* are the local alcoholic brews prepared by the *Angami* tribe and the *Ao* tribe of Nagaland respectively (Das and Deka, 2012). The starter cake used in the preparation of *zutho* is known as *piazu*. The latter is prepared by soaking un-hulled rice for about 3–4 days and the grains are allowed to germinate. After being dried in the air, the sprouted grains are pounded on a wooden mortar with a pestle. The powder obtained is known as *piazu*. For production of *zutho*, boiled rice is fermented by adding some quantity of *piazu*. After completion of fermentation (i.e., 3–4 days), some amount of water is added to the fermented mass (Plate 4, Figure 4.26). *Zutho* is filtered by using a bamboo or plastic mesh and usually served in bamboo cups (Das and Deka, 2012).

4.3.5 FOOD SYSTEMS AND CULTURE

Food, cooking, and eating habits play a central role in every culture. Habits of eating and drinking are invested with significance by the particular culture or sub-culture to which they belong. Food is an appropriate mediator because when we eat, we establish a direct identity between ourselves (culture) and our food (nature) (Leach, 1976). The food systems of Northeast India have a close association with the ethnic groups and describe their culture. Each of the cultural groups has their own way of food selection not only in the domestic region but even in the wild. Their ways and choice of cultivating food crops also differs to some extent. The ethnic communities practice unique culinary methods producing food with a different taste, color and odor. Basically, the traditional food systems of Northeast India are incomplete without a steaming platter of steamed rice, varied green vegetables and predominance of meat and fresh water fishes. Though Northeast states has its own identifiable culinary method, each of them has a taste for the pungent bamboo shoot, fermented soya beans, fermented fish and fermented meat amongst others. Bamboo shoot is a popular food material in almost every tribal food system and widely used as a souring agent in every tribal dish. Some notable fermented ethnic foods of NER include *akhuni* (Nagaland), *kinema* (Sikkim) and *tungrymbai* (Meghalaya). These (i.e., ethnic foods) are significant ingredients used to create a pungent aroma in various dishes; also used as a pickle with lots of chilies stuffed along with it. The world's hottest chilli popularly known as King Chilli (*Capsicum chinense* Jacq.) or *raja mircha*, variously referred as *u-morok* in Manipur and *bhoot jolokia* in Assam, is widely relished. None of the pork dishes in Nagaland is complete without this fiery chilli. Karbis of Assam maintain rich tradition and culture and introduction of their ethnic food generally begins with certain rituals. No ritual is complete without offering *hanmoi* and *hor* to local deities and ancestral spirits. A recipe which is practiced as an age-old tradition includes the use of rice flour during ritual (*seh-karkli*) when chicken is sacrificed to the deity and the meat is cooked with rice flour and served with banana leaves, much like the Bodos who prepares a stew out of chicken and rice called *onla-wangkhrai*. Rice is fundamental and apart from cooking rice in utensils, the tribals steam them in hollow bamboo tubes. Among the Karbis, rice cooked in bamboo tube is offered to deity during the ritual *Rek Anglong*. Karbis have a rice preparation, called *sayaa-an*, with the intestines of pork along with the blood and it is usually served during a ritual called *Cho-jun*. During this ritual pig's blood cooked with leaves of *suvat* (*Begonia* species) in a revered item. Also the Karbis do not cook sour dishes when member of a family dies on the belief that other members attending the dead rites will heap curse on them. Likewise, the tribes in Meghalaya also have a dish called *jadoh* prepared from rice and liver of pig. Despite predominance of meat in ethnic food, the people of Northeast are heavy vegetable consumers as well for the fact that vegetables grow naturally in abundance. In Assam, the ethnic food begins with a dish called *kolakhar*; the dish is prepared from papaya with additive called *khar* (alkali solution) derived from banana plants (*Musa* species) (Deka and Talukdar, 2006). Some women in rural Assam have been able to grow long and healthy hair using *kolakhar* alone (Anonymous, 2002; Deka and Talukdar, 2006). Likewise, the *khar*-based dish is also vibrant in the Karbi ethnic food system, where the food additive called *pholo* is cooked with vegetables, and few pieces of dry fish. *Pholo* is usually extracted from the burnt ashes of banana peels and other plants which are placed in a conical bamboo craft called *pholobisir* and water is poured into it. The drained solution collected from the craft is the ingredient *pholo* or *khar*.

In Sikkim, people ferment leafy vegetables like leaves of mustard, radish, cauliflower and sundried for future consumption. They call these preparations as *sinki*. Sikkim is also famous for cottage cheese, big momos and *thukpa* which are prepared from flat noodles along with meat and vegetables. Like pork, chicken, duck and other meat, fish is also very popular and prepared through varied methods. Fresh water fish is barbecued in banana leaves in Meghalaya, Assam and other states. Fish intestines are also relished along with fermented or dried fish and green chilies as *chutney*. The Reangs of Tripura love to cook their vegetables in hollow bamboo over charcoal fire. The preparation and consumption of food provides, moreover, a material means for expressing the more abstract significance of social systems and cultural values. It shows what people are prepared to take inside their bodies; it reflects their social identities, and their membership of social groups.

4.4 CONCLUSION

Based on the above information it can be said that the NER is a melting pot of high cultural and ethnic diversity. Wild plants continue to play vital role in food security and nutrition of the people. The NER display intricate link among four diversities- ethnic, cultural, dietary and linguistic. There is perfect exhibition of linguistic diversity with ethnic foods. It is amazing that the starter cakes which have almost same major components are referred by different names among the cultures. A supplement to this fact is soybean-based fermented foods being referred by varied names. They have knowledge of fermentation and the role of microbes in the process. Indigenous technology of alcoholic beverage production is an explicit expression of traditional knowledge and innovations of minds. Their practice is not without scientific reasoning. Old starter cakes which are added during preparation of fresh ones, is a source of inoculum and the various ingredients of starter cakes acts as medium for microbial growth. Preservation of the starter cakes (which is loaded with microbes) for years by keeping near fire place can be regarded synonymous with biological principle of maintaining microbial culture at a particular temperature. Starter cake is equivalent to microbial inoculum which is added to substrate before fermentation. The technology of extracting beer and liquor is an apt display of scientific principles of filtration and distillation. There is however, gradual dilution of ethnic food systems due to intrusion of modern foods and influence of modern culture.

The traditional foods consumed by the indigenous tribes of the NER is deeply associated with forest products and intimately connected to virtually all aspects of their socio-cultural, spiritual life and health. These indigenous communities now has undergone a rapid change by not only due to introduction of clothes but has also their diets have undergone change over the past few years due to intervention of modern crop varieties, materialistic life, awareness created by visitors and current trend towards increasing use of commercially processed foods. For the tribes, transformation of ethnic food system has been radical, as people have moved from a diet in which the majority of nutrients are drawn from local food, to more generic diet of store-bought food, most of which are produced and processed far away from their locality. More exploration, analysis and documentation of the ethnic foods consumed by the tribal communities of the NER can be undertaken along with its associated dynamics to understand food consumption pattern and availability, nutritional and medicinal values and associated cultural and social aspects of ethnic foods.

Continuation or maintenance of ethnic food systems or food culture poses a real challenge against the onslaught of globalization and climate change. Even rural markets around the globe have become flooded with factory-produced foods which are more palatable than less-processed ethnic foods. Availability of food plants is another cause of concern for preservation of food cultures. *Jhum* (slash and burn), particularly in Northeast India, have degraded large area of natural habitats of wild foods. Encroachment and agricultural expansion are other major factors that are threatening survival of wild foods. Nonetheless, ethnic foods provide multitude of opportunities for preservation of cultural heritage, research and development. The foods are purely organic and abound with many health benefits. Baruah and Bora (2009) suggested use of the rich nutritional profiles of indigenous vegetables of NER in nutritional schemes. The diverse ethnic foods provide a platform for ecotourism through which the local food systems can be popularized and promoted. This will encourage continuation of cultural practices and conservation of the associated indigenous knowledge. Ethnic food systems provide good scope for academic discourse covering scores of areas like traditional knowledge, wild foods, food security, management of plant resources, intellectual property, local development, etc. Research on ethnic foods and the ingredients can help in evaluation of the chemical constituents and food value. This in turn will be useful for validation of ethnic food systems. Being nutritious (as studies so far suggests) ethnic alcoholic beverages should be developed for local, national and international markets through value additions. Last but not the least, wild food plants are tolerable to environmental stress (Paul et al., 2011) and therefore this group of plants could form viable source of novel genes for improvement of conventional crops. Concerted multidisciplinary approach can help in realization of the value of ethnic food plants and food systems and present a case for their conservation.

ACKNOWLEDGEMENT

I am grateful to Miss Ni-et Teronpi and Shabana Hassan for their assistance in preparing this review.

KEYWORDS

- **conservation**
- **ethnic plants**
- **ethnobotany**
- **food systems**
- **North-east**
- **traditional knowledge**

REFERENCES

1. Agrahar-Murungkar, D., & Subbulakshmi, G. (2006). Preparation techniques and nutritive value of fermented foods from the Khasi tribes of Meghalaya. *Ecology of Food and Nutrition, 45*, 27–38.

2. Angami, A., Gajurel, P. R., Rethy, P., Singh, B., & Kalita, S. K. (2006). Status and potential of wild edible plants of Arunachal Pradesh. *Indian J. Trad. Knowl. 5(4)*, 541–550.

3. Annonymous (2002). *Aamar Axom*, an Assamese Daily published from Guwahati, July 13, 2002.

4. Arjun, J., Verma A. K., & Prasad, S. B. (2014). Method of preparation and biochemical analysis of local tribal wine Judima: an indigenous alcohol used by Dimasa tribe of North Cachar Hills District of Assam, India. *International Food Research J., 21(2)*, 463–470.

5. Arora, R. K. (1990). Native food plants of the tribals in northeast India. In: Jain, S. K. (ed.) Contribution to Ethnobotany of India. Scientific publishers, Jodhpur. pp. 137–152.

6. Baruah, A. M., & Borah, S. (2009). An investigation on on source of potential minerals found in traditional vegetables of North-eastern India. *Intern. J. Food Science and Nutrition. 60(S4)*, 111–115.

7. Bhutani, K. K. (2008). Herbal wealth of Northeast India, Database and Appraisal. National Institute of Pharmaceutical Science and Research, Punjab.

8. Blah, M. M., & Joshi, S. R. (2013). Nutritional content evaluation of traditional recipes consumed by ethnic communities of Meghalaya, India. *Indian J. Trad. Knowl. 12(3)*, 498–505.

9. Blandino, A., Al-Aseeri, M. E., Pandiella, S. S., Cantero, D., & Webb, C. (2003). Cereal-based fermented foods and beverages. *Food Res. Intern., 36*, 527–543.

10. Das, P. S., & Choudhury, M. D. (2003). A survey of non-conventional foods of southern Assam. *J. Econ. Taxon. Bot. 27(2)*, 416–420.

11. Das, A. J., & Deka, S. C. (2012). Mini Review Fermented foods and beverages of the North-East India, *Intern. Food Res. J., 19(2)*, 377–392.

12. Das, A. J., Deka, S. C., & Miyaji, T. (2012). Methodology of rice beer preparation and various plant materials used in starter culture preparation by some tribal communities of North-East India-A survey. *Intern. Food Res. J., 19(1)*, 101–107.

13. Deka, D., & Sarma, G. N. (2010). Traditionally used herbs in the preparation of rice-beer by the Rabha tribe of Goalpara, district, Assam. *Indian J. Trad. Knowl., 9(3)*, 459–462.

14. Deka, D. C., & Talukdar, N. N. (2006). Chemical and spectroscopic investigation of *Kolakhar* and its commercial importance. *Indian J. Trad. Knowl., 6(1)*, 72–78.

15. Deori, C., Begum, S. S., & Mao, A. A. (2007). Ethnobotany of *sujen*, a local rice beer of Deori tribe of Assam, *Indian J. Trad. Knowl. 6(1)*, 121–125.

16. Devi, A., Rakshit, K., & Sarania, B. (2014). Ethnobotanical notes on *Allium* species of Arunachal Pradesh, India. *Indian J. Trad. Knowl. 13(3)*, 606–612.

17. Devi, K. S., Devi, Y. S., & Singh, P. K. (2009). A census on edible flowers found in the valley districts of Manipur. *J. Econ. Taxon. Bot. 33*, 232–239.

18. Dung, N. T. P., Rhombouts F. M. & Nout, M. J. R. (2007). Characteristics of some traditional Vietnamese starch-based rice wine starters. *Food Microbiol., 23,* 331–340.

19. Dutta, B. K., & Dutta, P. K. (2005). Potential of ethnomedicinal studies in Northeast India: An overview. *Indian J. Trad. Knowl. 4(1),* 7–14.

20. FAO (1996). The state of food and agriculture. Rome, Italy.

21. Gajurel, P. R., Rethy, P., Singh, B. &Angami, A. (2006). Ethnobotanical studies on Adi tribes in Dehang Debang Biosphere Reserve in Arunachal Pradesh, Eastern Himalaya. *Ethnobotany 18,* 114–118.

22. Haridasan, K., Bhuyan, L. R., & Deori, M. L. (1990). Wild edible plants of Arunachal Pradesh. *Arunachal forest News 8,* 1–8.

23. Ingram, J., Ericksen, P., & Liverman, D. (2010). Preface. Food Security and Global Environmental Change. Published by Earthscan, UK. pp. 13–15.

24. Jain, S. K., & Shanpru, R. (1977). Survey of wild edible plants of bazar of Meghalaya. *Bull. Meghal. Sci. Soc. 2,* 29–34.

25. Jaiswal, V. (2010). Culture and ethnobotany of Jaintia tribal community of Meghalaya, Northeast India – A mini review. *Indian J. Trad. Knowl.,* 9 (1), 38–44.

26. Jana, J. C. (2007). Use of traditional and underutilized leafy vegetables of Sub-Himalayan Terai region of West Bengal. *Acta Hort. 752,* 571–575

27. Jeyaram, J., Singh, T. A., Romi, W., Devi, A. R., Singh, W. M., Dayanidhi, H., Singh, N. R. & Tamang, J. P. (2009). Traditional fermented foods of Manipur. *Indian J. Trad. Knowl. 8(1),* 115–121.

28. Jeyaram, K., Singh, W. M., Capece, A., & Romano, P. (2008). Molecular identification of yeast species associated with '*Hamei*': A traditional starter used for rice wine production in Manipur, India. *Intern. J. Food Microbiol. 124,* 115–125.

29. Kar, A. (2004). Common wild vegetables of *Aka* tribes of Arunachal Pradesh. *Arunachal For. News. 3(3),* 305–313.

30. Kuhnlein, H. V., & Receveur, O. (1996). Dietary change and traditional food systems of idegenous peoples. *Annu Rev Nutr. 16,* 417–442. doi: 10.1146/annurev. nu.16.070196.002221.

31. Lalramnghinglova, H. (1999). Ethnobotanical and agroecological studies on genetic resources of food plants in Mizoaram state. *J. Econ. Taxon. Bot. 23,* 737–644.

32. Lalramnghinglova, H. (2002). Ethnobotanical study on the edible plants of Mizoram. *Ethnobotany 14,* 23–33.

33. Leach, E. R. (1976). Culture and Communication. Cambridge: Cambridge University Press.

34. Lynn, K., Daigle, J., Hoffman, J., Lake, F., Michelle, N., Ranco, D., Viles, C., Voggesser, G., & Williams, P. (2013). The impacts of climatic change on tribal traditional foods. *Climate Change. 120,* 545–556.

35. Maikhuri, P. K. (1991). Nutritional value of some lesser-known wild food plants and their role in tribal nutrition: A case study in North east India. *Trop. Sci. 31,* 397–405.

36. Mao, A. A., & Odyou, M. (2007). Traditional fermented foods of the Naga tribes of North-eastern India. *Indian J. Trad. Knowl., 6 (1),* 37–41.

37. Mao, A. A., Hynniewta, T. M., & Sanjappa, M. (2009). Plant wealth of Northeast India with reference to ethnobotany. *Indian J. Trad. Knowl. 8(1),* 96–103.

38. Minis, P. E. (1991). Famine foods of the Northern American desert borderlands in historical context. *J. Ethnobiol.*, *11(2)*, 231–257.

39. Murtem, G. (2000). Common wild vegetable of Nyishi tribe of Arunachal Pradesh. *Arunachal For News 18*, 64–66.

40. Nabhan, G. P. (2010). Perspectives in ethnobiology: ethnophenology and climatic change. *J. Ethnobiol. 30*, 1–4.

41. Paul, A. K., Chakma, P., Nahar, N., Akber, M., Ferdausi, D. et al. (2011). A survey of non-conventional plant items consumed during times of food scarcity by the Chakma people of Hatimara village of Rangamati district, Bangladesh. *American-Eurasian J. Sustainable Agriculture*, *5(1)*, 87–91.

42. Pegu, R., Gogoi, J., Tamuli A. K. &Teron, R. (2013). *Apong*, an alcoholic beverage of cultural significance of the Mishing community of Northeast India. *Global J. Interdisciplinary Social Sci.*, *2(6)*, 12–17.

43. Saha, D., Sundriyal, M., & Sundriyal, R. C. (2014). Diversity of food composition and nutritive analysis of edible wild plants in a multi-ethnic tribal land, Northeast India: an important facet for food supply. *Indian J. Trad. Knowl. 13(4)*, 698–705.

44. Sahoo, U. K., Lalremruata, J., Jeeceelee, L., Lalremruati, J. H., Lalliankhuma, C., & Lalramnghinglova, H. (2010). Utilization of Non timber forest products by the tribal around Dampa tiger reserve in Mizoram. *The Bioscan 3*, 721–729.

45. Samant, S. S., & Dhar, U. (1997). Diversity, endemism and economic potential of wild edible plants of Indian Himalaya. *Int. J. Sustain Dev. World Ecol. 4*, 179–191.

46. Samati, H. (2004). Kitchen garden plants of Pnar tribe in Jaintia hills district, Meghalaya. *Ethnobotany 16*, 125–130.

47. Samati, H., & Begum, S. S. (2007). *Kiad*, a popular local liquor of *Pnar* tribe of Jaintia hills district, Meghalaya. *Indian J. Trad. Knowl.*, *6 (1)*, 133–135.

48. Shankar, R., & Rawat, M. S. (2006). Medicinal plants for change in the socio-economic status in rural areas of North East India. *Bulletin of Arunachal Forest Res.*, *22*, 58–63.

49. Sharma, T. C., & Mazumdar, D. N. (1980). Eastern Himalayas: A study on Anthropology and Tribalism. Cosmo Publications, New Delhi, 17–31.

50. Shrivastava, K., Greeshua, A. G. & Srivastava, B. (2012). Biotechnology in Tradition- A process technology of alcoholic beverages practiced by different tribes of Arunachal Pradesh, North East India. *Indian J.Trad. Knowl. 11(1)*, 81–89.

51. Singh, A., Singh R. K., & Sureja, A. K. (2007). Cultural significance and diversities of ethnic foods of Northeast India. *Indian J. Trad. Knowl.*, *6(1)*, 79–94.

52. Singh, P. K., & Singh, K. I. (2006). Traditional alcoholic beverage, *Yu* of *Meitei* communities of Manipur. *Indian J. Trad. Knowl. 5(2)*, 184–190.

53. Sohliya, I., Joshi, S. R., Bhagobaty, R. K., & Kumar, R. (2009). *Trungrymbai*: A traditional fermented soybean food of the ethnic tribes of Meghalaya. *Indian J. Trad. Knowl. 8(4)*, 559–561.

54. Sujaya, I. N., Antara, N. S., Sone, T., Tanura, Y, Aryanta, U.R, Yokota, A., Asano, K., & Tomita, F. (2004). Identification and characterization of yeasts in brem: a traditional Balinese rice wine. *World J. Microbiol. Biotech.*, *20*, 143–150.

55. Sundariyal, M., & Sundariyal, R. C. (2000). Potential of wild edible plants in the Sikkim Himalaya: Conservation concerns. *J. Non Timber forest Prod. 7*, 253–262.

56. Sundariyal, M., & Sundariyal, R. C. (2001). Wild edible plants of Sikkim Himalayas: Nutritive values of selected species. *Econ. Bot. 55(3)*, 377–390.

57. Tamang, J. P., Dewan, S., Tamang, B., Rai, A., Schilinger, U., & Holzapfel, W. H. (2007). Lactic acid bacteria in Hamei and Marcha of North East India. *Indian J. Microbiol., 47*, 119–125.

58. Tanti, B., Gurung, L., Sarma, H. K., & Buragohain, A. K. (2010). Ethnobotany of starter culture used in alcohol fermentation by a few ethnic tribes of Northeast India, *Indian J. Trad. Knowl., 9(3)*, 463– 466.

59. Terangpi, R., Basumatary, R., Tamuli, A. K., & Teron, R. (2013). Pharmacognostic and physicochemical evaluation of stem bark of *Acacia pennata* (L.) Willd., a folk plant of the Dimasa tribe of Assam. *J. Pharmacognosy and Phytochem., 2(2)*, 234–240.

60. Teron, R, (2006). *Hor*, the traditional alcoholic beverage of Karbi tribe in Assam, *Natural product Radiance, 5(5)*, 377–381.

61. Turner, N. J., & Davis, A. (1993). "When everything was scarce": The role of plants as famine foods in Northwestern North America. *J. Ethnobiol., 13(2)*, 171–201.

62. Wakefield, S, Yeudall, F., Taron, C., Reynolds, J., & Skinner, A. (2007). Growing urban health: Community gardening in South-East Toronto. *Health Promotion Intern., 22(2)*, 92–101.

63. Woodley, E., Crowdey, E., de Pryek, J. D., & A Carmen (2009). Cultural indicators of indigenous people's food and agro-ecological systems. Mountain Policy Project, United Nations.

CHAPTER 5

ETHNOMEDICINAL PLANTS OF NORTH-EAST INDIA

SUVASHISH CHOUDHURY,[1] BIR BAHADUR,[2] and T. PULLAIAH[3]

[1]*Central Instrumentation Laboratory, Assam University, Silchar – 788011, India, E-mail: shuvasish@gmail.com*

[2]*Department of Botany, Kakatiya University, Warangal – 506009, A.P., India*

[3]*Department of Botany, Sri Krishnadevaraya University, Anantapur – 515003, A.P., India, E-mail: pullaiah.thammineni@gmail.com*

CONTENTS

Abstract 93
5.1   Introduction 94
5.2   Ethnomedicinal Plants of NE India and Their Uses 97
Keywords 151
References 151

ABSTRACT

The North Eastern (NE) states of India harbors immense floral diversity and lies among the biodiversity hot spot regions of the world. The region houses considerable ethnic multiplicity, which largely differ in their traditions, customs and language. Majority of these tribes are rich in the utilization of plants for medicinal purposes. Several studies pertaining to the documentation of rich ethnomedicinal diversity of North East India have been conducted and the reports indicate vast diversity of plants that are used for treatment of diverse diseases and ailments. In this chapter, we emphasize on some selected ethnomedicinal plants and their uses in treatment of various ailments among tribes of NE India.

5.1   INTRODUCTION

Human use of plants as a source of medicine dates back to the paleolithic age, about 60,000 years ago (Solecki and Shanider, 1975). There are several evidences where plants and plant products have been used as the primary source of medicine to cure wide range of ailments. Plant parts/products constitute large variety of natural products like steroids, terpenoids, alkaloids, flavonoids, etc. that contribute to their healing ability and serves as a irreplaceable source of pharmaceuticals today. Our understanding and knowledge on medicinal use of plants is far from complete. Traditional systems of medicine have provided mankind with large variety of drugs and food products, which till today are used as a potential source of medicine. Majority of drugs that are being used in traditional system of medicine are crude, mostly in their natural states/crude preparations. They are complex potpourri of natural compounds, some of which are beneficial, while some may be harmful, some may be vitamins or some may be highly toxic if taken alone. When these crude components are mixed in a formulation or crude preparation, they act like a single chemical agent and exert tremendous curative property. It is possible that one component counter balances the negative impact of the other and when mixed together they exert synergistic effect to cure the ailment. It is the main reason why natural medicine has very little or no side effects. It is estimated that out of 4,22,000 flowering plants in the world, almost 50,000 are being used for medicinal purpose and India represent 43% of it (Pushpangadan, 1995; Schipmann et al., 2002).

In India, the utilization of plants for medicinal purposes have been documented in several ancient literature, however, organized studies began during mid 1950's and off late such studies gained significant popularity amongst plant biologists. The documentation of ethnic knowledge resulted in discovery of many new drugs or lead compounds and today almost 80% of the global population have direct dependency on plants as primary source of medicine (Farnsworth et al., 1985; Fabricant and Farnsworth, 2001).

According to the estimates of the World Health Organization (WHO), approximately 65% of the world populations are dependent on plants as primary source of medicine (Fabricant and Farnsworth, 2001). There have been a considerable development in the field of ethnobotany and medicinal plant research, as such several publications in terms of volumes, flora, research articles and reviews have come up. In North Eastern region of India, several researchers were engaged in this field and consequently many important publications have emerged.

The decade at the beginning of the year 1995 was observed as the *International Decade for World's Indigenous and Ethnic People*. A complex link has always existed between ethnic culture and botanical conservation. In almost all the parts of the world, the ethnic/tribal people have sincerely co-existed with nature and its resources. The agenda 21 of the Rio Earth Summit, 1992 states that indigenous people have a vital role in environmental management vis-à-vis sustainable development due to their knowledge about traditional practices and such practices enable them to have an effective participation in the achievement of sustainable development. The documentation of ethnic knowledge is not a new practice. It possibly existed with the advent of human civilization. Archeological records suggest that documentation of ethnic and traditional knowledge existed in ancient Greek, Egyptian, Chinese, Indian and perhaps other civilizations of the world. Ancient literature that exist today on the use of plants for medicinal purposes reflect a clear dependency of human on plants for their day-to-day needs. Plants like *Rawolfia serpentina*, *Papaver somniferum* and *Cinchona officinalis* were widely used and are being used till today as an excellent source of crude medicine. The time-tested traditional knowledge on the use of plants for medicinal and therapeutic purpose has opened a wider scope under different scientific themes, where traditional and indigenous knowledge can be explored and utilized in a sustainable manner. Traditional knowledge has a strong impact on modern day drug discovery pipeline. Many revolutionary drugs that we see now have their origin from plants that have traditional or folkloristic significance. Today, the ethnic ideas coupled with scientific inputs have revolutionized the drug discovery process.

It is estimated that there are approximately 4,22,000 higher (flowering) plants on this planet (Fabricant and Farnsworth, 2001), out of which only 6% have been screened for biological activity and 15% phytochemically (Fabricant and Farnsworth, 2001). It is, therefore, obvious that with such a huge diversity of plants existing on this planet, the proximity of finding new drugs and lead molecules is extremely high and traditional knowledge can strongly support such findings. Further, the use of plants based on traditional knowledge has got some major advantages. The medicinal property of plants used in ethnic culture is claimed on the basis of its long-term use, often hundreds and thousands of years and one can expect diverse chemical constituents present in that plant extract or formulation (Fabricant and Farnsworth, 2001). Thus, documentation and conservation of ethnic and traditional knowledge has immense significance on present day heath care system. Rapid industrialization and loss of ethnic culture has resulted in significant loss of such important knowledge and it is quite possible that in due course of time such knowledge will disappear. Till today, collection of ethnobotanical information remained as an academic endeavor, with very little or no interest on industrial/commercial aspects. Ancient civilizations of the world were dependent mainly on plants as their source of healthcare system. The Chinese, Egyptian, Greeks and Indian civilization have provided significant information on medicinal properties of plants, which are well reflected in their ancient writings and inscriptions. The extraordinary property of garlic is known for hundreds of years. In ancient China, *Artemisia annua* L. was used for treatment of fever and malaria and as such in 1972 anti-malarial drug 'artemisinin' was isolated from it. The medicinal property of ginseng (*Panax ginseng*) was also recognized by the ancient Chinese culture and today ginsenodies and associated flavonoids are well known for their potential curative properties. *Ginkgo biloba*, is used in traditional Chinese medicine to improve mental alertness and later ginkgolides and flavonoids were isolated from it. These are several examples of plants that have immense significance in our health care system and have roots from traditional knowledge. The medicinal property of a plant is unique, some are taken raw, some in the form of crude extracts or as formulation, while other are eaten either as vegetable or fruit. Their activity is dependent mainly on the characteristic chemical compound hidden inside or as a result of synergistic effect of the secondary metabolites present.

5.2 ETHNOMEDICINAL PLANTS OF NE INDIA AND THEIR USES

The North-Eastern region of India is one of the biodiversity hot spots, which harbors immense diversity of flora and fauna. The vast geographical area of North-East India is inhabited by large number of ethnic tribal groups, which largely differ in their traditional, lingual and cultural practices. The inhabitants are mostly aware of their surrounding and acquainted in utilizing their surrounding resources in their day-to-day life. The traditional knowledge of each of the tribes are unique and developed by trial and error method, which is further passed onto the next generation as a guarded secret and remains limited within the tribes. Efforts have been made by several investigators to document the ethnic knowledge on the use of plants for medicinal purpose and as results many significant publications have come up. The region is physiographically divided into distinct regions of Eastern Himalayas, Patkai – Naga Hills, Lushai Hills, Brahmaputra Valley and plains of Bark Valley. Out of 450 tribes of India, about 225 are found in North East (Lokho, 2012). The regions harbor almost 50% of the total biodiversity of India and being recognized as one of the major biomes of the world (Mao et al., 2009). The tribal communities of North East India are mainly concentrated in the hilly terrains and certain parts of the fertile alluvial plains of Brahmaputra and Barak valley, practicing agriculture, animal rearing and handloom as their primary occupation. North East India being a storehouse immense biological diversity and rich in ethnic culture has attracted several researchers to carry out comprehensive work on ethnobotanical aspects of several tribes. The emphasis on the ethnobotanical studies of North East India emerged in late 1970's and as such several major publications have emerged. Pioneering work on lesser-known medicinal plants among the Mikir tribes of North East India was done by Borthakur (1976). Hajra (1977) reported large number of traditionally used medicinal plants from Kamang district of Arunachal Pradesh. Several other important works that emerged on ethnomedicine of North East India include inclusive documentation of medicinal plants used by various tribes of Assam, Meghalaya, Arunachal Pradesh and Nagaland (Mazumder et al., 1978; Tiwary et al., 1978, 1979; Jain and Dam, 1979; Bhattacherjee et al., 1980). Beside these pioneering work, major work on ethnobotany of North East India included those reported by Kumar et al. (1980) on medicinal plants of Balphakrah Wildlife Sanctuary in Meghalaya, ethnomedicinal plants of Khasi and Jaintia Hills (Joshep and Kharkongor, 1980), ethnomedicinal aspects of Mikirs of North East India (Jain and Borthakur, 1980), ethnomedicinal plants of Nagaland (Rao and Jamir, 1982 a,b), medicinal plants used by Boros of Assam (Baruah and Sharma, 1984), anti-jaundice plants of Assam (Gogoi and Boissya, 1984), ethnomedicinal aspects of Reangs of Assam (Choudhury, 1999; Choudhury and Choudhury, 2002), ethnomedicinal aspects of Rongmai Naga of Southern Assam (Choudhury et al., 2005), ethnomedicinal aspects of Choreis of Southern Assam (Choudhury, 2007; Choudhury et al., 2012). Some folklore claims of Brahmaputra valley in Assam were recorded by Boissya and Majumdar (1980). Changkija and Kumar (1996) reported ethnobotanical folk practices of Ao-Naga and documented diverse uses of plants and formulations used in the treatment of various ailments. Neogi et al. (1989) investigated ethnobotany of some weeds of Khasi and Garo Hills of Meghalaya and reported 65 taxa. Changkija (1999) documented an account of 109 plant species that have medicinal uses among the tribes of Nagaland. Singh et al. (2001) gave the ethnobotanical uses of 14 species of Pteridophytes used by the ethnic tribes of Manipur. Gogoi and Borthakur (2001) reported 69 herbal recipes for 27 ailments involving 68 plant species prevalent among the Bodo tribe inhabiting Goreswar, Rangia and Jajikona Development blocks of Kamrup district of Assam. Tripathi and Goel (2001) gave an account of ethnobotanical diversity of Zingiberaceous plants in North-Eastern India and reported ethnobotanical uses of 43 taxa of Zingibers. Indigenous practice of treating human liver disorders in Assam was dealt by Das and Saikia (2001) and gave details of methods of treatment. Singh et al. (2002) reported 64 species of plants used as medicine among ethnic groups in Sikkim. Important ailments purportedly cured by these plants are epilepsy leprosy, paralysis, asthma, typhoid, diabetes, hemorrhages during child birth, cholera as well as other. Das and Saikia (2002) investigated the folk belief on plants used as abortifacient and antifertility. Bharadwaj and Gakhar (2003) carried out ethnobotanical studies in Mizoram and reported 25 plant species used by the native people for the cure of dysentery.

Ethnomedicinal uses of 33 plant species belonging to 22 families for various ailments among the Zeme Nagas, one of the prominent ethnic tribes of North Cachar Hills district of Assam was reported by Tamuli and Saikia (2004). Pfoze and Chhetry (2004) reported that 72 medicinal plants are being used by Shephoumaramth Nagas as folk medicines including rare species *Taxus baccata* and *Panax pseudoginseng.* Thirty nine hepatoprotective herbal recipes prevalent among different ethnic groups of Assam were reported by Borthakur et al. (2004) along with local names of the plant species, method of preparation and the dose-regime.

Ahmed and Borthakur (2005) gave an account of botanical wisdom of Khasis (Hynnew Treps) of Meghalaya. The usage of 17 wild plants by the native people for curing cuts and wounds was described by Bharadwaj and Gakhar (2005). Ethnobotanical studies carried out by Khmbongmayum et al. (2005) in the four sacred groves of Manipur revealed therapeutic applications of 120 plant species. Kala (2005) reported 158 medicinal plants belonging to 73 families and 124 genera used by Apatani tribe of Arunachal Pradesh. These studies laid one of the major foundations of ethnobotanical aspects of North East India by revealing huge datasets of plants and their medicinal properties. Some major notable studies on ethnomedicinal use of *Pinanga mannii* and cane among the Adi and Mishing were also reported from Arunachal Pradesh. An attempt has been made by Kalita et al. (2005) to study the plant and animal based folk medicine used by people of Dibrugarh district, Assam for treatment of eleven different diseases. Kayang et al. (2005) provided a list of the most frequently used medicinal plants in the tribal areas of Eastern and Western Khasi hills of Meghalaya, India and the diseases against which these plants are used.

Saikia (2006) described the traditional knowledge related to ethnomedicine of different communities (Assamese, Bodo, Mishing, Napali and Santhal) of Gohpur of Sonitpur district of Assam. All together 22 prescriptions were recorded from 20 plant species. Kalita and Deb (2006) listed 22 plant species used in folk medicine by the *Bejas* and *Bejins* in Lakhimpur district of Brahmaputra valley in Assam. The paper by Majumdar et al. (2006) deals with 33 medicinal plants along with their local name, parts and ethnomedicinal uses prescribed by tribal and non-tribal medicine men of Tripura state. Plants used by Garo, Khasi and Jaintia of Meghalaya was reported by Nath et al. (2007) which documented 65 weeds belonging to 26 families of angiosperms. Lafakzuala et al. (2007) enumerated and discussed the ethnobotanical aspect of the plants used by the tribal of Mizoram.

Pradhan and Badola (2008) recorded ethnomedicinal plant use by Lepcha tribe of Dzongu valley bordering Khangchendzonga Biosphere Reserve, in North Sikkim. This paper reports 118 species, belonging to 71 families and 108 genera, under ethnomedicinal utility by the Lepchas for curing approximately 66 ailments, which could be grouped under 14 broad categories. Zingiberaceae appeared as the most used family (8 species and 5 genera). A. K. Das et al. (2008) carried out a survey in different parts of Cachar district of Assam to gather information regarding the uses of medicinal plants by the different tribes/communities and reported 107 plant species. An ethnobotanical survey of East Khasi hills, West Khasi hills and Ri Bhoi districts of Meghalaya was conducted by Hynniewta and Kumar (2008) and reported 54 ethnomedicinal plants.

The major ethnic tribal groups inhabiting the North East regions of India have evolved several ways to utilize the plant resources (Das and Tag, 2005; Nima et al., 2009; Rethy et al., 2010). The uses of plants vary diversely among the tribes and recent studies have shown that mode of uses of the plants are considerably different (Tangjang et al., 2011). Influence of modern civilization has resulted in loss of traditional knowledge and younger generations have very little or no interest to preserve this rich folk culture. Namsa et al. (2009) reported 34 species of plants having anti-inflammatory properties. The study focused exclusively on use of plants in the management of inflammation related ailments by the Khampti tribe of Arunachal Pradesh (Namsa et al., 2009). The 34 plants species were distributed among 22 families and 32 genera, and similar uses were mentioned even in ancient system of medicine like the Ayurveda, Unani and Siddha (Namsa et al., 2009). With majority of the plants previously reported for similar uses, 13 species were reported for the first time with anti-inflammatory properties (Namsa et al., 2009). Bantawa and Rai (2009) discussed the traditional practices among Jhankri, Bijuwa and Phedangma on locally available plants material to cure various ailments and disorders. The study by Shil and Choudhury (2009) mainly focused on the ethnomedicinal importance of Pteridophytic flora used by the Reang tribes of Tripura state and presented 16 Pteridophyte species. Medhi and Chakrabarti (2009) described the information on the traditional knowledge of people of Northeastern region on wild orchids including ethnomedicinal uses. Mao et al. (2009) gave an account of plant wealth of Northeast India with special reference to ethnobotany. This included ethnomedicinal plants and threatened medicinal plants.

An ethno-medico-botanical survey was carried out by Kagyung et al. (2010) in Adi dominated areas of Dehang-Debang Biosphere reserve of Arunachal Pradesh. They recorded a total of 44 plant species belonging to 31 families. The tribes of North East India have utilized the plant/floral diversity of the region and preserved their traditional knowledge. Herbal medicine is considered as an integral part of traditional culture of North East India and traditional healers are given utmost respect. It is estimated that 2,416 plants have been documented in India for ethno-medicinal purposes out of which almost 1,953 plants were used by tribes of North East India (Sajem and Gosai, 2006; Tushar et al., 2010). Tushar et al. (2010) reported 37 species of plants belonging to Zingiberaceae that are used by tribes of North East India for treatment of multiple ailments. Almost 88% of Zingiberaceous plants are distributed in Arunachal Pradesh and majority of the crude preparations are obtained from rhizomes (Tushar et al., 2010). Rout et al. (2010), had revealed that the Zeme Naga from Assam are using 8 species of medicinal plants for the treatment of diarrhea. Saikia et al. (2010) carried out ethnobotanical survey work near the border area of Arunachal Pradesh. Totally, 20 plant species were collected and recorded for their use in various ailments. Jamir et al. (2010) dealt with first hand information on 55 plants used by the Lotha-Naga tribes in Wokha district, Nagaland for the treatment of various diseases and ailments. Rai and Lalramnghnglova (2010a) provided first-hand information of 57 ethnomedicinal plants from Mizoram. They also reported 159 ethnomedicinal plant species from tropical forests, home gardens, roadsides and University campus of Mizoram (Rai and Lalramnghnglova, 2010b). In another report Rai and Lalramnghnglova (2010c) gave an account of 54 ethnomedicinal plants from Agroforestry systems and home gardens of Mizoram.

The indigenous or traditional healers are solely dependent on plants for their medicinal preparations. They either use a single plant or mixture of plant parts to prepare the crude formulation. Ethnomedicinal practices among the Tai-Khamyangs of Sivassagar district of Assam were given by Sonowal and Barua (2011). Laloo and Hemalatha (2011) enlisted information regarding the traditional method of utilization of plant species that are used to treat and cure diarrhea and dysentery. A study by Devi et al. (2011) revealed that 73 plant species were used by local practitioners in Manipur for the treatment of diabetes. Tangjang et al. (2011) studied ethnomedicinal plants of Eastern Himalaya zone of Arunachal Pradesh and documented major differences in mode of use of plants among Nocte, Nishi and Adi tribes. They documented 74 plant species belonging to 41 families and 61 genera that are being used to treat 25 different diseases (Tanganj et al., 2011). An ethnobotanical study focused on medicinal utility of plants was carried out by Buragohain (2011) among the ethnic communities of Tinsukia district of Upper Assam. A total of 175 plant species were described which have been used in the treatment of about 56 diseases. Studies on the medicinal plants used by Tangkhul Nagas of Nagaland reveled 36 different species of plants used by the tribe for treatment of diverse ailments (Salam et al., 2011). Namsa et al. (2011) documented 50 plants species used for treating 22 human ailments by Monpa ethnic group at Arunachal Pradesh. They also documented plants used for dietary supplements, religious purpose, local beverage and plants used to poison fish and wild animals. Deb et al. (2011) reported the ethnomedicinal uses of the following plants: *Zingiber officinale* as anticough, antifever, antidiabetic, anticancer, *Zingiber cassumunar* as anticough, antidiabetic, *Zingiber zerumbet* as anticough, antifever, *Clerodendrum colebrookianum* as hypertensive, *Oroxylum indicum* as antipiles, *Eupatorium nodiflorum* as anti-diarrheal, *Annesia fragrans* for treatment of kidney stone and *Prunus persica* as antihypertensive. Rai and Lalramnghinglova (2011b) studied threatened and less known medicinal plants and their ethnomedicinal importance from Indo-Burma hotspot region. They reported 40 plant species out of which 17 belong to the threatened category (Rai and Lalramnghinglova, 2011b). The ethnomedicinal aspects of different tribes of North East India have been reported by various workers. It is now well known that the diverse plant species have potential curative properties against several human diseases. Being ethnically diverse, the North East India harbors the storehouse of immense ethnobotanical information on the therapeutic uses of plants against large number of diseases. The immense biological diversity also contributes significantly to the knowledge of ethnic people about plants and their medicinal properties. Choudhury et al. (2011) documented traditional knowledge of 22 medicinal plant species that are used in the treatment of different reproductive health related disorders and diseases by the rural people of Rungia subdivision of Kamrup district, Assam.

Studies conducted by Tag et al. (2012) in Lohit district of Arunachal Pradesh documented 46 plant species used for management and treatment of diabetes. They reported 11 species that are new in treatment of diabetes, which include *Begonia roxburghii, Calamus tenuis, Callicarpa arborea, Cuscuta reflexa, Dillenia indica, Diplazium esculentum, Lactuca gracilis, Millingtonia hortensis, Oxalis griffithii, Saccharum spontaneum*, and *Solanum viarum* and few of these plants also showed efficacy or antidiabetic activity in rodent models (Tag et al., 2012). Das et al. (2012) reported a large number of plants, plant extracts, and decoctions used by ethnic and rural people of Eastern Sikkim Himalayan region in treatment of various ailments. The variety of plants used for treatment of diabetes in Arunachal Pradesh clearly indicated the significance of plants in primary health care system and dependency of tribal people on plants as source of medicine. Such studies clearly indicated the importance of ethnobotanical studies and traditional knowledge. Sharma et al. (2012) reported medico-religious plants used by Hajong community of Assam. Hajongs uses various plants species for medicinal purpose and different rituals. The study documented 36 plant species that are used for treatment of 51 different diseases with 63 formulations (Sharma et al., 2012). The study clearly reflected that social, economic and religious significance of plants within the Hajong community (Sharma et al., 2012). However, with immense influence of urban life, traditional knowledge among the Hajong youth is very limited and conservation of cultural diversity needs urgent attention (Sharma et al., 2012). An ethnobotanical survey was conduced in river island Majuli aimed at identifying the plants used in the treatment of Jaundice in the Satra culture people in Assam. Yumnam et al. (2012) investigated the ethnomedicinal uses of plants used by people of Manipur. A total of

41 plant species have been mentioned as folkloric treatment with herbal material that are being used by the people of Manipur. Shankar et al. (2012) surveyed folk medicinal plants used by folk healers of Mishing tribe in few places of Lakhimpur and Dhemaji district of Assam and East Siang district of Arunachal Pradesh for the malaria, jaundice and female menstruation problems which are the prominent diseases in the community. The rural populations among the Monpa ethnic group in Arunachal Pradesh have a rich knowledge of forest-based natural resources and consumption of wild edible plants as an integral part of selecting socio-cultural life. Rout et al. (2012) surveyed and collected information on traditional uses of plants by the Dimasa tribe of Assam for curing and treating different diseases like urinary disorder, diarrhea, malaria, etc. Among the plant types, like herbs were the most frequently used, ferns and Cycads also find usage in their traditional healing. Panda (2012), found that the traditional healers act as health care actors for treating arthritis, fracture, jaundice, diarrhea and respiratory diseases of children with other persistence, long lasting chronic health conditions with the use of medicinal plants. 52 species of medicinal herbs being used in a wide range by various Naga tribes have been recorded by Jamir et al. (2012).

Traditional medicines are used in the form of diverse preparations. Some are chewed directly, some are taken in the form aqueous extracts while others are taken in the form of dry powder, formulation, etc. Ningthoujam et al. (2013) reported the use of vapor-based medicine among the Meithei Manipuris of North East India. They reported 13 distinctive route of administration of both mono and multi-ingredient composition for treatment of 41 diseases (Ningthoujam et al., 2013). Lalmuanpuii et al. (2013) documented the traditional practice and knowledge of medicines/naturopathy among the Mizo ethnic group of Lunglei district. A total of 82 medicinal plant species belonging to 42 families and 76 genera were documented along with their parts used, methods of preparation and types of ailments treated. It was revealed that there is a positive relationship between age and traditional knowledge and practice; while a negative relationship between educational level and traditional knowledge and practice was observed. Sharma (2013) carried out an ethnobotanical study in Darjeeling Himalayas to document plants used against skin diseases. During the field survey, ethnomedicinal information of 91 species of medicinal plants belonging to 53 families was compiled from different habitats of the study area. Application of plants against skin diseases included various forms of preparation. Shankar and Rawat (2013) recorded 37 folklore claims of traditional healing herbs used by Mizo tribe in the treatment of several ailments. Mao et al. (2013) discussed ethnobotany of *Rhodoedron* species in North-East India and gave ethnomedicinal uses of *Rhododendron* species. 50 ethnomedicinal plant species used for traditional herbal formulation by different tribes in Tripura were given by Majumdar and Datta (2013) with scientific name, vernacular name(s), part(s) used, availability status, ailments and mode of administration.

The diversity of traditional used of plants in North East India is massive, which makes this region an important hot-spot of ethnobotanical information. It is, therefore, essential to gather and document unique information on the use of plants. Deb et al. (2012) reported customary usage of 39 plant species by the Darlong tribes in Tripura. Bhuyan et al. (2014) reported that an extensive study on Traditional practice of medicinal plants by four major tribes of Nagaland was conducted in different localities from districts of the state. The tribes undertaken for study were Ao, Angami, Lotha, Sema, residing in Nagaland. The study comprises 257 species of ethnomedicinal plants belonging to 85 families. Shil et al. (2014) reported 125 different species of plans belonging to 59 families comprising 116 genera used by the Reang tribe of Tripura for the treatment of 42 different ailments. They reported that the traditional remedies are generally taken orally and the leaves are the major component of plant part used to prepare the crude drugs (Shil et al., 2014). The use of plant species by the Reang people is strictly based on the flora available locally and their knowledge is passed on to the next generation through oral traditions without any written documentation (Shil et al., 2014). Chettri et al. (2014) documented the use of thirty medicinal plants, nineteen food and fodder plants by the workers of the tea gardens comprising of different traditional communities like Tamang, Limboo, Dupka and Lepchas. Singh et al. (2014) documented pharmaceutically important plant resources used in primary health care of ethnic Garo tribes from Eastern Himalayas (Nokrek Biosphere Reserve [NBR], India) in order to document information on medicinal plants and to maximize the collection of indigenous knowledge of Garo tribes. A total of 157 plant species representing 134 genera and 81 families were found to be commonly used in the treatment of 67 health-problems. Pandey and Mavinkurve (2014) prepared an inventory of ethnomedicinal plants used by the Chakma tribe of Tripura state, India. Chakma people are mostly residing in deep forest and depend on their own traditional health care system. The survey was conducted during 2012 in Agartala, Tripura by interviewing the local health practitioners of the different villages of the state, a total of 19 angiosperms and one pteridophyte have been documented for folklore medicinal plants used by Chakma tribes of Tripura. A field survey was performed by Debnath et al. (2014) over Mog and Reang communities of Sabroom and Santirbazal subdivision of Tripura to find out ethnomedicinal knowledge and plant parts utilized in their various ailments and identified 51 species.

In Unakoti district, Tarafdar et al. (2015) reported 39 species of plants belonging to 28 families and 37 genera that are used by tribes against diabetes. The study revealed commonness in use of the plants among different tribes groups of North East India and other parts of the world (Tarafdar et al., 2015). The mode of use *Syzygium cumini* L. by Reangs for treatment of diabetes is common with some major tribes of Southern Assam and Manipur (Banik et al., 2010; Devi, 2011; Tarafdar et al., 2015). Many of the plants documented in the study also possess hepatoprotective, antioxidant, antimicrobial, anticancerous, hypotensive and nematicidal activities that were previously reported (Tarafdar et al., 2015). In North Tripura district of Tripura, 75 different plants species belonging to 43 families have been reported to be used by various ethnic communities as an effective crude drug against 15 disease categories (Choudhury et al., 2015). Most of these plants were administered orally in the form of crude extracts against gastrointestinal and respiratory disorders (Choudhury et al., 2015). Kichu et al. (2015) reported 135 plant species belonging to 69 families and 123 genera from Chungtia village of Nagaland used by the Ao Naga tribes. As per the ethnic classification, the plants are used to treat 13 categorized ailments with most frequent use against gastrointestinal ailments and dermatological disorders (Kichu et al., 2015). The study revealed that the Ao Naga tribes have strongly preserved their ethnic traditions of use of plants and vis-à-vis conserved the floral biodiversity in the vicinity. Choudhury et al. (2012) reported 53 different plants used by Chorei tribe of Southern Assam for 9 disease categories. Most of the plants species were used against skin or related infections, followed by jaundice, constipation, dysentery, cough-cold and diabetes (Choudhury et al., 2012). Jamir (2012) discussed traditional knowledge of medicinal plants used by Ao-Naga tribes of Mokokchung district, Nagaland and reported 38 species of medicinal plants for treatment of various diseases and ailments.

Lokho and Narasimhan (2013) gave ethnobotanical descriptions of 63 taxa, citing their local names, medicinal uses, culinary and ritualistic uses. The paper also sheds light on indicator plants which are used y the tribe for *jhum* cultivation and other agricultural practices. In another study, survey was done by Singh and Huidrom (2013) in Central Valley of Manipur. It was found that Meitei community in the study area extensively used *Justicia adhatoda* L., as ethno-medicine as well as food plant. Parkash et al. (2013) documented the hidden traditional medicinal usage of 35 wild plants by Khasi tribe of Nonghkyllem Reserve Forest, Nongpoh, Meghalaya.

Basumatary et al. (2014) documented the indigenous knowledge pertaining to the utilization of 44 medicinal plant species used by the Bodo-Kachari tribes of Karbi Anglong district of Assam. Das et al. (2014) documented a total of 55 ethnomedicinal plants belonging to 42 families and 49 genera having antifertility property. Gurumayum and Soram (2014) recorded 45 plant species used by Mao Naga tribe community of Mao, Senapati district, Manipur for treating diarrheas and dysentery. Leishingthem and Sharma (2014) recorded 50 ethnomedicinal plants for the treatment of different diseases, viz., asthma, arthritis, cough, fever, diabetes, dysentery, gastric and indigestion, jaundice, toothache, skin diseases, etc. Details of 52 plant species used by Hmar, Manipuri and Barman community of Hailakandi district of Assam (India) for the treatment of diabete were given by Khan et al. (2014). An investigation by Ningombam et al. (2014) on 41 local Maiba and Maibi of Meetei community of Manipur is carried out to find reliability of their knowledge and tested if these were related to significantly to age, literacy, hesitation, results of their treatment, doses and to document such knowledges based on a total of 205 locally available medicinal plant species used for treating 18 major diseases classes. Mir et al. (2014) listed 131 medicinal plant species used by ethnic tribes in Meghalaya used for curing different ailments.

Jamir et al. (2015) carried out study on ethnomedicinal plants in Zumheboto district, Nagaland and documented 59 medicinal plants and their uses. A study was carried out by Zhasa et al. (2015) to explore indigenous knowledge on utilization of available plant biodiversity which have been utilized for treatment and cure of human ailments by eight Naga tribes, i.e., Angami, Zeliang, Ao, Lotha, Sangtam, Konyak, Chakhesang, Rengma and Khaimniungam in Nagaland. About 241 plant species were recorded for traditional medicine used by the eight Naga tribes. Gohain et al. (2015) conducted an ethnobotanical survey of potent antimalarial plants used by different tribes and communities of highly malaria affected seven districts of Assam. A total of 22 plant species have been recorded. These include *Ageratum conyzoides, Alpinia nigra, Asparagus racemosus, Caesalpinia bonduc, Cedrus deodora, Clerodendrum infortunatum, Coptis teeta, Cucumis sativus, Curanga amara, Dillenia indica, Flemingea strobilifera, Ichnocarpus frutescens, Impatiens balsamina, Ocimum gratissimum, Phlogacanthus thyrsiformis, Piperr longum, Rubus rugossus, Solanum myriacanthum, Spilanthes acmella, Stemona tuberosa, Swertia chirata* and *Vitex negudo*. Bhuyan (2015) listed 20 ethnomedicinal plants used by the ethnic tribes of North East India. Several PhD theses have been submitted by different research scholars working on ethnobotany of Northeast India and these include Choudhury (1999) and Dutta (2000).

Other publications on Ethnomedicobotany of North East India include Baruah and Sarma (1987), Bora (1999), Borthakur (1976, 1981, 1992), Borthakur and Goswami (1995), Chhetri (1994), Choudhury et al. (2005), Choudhury and Neogi (2003), Dam and Hajra (1997), Das et al. (2007), Das and Sharma (2003), Hajra and Baishya (1981), Idrisi et al. (2012), Islam (1996), Jamir (1990, 1991, 1999, 2006), Kharkongor and Joseph (1981), Kumar et al. (1987), Lalrammghinglova (2003), Lunusnep and Jamir (2010), Maiti et al. (2003), Majumdar (2007a,b), Mao (1993), Megoneitso and Rao (1983), Moktan and Das (2013), Rai et al. (1998), Rao (1981, 1997), Rao et al. (1989), Rawat and Choudhury (1998), Sanjem et al. (2008), Schipman et al. (2002), Singh et al. (1996), Singh et al. (2015), Sinha (1987), Sumitra and Jamir (2009), and Tiwari et al. (2009).

A list of ethnomedicinal plants used by various tribes of North-East India is given in Table 5.1.

TABLE 5.1   Ethnomedicinal Plants Used By Tribes of North East India

S. No.	Name of the plant species	Parts Used	Purpose	Reference(s)
1	*Abies densa* Griff.	Leaf	Asthma, stomach pain, bronchitis,	Badola and Pradhan, 2013
2	*Abrus precatorius* L.	Fruit, root	Throat pain	Badola and Pradhan, 2013
3	*Abroma augusta* (L.) L.	Stem bark and leaf	Anti-diabetic	Chhetri et al., 2005
4	*Abutilum indicum* (L.) Sw.	Stem bark	Anti-diabetic	Chhetri et al., 2005
5	*Acacia pennata* (L.) Willd.	Leaf	Bleeding gums, indigestion in infants	Badola and Pradhan, 2013
6	*Achyranthes aspera* L.	Leaves	Wounds, injuries, diabetes, painful urination	Salam et al., 2011
7	*Achyranthes bidentata* Blume	Leaf	Water borne foot disease	Shil et al., 2014
8	*Aconitum ferox* Wall. ex Seringe	Rhizome	Diarrhea, cough, cold	Badola and Pradhan, 2013
9	*Aconitum heterophyllum* Wall. ex Royle	Root	Rheumatism	Chhetri, 2005
10	*Aconitum palmatum* D. Don.	Root	Anti-diabetic	Chhetri et al., 2005
11	*Aconitum spicatum* Stapf	Rhizome, leaf	Diarrhea, cough, cold, fever, headache	Badola and Pradhan, 2013
12	*Acorus calamus* L.	Rhizome	Cough, cold, snake bite, asthma, fever, rheumatism, bronchitis, toothache, throat pain, headache, heart complaints, hemorrhoids	Jamir et al., 2011; Khongsai et al., 2011; Nath et al., 2011; Ringmichon et al., 2011; Badola and Pradhan, 2013; Ningthoujam et al., 2013
13	*Adhatoda vasica* Nees	Leaves	Cough, cold, fever, itching	Choudhury et al., 2008; Ringmichon et al., 2011; Singh et al., 2011; Choudhury et al., 2012

TABLE 5.1   (Continued)

S. No.	Name of the plant species	Parts Used	Purpose	Reference(s)
14	*Adiantum capillus-veneris* L.	Fronds	Stimulant, febrifuge, expectorant, purgative, demulcent, respiratory problems, menstrual disorders	Benniamin, 2011; Sen and Ghosh, 2011
15	*Adiantum caudatum* L.	Fronds, rhizome	Fever, cough, skin diseases, diabetes	Benniamin, 2011; Sen and Ghosh, 2011
16	*Adiantum lunulatum* Burm.	Rhizome, fronds	Fever, itch, epileptic fits, rabies	Benniamin, 2011
17	*Adiantum philippense* L.	Fronds, rhizome	Fever, dysentery	Sen and Ghosh, 2011
18	*Aegle marmelos* (L.) Correa.	Fruit, leaves, root	Constipation, indigestion, body ache, diarrhea, dysentery, fever, acidity, urine infection, nephritis,	Choudhury et al., 2008, 2012; Deb et al., 2012; Sharma et al., 2012; Nath et al., 2013; Ningthoujam et al., 2013; Shil et al., 2014
19	*Aesculus assamica* Griffith	Leaves	Skin infection, backache	Khongsai et al., 2011
20	*Ageratum conyzoides* L.	Flower, tender plant tip, leaves, whole plant, roots	Throat pain, cuts, wounds, diarrhea, dysentery, stomach disorder, rheumatic swelling, arthritis, anthelmintic, blood coagulant, fever, malaria, liver problems	Jamir et al., 2008a, 2011; Namsa et al., 2009; Khongsai et al., 2011; Ringmichon et al., 2011; Salam et al., 2011; Deb et al., 2012; Badola and Pradhan, 2013; Shil et al., 2014
21	*Ajuga macrosperma* Wall. ex Benth.	Leaves	Earache, cough, fever, lice	Khomdram et al., 2011
22	*Albizia chinense* (Osb.) Merr.	Stem bark	Snake and spider bites	Jamir et al., 2008a

TABLE 5.1 (Continued)

S. No.	Name of the plant species	Parts Used	Purpose	Reference(s)
23	*Albizia procera* (Roxb.) Benth.	Bark	Fever	Badola and Pradhan, 2013
24	*Albizia lebbeck* Benth.	Bark	Skin diseases	Choudhury et al., 2008
25	*Aleuritopteris tenuifolia* (Burm.f.) Sw.	Fronds	Antiseptic	Sen and Ghosh, 2011
26	*Allium ascalonicum* L.	Bulb	Paralysis	Jamir et al., 2011
27	*Allium cepa* L.	Leaves, bulb	Boils, sprained muscles and joints, insect bites, indigestion	Choudhury et al., 2008; Jamir et al., 2008a, 2011; Salam et al., 2011; Badola and Pradhan, 2013
28	*Allium hookeri* Thw.	Leaves	Bodyache	Jamir et al., 2011
29	*Allium odorum* L.	Whole plant	Fever	Ringmichon et al., 2011
30	*Allium sativum* L.	Bulb	Backache, lumbago, altitude sickness, blood pressure, injuries, paralysis, heart problems	Choudhury et al., 2008; Nath et al., 2011; Singh et al., 2011; Badola and Pradhan, 2013
31	*Alnus nepalensis* D.Don	Root and stem bark, fruits	Diarrhea, dysentery, stomachache, joint pains, rheumatism	Jamir et al., 2008a, 2011
32	*Alocasia indica* Schott	Tuber, stem	Jaundice, wounds	Choudhury et al., 2012; Deb et al., 2012
33	*Aloe vera* (L.) Burm.f. (Syn.: *Aloe barbadensis* Mill.)	Leaves	Burnt wounds, cuts, dermatitis, fever, jaundice, ulcers,	Jamir et al., 2011; Ringmichon et al., 2011; Badola and Pradhan, 2013
34	*Alpinia allughas* (Retz.) Roscoe	Fruit and Rhizome	To treat ring worm., Antipyretic	Tushar et al., 2010
35	*Alpinia nigra* (Gaertn.) Burtt	Rhizome	Carbuncle; Diabetes	Shil et al., 2014; Choudhury et al., 2012

TABLE 5.1 (Continued)

S. No.	Name of the plant species	Parts Used	Purpose	Reference(s)
36	*Alsophila contaminans* Wall. Ex Hook.	Apex of caudex	Cuts, wounds	Sen and Ghosh, 2011
37	*Alsophila spinulosa* (Wall. Ex Hook.) R. M.Tryon	Rhizome	Cuts, wounds	Sen and Ghosh, 2011
38	*Alstonia scholaris* (L.) R.Br	Leaves, latex, flower, bark	Stomach disorder, snake bite, boils, lactation	Choudhury et al., 2008, 2012; Nath et al., 2013; Shil et al., 2014
39	*Alternanthera paronychioides* A. St.-Hil	Leaf	Cut and wound	Shil et al., 2014
40	*Amaranthus gracilis* Desf.	Whole Plant	Allergic swelling	Shil et al., 2014
41	*Amaranthus spinosus* L.	Whole plant, roots	Gastric disorders, laxative, appetizer, tonic, skin infection	Jamir et al., 2008a, 2011; Khongsai et al., 2011
42	*Amischotolype hookeri* (Hassk.) Hara	Leaf	Naval Pain	Shil et al., 2014
43	*Amomum subulatum* Roxb.	Seed	Teeth and gum infection	Badola and Pradhan, 2013
44	*Ampelocissus barbata* (Wall.) Planch.	Plant juice	Sores in mouth and tongue of milk sucking baby	Badola and Pradhan, 2013
45	*Ampelocissus divaricata* (Wall. ex Laws.) Planch.	Leaf	Cuts, wounds	Shil et al., 2014
46	*Amphineuron extensus* (Bi.) Holtt.	Frond	Diarrhea, malaria, abnormal menstruation	Das, 1997
47	*Amphineuron poulentum* Kauf.	Leaf	Anti-poison	Tangjanj et al., 2011
48	*Ananas comosus* (L.) Merr.	Roots	Diarrhea, stomachache, indigestion, anti-inflammatory, gout, rheumatism, cough	Jamir et al., 2008a, 2011; Nath et al., 2011; Tangjang et al., 2011

TABLE 5.1 (Continued)

S. No.	Name of the plant species	Parts Used	Purpose	Reference(s)
49	*Anacolosa ilicoides* Mast.	Leaf	Cuts, wounds	Shil et al., 2014
50	*Ananas comosus* (L.) Merr.	Fruit, leaves	Diuretic, blood purifier, cardiac problems, cough, cold, breathing problems, urinary tract stones	Jamir et al., 2011; Salam et al., 2011; Singh et al., 2011; Deb et al., 2012
51	*Andrographis paniculata* (Burm. f.) Wall. exNees	Leaves, whole plant, stem	Stomachic, malaria, jaundice, diabetes, small worms, stomach problem, fever, cough, liver troubles, gastritis	Choudhury et al., 2012; Khongsai et al., 2011; Singh et al., 2011; Deb et al., 2012; Nath et al., 2013; Shil et al., 2014
52	*Angiopteris evecta* (G.Forst.) Hoffm.	Fronds, rhizome	Dysentery, leprosy, bodyache, piles	Benniamin, 2011; Sen and Ghosh, 2011
53	*Anisomeles indica* (L.) O.Kuntze	Leaves, seeds, seed oil	Carminative, laxative, dysentery, urinary tract infections, bowel complaints	Khomdram et al., 2011; Nath et al., 2013
54	*Annona squamosa* L.	Root, seed paste	Headache	Badola and Pradhan, 2013
55	*Anthcephalus chinensis* (Lam.) Rich. ex Walp.	Fruit	Stomachache	Badola and Pradhan, 2013
56	*Aphanamixis polystachya* (Wall.) R. Parker	Leaf	Chronic asthma	Ningthoujam et al., 2013
57	*Ardisia paniculata* Roxb	Bark	Burns	Shil et al., 2014
	Areca catechu L.	Leaf	Toothache	Choudhury et al., 2012
58	*Argyreia nervosa* (Burm. f.) Bojer	Root	Sprain	Shil et al., 2014
	Aristida adscensionis L.	Root	Cancer	Choudhury et al., 2012
59	*Arisaema tortuosum* (Wall.) Schott.	Corm	Insect repellent	Jamir et al., 2011

TABLE 5.1   (Continued)

S. No.	Name of the plant species	Parts Used	Purpose	Reference(s)
60	*Artemisia indica* Willd.	Young shoot, leaves	For easy delivery, itching	Jamir et al., 2011
61	*Artemisia maritima* L.	Leaves	Fever	Ringmichon et al., 2011;
62	*Artemisia nilagirica* (C. B.Clarke) Pamp	Leaves	Hemostatic, fever, stomach problems	Jamir et al., 2008a, 2011; Ringmichon et al., 2011; Salam et al., 2011
63	*Artemisia vulgaris* L.	Leaves	Nose bleeding, mouth ulcers, skin allergy	Badola and Pradhan, 2013
64	*Artocarpus heterophyllus* Lam.	Seeds, latex, fruit	Urinary disorders, boils, bone fracture, laxative	Jamir et al., 2008a; Choudhury et al., 2012; Badola and Pradhan, 2013
65	*Artocarpus lakoocha* Roxb.		Boils, bone fracture	Badola and Pradhan, 2013
66	*Asclepias curassavica* L.	Leaves, root	Tumors, blood coagulation	Choudhury et al., 2012; Shil et al., 2014
67	*Asparagus racemosus* Willd.	Root, fruits	Kidney problems, fever, cold, cough, pimples	Jamir et al., 2011; Badola and Pradhan, 2013
68	*Asphodelus tenuifolius* Cav.	Whole plant	Burns	Deb et al., 2012
69	*Asplenium nidus* L.	Leaves	Fever, elephantiasis, lice, jaundice	Benniamin, 2011; Yumkham and Singh, 2011; Sen and Ghosh, 2011
70	*Astilbe rivularis* Ham.	Root, leaf	Back pain, toothache	Badola and Pradhan, 2013
71	*Averrhoa carambola* L.	Fruit	Jaundice, liver problems	Jamir et al., 2008a; Namsa et al., 2009
72	*Azadirachta indica* A.Juss.	Leaf	Diabetes	Badola and Pradhan, 2013
73	*Baccaurea ramiflora* Lour.	Root	Insect Sting	Shil et al., 2014

TABLE 5.1 (Continued)

S. No.	Name of the plant species	Parts Used	Purpose	Reference(s)
74	*Bambusa balcooa* Roxb.	Shoots	Sprain	Nath et al., 2011
75	*Bambusa tulda* Roxb.	Wax and hair; Leaf ash	Check bleeding; Vermifuge	Singh et al., 2011; Kichu et al., 2015
76	*Basella alba* L.	Leaf	Stomach disorders laxative	Choudhury et al., 2012; Kichu et al., 2015
77	*Bauhinia iliate* L.	Leaf	Bone fracture; gastro-intestinal problems	Jamir et al., 2008a; Shil et al., 2014; Kichu et al., 2015
78	*Bauhinia purpurea* L.	Bark	Insect bites, irregular mensuration, chest pain, diarrhea, boils	Purkayastha et al., 2005; Badola and Pradhan, 2013
79	*Bauhinia tenuiflora* Watt. ex Cl.	Leaves	Heart disease	Jamir et al., 2011
80	*Bauhinia variegata* L.	Stem bark	Dysentery, stomachache	Jamir et al., 2008a
81	*Begonia picta* Smith	Leaf	Hand sanitizer	Kichu et al., 2015
	Begonia roxburghii (Miq.) DC.	Root	Blood dysentery	Nath et al., 2013
82	*Begonia thomsonii* A.DC.	Root	Diarrhea, skin rashes and infections	Shil et al., 2014; Choudhury et al., 2012
83	*Berberis aristata* DC.	Stem, root	Bitter tonic, fever	Khongsai et al., 2011
84	*Berberis asiatica* DC.	Fruit, leaf, bark, root	Diarrhea, dysentery, jaundice, fever; anti-diabetic	Badola and Pradhan, 2013; Chhetri et al., 2005
85	*Bergenia ciliata* (Haw.) Sternb.	Root	Bone fracture, wounds, diarrhea, dysentery, cough, cold	Badola and Pradhan, 2013

TABLE 5.1   (Continued)

S. No.	Name of the plant species	Parts Used	Purpose	Reference(s)
86	*Bergenia purpurascens* (Hook.f. & Thoms.) Engl.	Roots	Body ache	Badola and Pradhan, 2013
87	*Betula utilis* D.Don	Bark	Antiseptic	Badola and Pradhan, 2013
88	*Bidens pilosa* L.	Leaves	Wounds, ulcers, ear and eye problems, pain	Khongsai et al., 2011; Badola and Pradhan, 2013
89	*Bidens tripartita* (D.Don) Sheritt.	Leaves	Malaria	Jamir et al., 2008a
90	*Blechnum orientale* L.	Pinnae	Boils, urinary disorders, cuts, wounds, abscess	Sen and Ghosh, 2011; Shil et al., 2014
91	*Blumea lanceolaria* (Roxb.) Druce	Leaf	Vaginal protrusion	Shil et al., 2014
92	*Blumeopsis flava* (DC.) Gagnep	Leaves	Dry cough, cuts and wounds, bleeding, joint pains, cold	Salam et al., 2011; Ningthoujam et al., 2013
93	*Boehmeria macrophylla* Horn.	Leaves	Cancers	Choudhury et al., 2012
94	*Boenninghausenia albifolia* (Hook. F.) Reich ex. Meissn	Whole plant	Anti-diabetic	Chhetri et al., 2005
95	*Bombax ceiba* L.	Stem bark, root bark, gum, flower	Bone fracture, skin diseases, diarrhea, dysentery, small pox in children	Jamir et al., 2008a; Badola and Pradhan, 2013
96	*Bombax malabaricum* DC.	Bark	Menstrual problems	Choudhury et al., 2012
97	*Bougainvillea spectabilis* Willd.	Leaves	Laxative	Jamir et al., 2008a
98	*Brassaiopsis polyacantha* (Wall.) Banerjee	Leaves	Kidney troubles	Salam et al., 2011

TABLE 5.1 (Continued)

S. No.	Name of the plant species	Parts Used	Purpose	Reference(s)
99	*Brassica campestris* L.	Seed oil	Muscular pain, joint pain, dandruff, cold	Badola and Pradhan, 2013
100	*Brassica mitis* C. B. Clarke	Roots	Dysentery	Badola and Pradhan, 2013
101	*Brassica nigra* (L.) Koch	Seed oil	Rheumatism	Nath et al., 2011
102	*Bridelia retusa* (L.) Spreng.	Bark	Cuts and wounds	Badola and Pradhan, 2013
103	*Bryophyllum calycinum* (Lamk.) Pers.	Leaves	Kidney and gallbladder stones	Deb et al., 2012
104	*Bryophyllum pinnatum* Kurz.	Leaf	Cough, cold	Choudhury et al., 2012
105	*Buddleja asiatica* Lour.	Leaves	Skin rashes, allergy	Badola and Pradhan, 2013
106	*Caesalpinia pulcherrima* (L.) Sw.	Root	Malarial Fever	Shil et al., 2014
107	*Cajanus cajan* (L.) Millsp.	Leaves, roots, pods	Wound, jaundice, stomach ulcers, skin infections	Choudhury et al., 2012; Jamir et al., 2011; Salam et al., 2011; Deb et al., 2012
108	*Calamus rotang* L.	Raw fruit	Anti-diabetic	Chhetri et al., 2005
109	*Callicarpa arborea* Roxb	Tender shoots, root, stem bark, leaf, fruit	Gastric problems, leucorrhoea, gastritis; skin diseases, fever, indigestion, gastric problems, scorpion sting, carminative	Jamir and Rao, 1990; Chaturvedi and Jamir, 2007Jamir et al., 2008a; Devi and Singh, 2008; Khongsai et al., 2011; Choudhury et al., 2012; Badola and Pradhan, 2013; Shil et al., 2014
110	*Callicarpa macrophylla* Vahl	Leaves	Bodyache	Devi and Singh, 2008

TABLE 5.1 (Continued)

S. No.	Name of the plant species	Parts Used	Purpose	Reference(s)
111	*Callicarpa rubella* Lindl.	Leaves	To stop bleeding	Devi and Singh, 2008
112	*Calotropis procera* (Aiton) W. T.Aiton	Latex, plant juice	Skin diseases, gastric problems, diarrhea, stomach ulcer, urinary tract infections	Singh et al., 2011
113	*Calotropis gigantea* L.	Stem	Headache	Ningthoujam et al., 2013
114	*Campylandra aurantiaca* Baker	Flower	Anti-diabetic	Chhetri et al., 2005
115	*Cannabis sativa* L.	Leaves, seeds	Pain killer, stomach disorder, dysentery, diarrhea, body pain	Jamir et al., 2008; Khongsai et al., 2011; Badola and Pradhan, 2013
116	*Canarium resiniferum* Bruce ex King	Oleoresin	Hemorrhoids	Ningthoujam et al., 2013
117	*Capsicum frutescens* L.	Fruit	Menstrual excess bleeding, pain due to bee sting	Choudhury et al., 2012; Jamir et al., 2011
118	*Cardamine hirsuta* L.	Leaves	Typhoid	Jamir et al., 2011
	Cardiospermum halicacabum L.	Leaves	Skin diseases	Singh et al., 1997
119	*Carica papaya* L.	Fruit, leaves, latex, seeds, fruits	Liver disorders, stomachache, heart problems, skin diseases, dog bite, bone fracture, burns, cuts, wounds, heels crack, tape worm infection, jaundice	Jamir et al., 2008, 2011; Khongsai et al., 2011; Choudhury et al., 2012; Badola and Pradhan, 2013
120	*Caryota urens* L.	Nut	Cuts and wounds	Jamir et al., 2011
121	*Cassia alata* L.	Leaves	Ringworm, white patches	Deb et al., 2012
122	*Cassis fistula* L.	Fruit	Acidity, tapeworm	Nath et al., 2013; Shil et al., 2014
123	*Cassia tora* L.	Leaf	Ringworm	Shil et al., 2014

TABLE 5.1 (Continued)

S. No.	Name of the plant species	Parts Used	Purpose	Reference(s)
124	*Ceiba pentandra* (L.) Gaertn	Root	Carbuncle	Shil et al., 2014
125	*Celastrus paniculatus* Willd.	Leaves	Cancerous growth	Choudhury et al., 2012
126	*Celosia argentea* L.	Leaves	Fever, diarrhea, dysentery	Badola and Pradhan, 2013; Shil et al., 2014
127	*Celosia cristata* L.	Flower; leaf	Urinary tract infection; cuts and wounds	Kichu et al., 2015
128	*Centella asiatica* L.	Whole plant, leaves, plant	Cough, fever, cholera, stomachache, boil, rheumatism, skin disease, fractures, leprosy, asthma, tuberculosis, skin infections, dysentery, digestive problems, jaundice	Choudhury et al., 2012; Jamir et al., 2008, 2011; Khongsai et al., 2011; Singh et al., 2011; Deb et al., 2012
129	*Centipeda minima* (L.) Br. & Aeschers	Leaves	Cold	Saikia et al., 2010
130	*Cheilanthes tenuifolia* (Burm. f.) Sw	Fronds	Abscess	Shil et al., 2014
131	*Chenopodium album* L.	Plant, leaves	Common worms, back pain, constipation, acidity, diarrhea, dysentery, laxative	Saikia et al., 2010; Jamir et al., 2011; Badola and Pradhan, 2013; Nath et al., 2013
132	*Chonemorpha fragrans* (Moon) Alston	Leaf	Blood Coagulation	Shil et al., 2014
133	*Christella parasitica* (L.) Lev.	Frond	Numbness	Saikia et al., 2010
134	*Chukrasia tabularis*	Bark	Astringent, back pain	Khumbongmayum et al., 2005

TABLE 5.1 (Continued)

S. No.	Name of the plant species	Parts Used	Purpose	Reference(s)
135	*Chrysanthemum indicum* L.	Flowers	Stomach ache	Badola and Pradhan, 2013
136	*Cinnamomum camphora* (L.) Siebold	Bark	Cardiac Problem	Shil et al., 2014
137	*Cinnamomum tamala* (Buch.-Ham.) Nees & Eberm.	Bark, leaf	Intestinal disorder, diarrhea	Badola and Pradhan, 2013
138	*Cinnamomum zeylanicum* Breyn	Bark	Cuts, injury	Salam et al., 2011
139	*Cissampelos pareira* L.	Leaf, root	Bone Facture, anti-diabetic, high blood pressure, malaria, dysentery, piles, gastric problems	Shil et al., 2014; Chhetri et al., 2005; Kichu et al., 2015
140	*Cissus adnata* Roxb.	Tubers	Carbuncle	Shil et al., 2014
141	*Cissus assamica* (Laws.) Craib	Root	Carbuncle	Shil et al., 2014
142	*Cissus discolor* Bl.	Leaves	Kidney stones	Salam et al., 2011
143	*Cissus quadrangularis* L.	Stem	Rheumatism	Nath et al., 2011
144	*Cissus repens* Lam.	Leaf	High blood pressure; urinary and kidney disorders	Kichu et al., 2015
145	*Citrus limon* (L.) Burm.f.	Fruit, seed	Snake bite, inflammation of joint, laxative, stimulant,	Nath et al., 2011
146	*Citrus maxima* Merr.	Fruit, seed	Diabetes, worm infestation	Jamir et al., 2008; Nath et al., 2013
147	*Citrus medica L.*	Fruit, leaves	Malaria, indigestion, epilepsy, cardiotonic, cough, vomiting, jaundice typhoid, dysentery, nausea, mental disorder	Singh et al., 1997; Jamir et al., 2008; Choudhury et al., 2012; Khongsai et al., 2011; Badola and Pradhan, 2013

TABLE 5.1   (Continued)

S. No.	Name of the plant species	Parts Used	Purpose	Reference(s)
148	*Citrus reticulata* Blanco	Fruit skin	Softens and cleans skin	Badola and Pradhan, 2013
149	*Clausena heptaphylla* (Roxb.) Wt. & Arn	Leaves, fruit	Dysentery, cough and Asthma	Deb et al., 2012; Shil et al., 2014
150	*Clematis buchananiana* DC.	Roots, leaves	Sinusitis, nose blocks	Badola and Pradhan, 2013
151	*Clerodendrum cecil-fischeri* A. Rajendran & Daniel	Leaves	Asthma, sinus	Devi and Singh, 2008
152	*Clerodendum colebrookianum* Walp.	Leaves, bark	Malaria, rheumatism, gout, high blood pressure, diabetes, malaria, cough, dysentery, skin diseases	Gajurel et al., 2006; Jamir et al., 2008, 2011; Devi and Singh, 2008; Khongsai et al., 2011; Salam et al., 2011
153	*Clerodendron cordatum* D.Don	Leaves	Fever, bowel complaints	Devi and Singh, 2008
154	*Clerodendrum indicum* (L.) O. Kuntze	Root, stem, leaves	Swellings, syphilis, cough, fever, dysentery, asthma, bronchitis,	Devi and Singh, 2008; Deb et al., 2012; Ningthoujam et al., 2013
155	*Clerodendrum kaempferi* (Jacq.) Siebold	Leaves	High blood pressure	Devi and Singh, 2008
156	*Clerodendrum paniculatum* L.	Root	Typhoid	Shil et al., 2014
157	*Clerodendrum squantum* Vahl	Leaves	High blood pressure	Choudhury et al., 2012
158	*Clerodendrum serratum* (L.) Moon	Leaves	Cold, cough, jaundice, stomach disorders	Devi and Singh, 2008

TABLE 5.1   (Continued)

S. No.	Name of the plant species	Parts Used	Purpose	Reference(s)
159	*Clerodendrum viscosum* Vent.	Root, leaves	Inflated body, diarrhea, dysentery, high blood pressure	Saikia et al., 2010; Khongsai et al., 2011; Deb et al., 2012; Nath et al., 2013; Shil et al., 2014
160	*Clitoria ternatea*	Leaves	Blood dysentery	Nath et al., 2013
161	*Coccinea grandis* (L.) Voigt.	Root	Anti-diabetic	Chhetri et al., 2005
162	*Cochlospermum religiosum* (L.) Alst.	Root	Urinary infection	Shil et al., 2014
163	*Codariocalyx motorius* (Houtt.) H. Ohashi	Leaf	Health Tonic	Shil et al., 2014
164	*Coix lacryma-jobi* L.	Fruit, leaf	As a source of vitamins	Kichu et al., 2015
165	*Colebrookea oppositifolia* Smith	Leaf	Dysentery	Badola and Pradhan, 2013
166	*Colocasia esculenta* (L.) Schott.	Petiole, rhizome	Minor cuts, burns, hemostatic, bee stings	Saikia et al., 2010; Jamir et al., 2011
167	*Combretum album* Pers.	Leaves	Anthelmintic, dysentery	Nath et al., 2013
168	*Combretum decundrum* Roxb.	Leaves, root	Diarrhea, malarial fever	Deb et al., 2012; Shil et al., 2014
169	*Coptis teeta* Wall.	Leaves, rhizome	Malarial fever, body ache, stomach trouble, dandruff, dysentery, diarrhea	Gajurel et al., 2006; Khongsai et al., 2011
170	*Corchorus olitorius* L.	Leaves	Increase appetite	Nath et al., 2013
171	*Cordyline fruticosa* (L.) A. Chev.	Root	Malarial Fever	Shil et al., 2014

TABLE 5.1 (Continued)

S. No.	Name of the plant species	Parts Used	Purpose	Reference(s)
172	*Costus speciosus* (Koenig ex. Retz) JE Smith	Roots, stems, rhizome	Piles, toothache, respiratory blockage, urinary disorder, ear pain, toothache, vermifuge	Jamir et al., 2011; Khongsai et al., 2011; Badola and Pradhan, 2013; Kichu et al., 2015
173	*Crassaocephalum crepidioides* (Benth.) Moor	Leaves, young shoots, flowers	Diarrhea, dysentery, fever, stomach ulcers, piles, dizziness, high blood pressure, hemostatic, gastroenteritis	Gajurel et al., 2006; Jamir et al., 2008; Ringmichon et al., 2011; Salam et al., 2011
174	*Crataeva nurvala* Buch-Ham.	Leaf	Relieving pain, body swelling, liver tonic	Kichu et al., 2015
175	*Crinum asiaticum* L.	Bulb	Rheumatic pain	Saikia et al., 2010;
176	*Crotalarias spectabilis* Roth	Root and Leaf	Health tonic; ring worm infection	Shil et al., 2014
177	*Crotalaria verrucosa* L.	Root	Rheumatism	Shil et al., 2014
178	*Croton caudatus* Gieseler	Leaf, root	Anti-cancer	Kichu et al., 2015
179	*Cucumis melo* Roxb.	Seed	Fever	Shil et al., 2014
180	*Cucurbita maxima* Duch.	Leaves	Boils	Choudhury et al., 2012
181	*Cucurbita pepo* L.	Seed	Vermifuge	Badola and Pradhan, 2013
182	*Curanga amara* Juss. (Syn. *Picria fel-terrae*)	Leaf	Dysentery, high blood pressure, gastric problems	Kichu et al., 2015
183	*Curculigo capitulata* (Lour.) O. Kuntze	Rhizome	Eyeache, venereal diseases, gastroenteritis	Jamir et al., 2008;
184	*Curcuma amada* Roxb.	Rhizome	Carminative, bronchiolytic, skin allergy, body itching, sprained joints, vulnerary	Tushar et al., 2010; Badola and Pradhan, 2013

TABLE 5.1 (Continued)

S. No.	Name of the plant species	Parts Used	Purpose	Reference(s)
185	*Curcuma caesia* Roxb.	Rhizome	Gout, malarial fever, fever, gastric problems, vomiting, injury	Nath et al., 2011; Ringmichon et al., 2011; Salam et al., 2011; Shil et al., 2014
186	*Curcuma longa* L. (Syn.: *C.domestica* Valet)	Rhizome	Rheumatism, piles, dyspepsia, vasodilator, urinary tract infections, fever, cuts, wounds	Tushar et al., 2010; Nath et al., 2011, 2013; Ringmichon et al., 2011; Singh et al., 2011; Deb et al., 2012
187	*Curcuma zedoaria* Rosc.	Rhizome	Bad breath	Badola and Pradhan, 2013
188	*Cuscuta reflexa* Roxb.	Whole plant	Jaundice	Shil et al., 2014
189	*Cyathea contaminans* (Wall. ex Hook.) Copel.	Leaves, young apex of the caudex	Eczema, antiseptic	Choudhury et al., 2012; Shil et al., 2014
190	*Cyclea peltata* Diels.	Leaf	Abscesses, boils	Kichu et al., 2015
191	*Cymbopogon citratus* (DC.) Stapf	Leaves	Fever, influenza, insect repellant, cough, cold	Jamir et al., 2008; Shil et al., 2014
192	*Cymbopogon nardus* (L.) Rendle	Root, leaves	Bleeding of nose	Saikia et al., 2010
193	*Cynodon dactylon* (L.) Pers.	Plant	Nasal bleeding, cuts and wounds, blood dysentery	Salam et al., 2011; Badola and Pradhan, 2013; Nath et al., 2013
194	*Dactylorhiza hatagirea* (D.Don) Soo	Rhizome	Cuts and wounds	Badola and Pradhan, 2013
195	*Daiswa polyphylla* Rafin.	Root	To treat alcoholism	Jamir et al., 2011
196	*Daphne cannabina* Wall.	Root	To remove poison	Badola and Pradhan, 2013

TABLE 5.1 (Continued)

S. No.	Name of the plant species	Parts Used	Purpose	Reference(s)
197	*Datura fastuosa* L.	Leaves, seeds, fruits	Joint pain, asthmatic fits, mad dog bites	Badola and Pradhan, 2013
198	*Datura innoxia* Mill.	Leaves	Joint pain	Choudhury et al., 2012
199	*Datura stramonium* L.	Leaves, fruit	Bronchitis, chest congestion, swellings, skin diseases	Salam et al., 2011; Choudhury et al., 2012
200	*Debregeasia longifolia* (Burm. f.) Wedd.	Root, leaf	Insomnia, anti-diabetic, fever, high blood pressure	Jamir et al., 2011; Kichu et al., 2015
201	*Dendrobium ariaefolium* Griff.	Plant	Narcotic	Lalramnghinglova and Jha, 1999
202	*Dendrobium nobile* Lindl.	Seeds	Hemostatic	Jamir et al., 2011
203	*Dendrocnide sinuata* Bl.	Stem	Cut and wounds, painful sting	Kichu et al., 2015
204	*Desmos longiflorus* (Roxb.) Safford	Bark	Toothache	Shil et al., 2014
205	*Dicranopteris linearis* (Burm. F.) Underwood	Fronds	Toothache	Shil et al., 2014
206	*Dicentra scandens* (D.Don) Walp.	Root	Gastritis	Badola and Pradhan, 2013
207	*Dichroa febrifuga* Lour.	Leaf	Fever	Badola and Pradhan, 2013
208	*Dicrocephala integrifolia* (D.Don) O. Kuntze	Leaves	Fever, stomach upsets,	Salam et al., 2011
209	*Dillenia indica* L.	Fruits	Cough, fever	Khongsai et al., 2011
210	*Dioscorea bulbifera* L.	Tuber	Health Tonic	Shil et al., 2014
211	*Dioscorea floribunda* M.Martin & Galeotti	Tuber	Vitalizer	Khongsai et al., 2011

TABLE 5.1 (Continued)

S. No.	Name of the plant species	Parts Used	Purpose	Reference(s)
212	*Disopyros lanceifolia* Roxb.	Fruit, root	Fish poison	Kichu et al., 2015
213	*Diospyros toposia* F. Ham.	Bark	Toothache, foul smell	Deb et al., 2012
214	*Dipteris wallichii* (R.Br.) Moore	Rhizome	Jaundice	Sen and Ghosh, 2011
214	*Dischidia nummularia* R.Br.	Leaves	Skin disease	Deb et al., 2012
216	*Dolichos lablab* L.	Leaf, pod	Diarrhea, nausea, vomiting, poor appetite, poisonous bites, dog bite	Kichu et al., 2015
217	*Dolichos uniflorus* L.	Plant	Kidney stone	Badola and Pradhan, 2013
218	*Drymaria cordata* Willd. ex Roem. & Schult.	Twigs, leaves	Stomach disorder, chest pain, head ache, sinusitis, cold, fever, skin diseases, itching, snake and spider bites, gastrointestinal disorders, asthma	Majumdar et al., 1978; Gajurel et al., 2006; Jamir et al., 2008; Saikia et al., 2010; Ringmichon et al., 2011; Badola and Pradhan, 2013
219	*Drymaria diandra* Bl.	Plant	Wounds	Jamir et al., 2011
220	*Drymoglossum heterophyllum* (L.) Trimen	Pinnae	Skin diseases, bone fracture	Choudhury et al., 2008; Shil et al., 2014
221	*Drynaria quercifolia* (L.) J.Smith	Rhizome, fronds	Tuberculosis, throat infection	Sen and Ghosh, 2011
222	*Duabanga grandiflora* (Roxb. Ex DC) Walp.	Stem bark	Skin infection, cut and wounds	Kichu et al., 2015
223	*Eclipta prostrata* (L.) L.	Twig, leaf	Conjunctivitis, cuts and Wounds	Saikia et al., 2010; Shil et al., 2014
224	*Ehretia acuminata* R.Br.	Leaf	Bone Facture	Shil et al., 2014

TABLE 5.1   (Continued)

S. No.	Name of the plant species	Parts Used	Purpose	Reference(s)
225	*Elaeocarpus sphaericus* K.Schum.	Seed	Cough	Badola and Pradhan, 2013
226	*Elatostema platyphyllum* Wedd.	Shoot	Gastritis	Badola and Pradhan, 2013
227	*Elephantopus scaber* L.	Leaves	Diarrhea, dysentery	Gajurel et al., 2006
228	*Elsholtzia blanda* Benth.	Leaves, inflorescence	Hypertension, piles, cough, cold, fever, sinusitis, tonsillitis, throat trouble, cuts	Khomdram et al., 2011; Salam et al., 2011; Kichu et al., 2015
229	*Elsholtzia communis* (Coll. & Hemsl.) Diels	Plant, leaves, inflorescence	Sore throat, tonsillitis, cough, fever, diarrhea, menstrual disorders,	Khomdram et al., 2011; Salam et al., 2011
230	*Emblica officinalis* Gaertn.	Fruit	Liver tonic, diabetes, jaundice, heart problems	Khongsai et al., 2011
231	*Emilia sonchifolia* (L.) DC.	Plant, root	Cuts, wounds, diarrhea	Salam et al., 2011
232	*Engelhardtia spicata* Bl.	Leaves, inflorescence	Scabies, skin diseases	Chhetri, 1994
233	*Entada phaseoloides* (L.) Merr.	Seeds	Arthritis, paralysis, mumps	Deb et al., 2012
234	*Entada pursaetha* ssp. *sinohimalensis* Grierson & Long	Seed	Mumps, lice, dandruff	Badola and Pradhan, 2013; Kichu et al., 2015
235	*Entada scandens* Benth.	Seed	Fever	Ringmichon et al., 2011;
236	*Ephedra gerardiana* Wall. ex Stapf	Ripe fruit, stem	Altitude sickness, indigestion, head ache	Badola and Pradhan, 2013
237	*Equisetum diffusum* D.Don	Leaves	Back pain	Yumkham and Singh, 2011

TABLE 5.1   (Continued)

S. No.	Name of the plant species	Parts Used	Purpose	Reference(s)
238	*Equisetum ramosissimum* Desf.	Root, plant	Fever in infants, bone fracture	Jamir et al., 2011; Salam et al., 2011
239	*Eranthemum nervosum* R.Br.	Leaves	Tumorous growth	Choudhury et al., 2008
240	*Eryngium foetidum* L.	Leaves	Indigestion	Kichu et al., 2015
241	*Erythrina stricta* Roxb.	Root, stem bark	Gout, dermatitis, eczema, skin infections	Nath et al., 2011; Kichu et al., 2015
242	*Eucalyptus globulus* Labill.	Leaves	Respiratory problems	Choudhury et al., 2008
243	*Eupatorium adenophorum* Spreng.	Leaves, tender shoot, seed	Fever, cuts, wounds, malaria, antiseptic, mumps, bleeding, dysentery	Jamir et al., 2008; Ringmichon et al., 2011; Salam et al., 2011; Badola and Pradhan, 2013
244	*Eupatorium cannabinum* L.	Leaves	Fever	Ringmichon et al., 2011
245	*Eupatorium nodiflorum* Wall. ex DC.	Leaves	Fever	Ringmichon et al., 2011
	Eupatorium odoratum L.	Leaves	Cuts, wounds	Deb et al., 2012
246	*Euphorbia hirta* L. [Syn.: *Chamaesyce hirta* (L.) Millsp.]	Plant, leaves	Bronchial, asthma, cough, anthelmintic, toothache, cuts and wounds	Khongsai et al., 2011; Salam et al., 2011; Shil et al., 2014
247	*Euphorbia ligularia* Roxb.	Leaf	Rheumatism	Nath et al., 2011
248	*Euphorbia royleana* Boiss.	Latex	Dysentery	Jamir et al., 2011;
249	*Eurya acuminata* DC.	Fruit, leaves	Dysentery, diarrhea, cholera, cuts and wounds, anti-gas	Jamir et al., 2011; Kichu et al., 2015
250	*Evodia fraxinifolia* Hook.f.	Seeds	Indigestion	Badola and Pradhan, 2013

TABLE 5.1 (Continued)

S. No.	Name of the plant species	Parts Used	Purpose	Reference(s)
251	*Fagopyrum esculentum* Moench	Leaf	Cold, cough, stomach ache and gastritis	Jamir et al., 2008; Badola and Pradhan, 2013
	Ficus hirta Vahl	Root	Tumorous growth	Choudhury et al., 2008;
252	*Ficus hispida* L.	Hypanthodium	Cough	Shil et al., 2014
253	*Ficus pumila* L.	Leaf	Anti-lice	Shil et al., 2014
254	*Ficus racemosus* L.	Fruit	Anti-diabetic	Chhetri et al., 2005
255	*Fragaria nubicola* Lindl. ex Lacaita	Root	Bleeding, cough, cold	Badola and Pradhan, 2013
256	*Galinsoga parviflora* Cav.	Leaves	Fever	Ringmichon et al., 2011
257	*Garcinia cowa* Roxb.	Fruit, stem bark, seed	Stomach disorders, dysentery, diarrhea	Gajurel et al., 2006; Kichu et al., 2015
258	*Garcinia lancifolia* Roxb.	Fruit	Stomach disorders	Gajurel et al., 2006
259	*Garcinia pendunculata* Roxb. ex. Buch.-Ham.	Stem bark, seed	Dysentery, diarrhea	Kichu et al., 2015
260	*Geum elatum* Wall.	Whole plant	Throat pain	Chhetri et al., 2005
261	*Girardiana heterophylla* Decne	Root	Anti-diabetic	Chhetri et al., 2005
262	*Girardinia palmata* (Forssk.) Gaudich	Root	Skin diseases, kidney problems, toothache	Badola and Pradhan, 2013
263	*Gmelina arborea* Roxb.	Root, bark, leaves, fruit	Snake bite, scorpion sting, blood purifier, stomach trouble, gonorrhea, cough, skin disease	Devi and Singh, 2008; Khongsai et al., 2011; Deb et al., 2012
264	*Gossypium herbaceum* L.	Leaves	Anti-inflammatory	Nath et al., 2011

TABLE 5.1 (Continued)

S. No.	Name of the plant species	Parts Used	Purpose	Reference(s)
265	*Gonatanthus pumilus* (D. Don) Engler & Krause	Leaf, stem	Vermifuge for veterinary use only (extremely poisonous for humans)	Kichu et al., 2015
266	*Gynocardia odorata* R.Br.	Seed; fruit	Massaging of infants; anti-diabetic	Badola and Pradhan, 2013; Chhetri et al., 2005
267	*Gynura crepidioides* Benth.	Leaves	Anti-diabetic	Kichu et al., 2015
268	*Gynura nepalensis* DC.	Leaves	Blood pressure, intestinal problems	Jamir et al., 2008
269	*Hedychium coronarium* Koenig	Rhizome	Fever	Ringmichon et al., 2011
270	*Hedychium spicatum* Buch.-Ham.	Rhizome	Fever	Ringmichon et al., 2011
271	*Hedyotis scandens* Roxb.	Leaf, root	Cut and wounds, urinary tract infection, piles, gastro-intestinal problems, laxative	Kichu et al., 2015
272	*Heliotropium indicum* L.	Leaves	Fever	Ringmichon et al., 2011
273	*Helminthostachys zeylanica* (L.) Hook.	Rhizome	Whooping cough, impotency	Sen and Ghosh, 2011
274	*Hemidesmus indicus* R.Br.	Root	Blood purifier in rheumatism	Nath et al., 2011
275	*Hemiphragma heterophyllum* Wall.	Fruit juice	Sore throat	Badola and Pradhan, 2013
276	*Heracleum wallichii* DC.	Plant	Digestion, vomiting, stomachache	Badola and Pradhan, 2013
277	*Hibiscus sabdariffa* L.	Flowers	Dyspepsia, food poisoning	Jamir et al., 2011

TABLE 5.1 (Continued)

S. No.	Name of the plant species	Parts Used	Purpose	Reference(s)
278	*Hodgsonia macrocarpa* (Blume) Cogn.	Roots, leaf, seed	Typhoid, laxative gastrointestinal problems, body pain,	Jamir et al., 2008; Kichu et al., 2015
279	*Holboellia latifolia* Wall.	Leaf	Burns	Kichu et al., 2015
280	*Holarrhena pubescens* (Buch.-Ham.) Wall. ex G.Don	Bark	Rheumatism	Nath et al., 2011
281	*Holboellia latifolia* Wall.	Leaves, root	Mouth infection, piles	Jamir et al., 2011
	Holmskioldia sanguinea Retz.	Leaves	Headache, dizziness, rheumatic arthritis	Devi and Singh, 2008
282	*Houttuynia cordata* Thunb.	Leaves, stems, whole plant rhizome, roots	Stomach disorders, dysentery, measles, gonorrhea, cough, skin troubles, stomach disorder, cholera, diuretic, snake, dog and cat's bite, high blood pressure	Gajurel et al., 2006; Jamir et al., 2008; Jamir et al., 2011; Khongsai et al., 2011; Nath et al., 2013; Kichu et al., 2015
283	*Hydrocotyle asiatica* L.	Plant, leaf	Pneumonia, skin diseases, toothache, indigestion, dysentery, sore throat, cough, fever	Ringmichon et al., 2011; Badola and Pradhan, 2013
284	*Hyptis suaveolens* Poit.	Seeds, leaf, inflorescence	Colic, impotency, migraine, boils, antidiabetic, stomach complaints	Khomdram et al., 2011; Nath et al., 2013
285	*Imperata cylindrica* (L.) P.Beauv.	Roots, leaves	Anthelmintic	Jamir et al., 2008
286	*Ipomoea aquatica* Forssk.	Twig, leaves	Impotency, bowel complaints	Saikia et al., 2010; Nath et al., 2013
287	*Ipomoea batatas* (L.) Lamk.	Aerial part	Anti-diabetic	Chhetri et al., 2005

TABLE 5.1   (Continued)

S. No.	Name of the plant species	Parts Used	Purpose	Reference(s)
288	*Ipomoea nil* (L.) Roth	Whole plant	Dysentery, diarrhea, vermifuge	Kichu et al., 2015
289	*Isodon coetsa* (Buch.-Ham. ex D.Don) Kudo	Seeds	Repel insects	Khomdram et al., 2011
290	*Isodon ternifolius* Kudo	Plant, leaves	Fumigant, antiseptic, insect repellent, headache, skin disease	Khomdram et al., 2011
291	*Jatropha curcas* L.	Latex, roots	Toothache, gout, burns, dysmenorrhea	Choudhury et al., 2008; Nath et al., 2011; Deb et al., 2012; N. J.Das et al., 2005
292	*Jatropha gossypifolia* L.	Leaf	Rheumatism	Nath et al., 2011
293	*Juglans regia* L.	Stem bark	Arthritis, rheumatism, skin diseases, toothache, anthelmintic	Badola and Pradhan, 2013
294	*Juniperus indica* Bertol.	Fruit	Headache, blood pressure	Badola and Pradhan, 2013
295	*Justicia adhatoda* L. (Syn.: *Adhatoda zeylanica* Medik.)	Leaves, root bark	Bronchitis, asthma, cough, antiseptic, rheumatism, bodyache, cold, cough, tumor, uterine problems	Jamir et al., 2008; Khongsai et al., 2011
296	*Kaempferia sikkimensis* (King ex Baker) K. Larsen	Rhizome	Bone fracture, sprained joints, on burns	Badola and Pradhan, 2013
297	*Lagenaria siceraria* (Molina) Standl.	Leaves	Boils, skin disease, inflammation	Singh et al., 2011; Kichu et al., 2015
298	*Lantana camara* L.	Leaves	Diarrhea, cuts, wounds, antiseptic, constipation, control bleeding	Devi and Singh, 2008; Salam et al., 2011; Badola and Pradhan, 2013

TABLE 5.1   (Continued)

S. No.	Name of the plant species	Parts Used	Purpose	Reference(s)
299	*Lasia spinosa* (L.) Thwaites	Leaf, stem	Vermifuge, skin diseases	Kichu et al., 2015
300	*Leonurus japonicas* Houtt.	Leaves	Cough and stomach disorders	Khomdram et al., 2011
301	*Leucas aspera* (Willd.) Link	Leaves, flower	Cough, sinusitis, menstrual problem	Choudhury et al., 2008; Khomdram et al., 2011; Tangjang et al., 2011
302	*Leucas decemdentata* (Willd.) R.Br. ex Sm.	Plant	Sinusitis	Khomdram et al., 2011
	Leucas plukenetii (Roth) Spreng.	Leaves	Diarrhea, dysentery	Nath et al., 2013
303	*Leucosceptrum canum* Sm.	Leaves, inflorescence	Hemostatic, astringent	Jamir et al., 2011
304	*Limnophyton obtusifolium* Miq.	Root	Cancerous growth	Choudhury et al., 2008
305	*Litchi chinensis* (Gaertn.) Son.	Bark	Dysentery	Nath et al., 2013
306	*Litsea citrata* Blume	Fruits	Nausea, giddiness	Badola and Pradhan, 2013
307	*Litsea cubeba* Pers.	Fruit	Anti-diabetic	Chhetri et al., 2005
308	*Luffa acutangula* L.	Flower, fruit, leaf	Laxative	Kichu et al., 2015
309	*Lycopodiella cernua* (L.) Pic.-Ser.	Whole plant	Beriberi, cough, chest infections	Sen and Ghosh, 2011
310	*Lycopodium clavatum* L.	Spores	Wounds	Badola and Pradhan, 2013
311	*Lygodium felxuosum* Sw.	Fronds	Expectorant in cough, jaundice	Salam et al., 2011; Sen and Ghosh, 2011

TABLE 5.1   (Continued)

S. No.	Name of the plant species	Parts Used	Purpose	Reference(s)
312	*Lygodium japonicum* (Tb.) Sw.	Root, fronds	Against food poisoning, diabetes, wounds, ulcers	Sen and Ghosh, 2011; Yumkham and Singh, 2011
313	*Lygodium microphyllum* (Cav.) R.Br.	Fronds	Dysentery	Sen and Ghosh, 2011
314	*Machilus villosa* Hook.f.	Leaf	Intestinal worms	Jamir and Rao, 1990
315	*Macropanax undulatus* (Wall. ex G. Don) Seem.	Leaf	Common cold, fever	Kichu et al., 2015
316	*Maesa indica* Roxb.	Fruit, leaf	Body temperature, homeostatic	Khongsai et al., 2011; Kichu et al., 2015
317	*Mahonia napaulensis* DC	Fruit, bark	Gastric problems, eye inflammation	Jamir et al., 2011; Badola and Pradhan, 2013
318	*Mallotus philippensis* (Lamk.) Mull. Arg.	Leaves	Sinus problems	Deb et al., 2012
319	*Mangifera indica* L.	Stem bark, tender shoots, leaves	Cholera, dysentery, fever, cough, sore throat	Jamir et al., 2008; Deb et al., 2012; Badola and Pradhan, 2013; Nath et al., 2013
320	*Manihot esculenta* Crantz.	Tuber	Sores and skin rashes	Jamir et al., 2008
321	*Maranta arundinacea* L.	Root	Tumorous growth	Choudhury et al., 2008
322	*Marsilea minuta* L.	Fronds	Insomnia, mental problems	Sen and Ghosh, 2011
323	*Melastoma malabathricum* L.	Leaves	Fever	Ringmichon et al., 2011
324	*Melia azadirachta* A.Juss.	Leaves	Skin disease	Choudhury et al., 2008
325	*Melia composita* Willd.	Fruit, leaves	Expel gas from stomach	Kichu et al., 2015

TABLE 5.1   (Continued)

S. No.	Name of the plant species	Parts Used	Purpose	Reference(s)
326	*Melia superba* Roxb.	Leaves	Malaria, lice	Khongsai et al., 2011
327	*Melothria perpusilla* (Blume) Cogn.	Whole plant	Jaundice	Salam et al., 2011
328	*Mentha arvensis* L.	Leaves, root, whole plant	Jaundice, gastritis, acidity, stomach disorder, influenza, cough, cold, fever, stomach complaint	Saikia et al., 2010; Khomdram et al., 2011; Khongsai et al., 2011; Ringmichon et al., 2011; Badola and Pradhan, 2013
329	*Mentha longifolia* (L.) Hud	Leaves	Jaundice, constipation, stomachache, hemostatic	Jamir et al., 2008
330	*Mentha spicata* L.	Plant, leaves	Stomach complaints, flatulence, diabetes, hiccough, irregular menstruation, tooth ache, liver complaints, diarrhea, dysentery	Choudhury et al., 2008; Khomdram et al., 2011; Salam et al., 2011
331	*Meriandra bengalensis* Benth.	Leaves	Fever	Ringmichon et al., 2011
332	*Michelia champaca* L.	Leaves	Skin infections	Choudhury et al., 2012
333	*Microsorium superficialae* (Bl.) Ching	Rhizome	Cough, cold	Sen and Ghosh, 2011
334	*Microtoena patchouli* (Clarke ex Hook.) Wu & Hsuan	Plant, root	Menstrual disorder, fever, dizziness, asthma, coughs, colic, piles	Khomdram et al., 2011
335	*Mikania micrantha* Kunth.	Tender leaf	Cuts, wounds, ringworm, skin infections	Singh et al., 2011; Choudhury et al., 2012; Deb et al., 2012

TABLE 5.1   (Continued)

S. No.	Name of the plant species	Parts Used	Purpose	Reference(s)
336	*Mikania scandensa* (L.) Wild.	Leaves	Cuts, wounds, diarrhea	Khongsai et al., 2011; Tangjang et al., 2011
337	*Millettia cinerea* Benth.	Root, leaf	Body pain	Kichu et al., 2015
338	*Mimosa pudica* L.	Root, leaves, whole plant	Boils, diarrhea, gall bladder and kidney problems, micturition, skin infections, worms, antiseptic, blood purifier, contraceptive, toothache, boil	Choudhury et al., 2008; Jamir et al., 2008; Saikia et al., 2010; Jamir et al., 2011; Khongsai et al., 2011; Choudhury et al., 2012; Deb et al., 2012; Nath et al., 2013
339	*Molineria capitulata* (Lour.) Herb	Rhizome	Eye infection, gastric problems	Jamir et al., 2011
340	*Momordica charantia* L.	Fruit, leaf	Blood purification, diabetes, fever,	Singh et al., 2011; Badola and Pradhan, 2013; Chhetri et al., 2005
341	*Moringa oleifera* (Lam.) Reseda	Bark, seed oil, leaves, fruit	High blood pressure, rheumatic pain, anemia	Choudhury et al., 2008; Nath et al., 2011; Tangjang et al., 2011
342	*Morus indica* L.	Tender leaves	Inflammation of vocal cord, hoarse voice	Badola and Pradhan, 2013
343	*Mucuna macrocarpa* Wall.	Seed	Tumorous growth	Choudhury et al., 2008
344	*Mucuna monosperma* Wall.	Seeds	Expectorant in cough	Badola and Pradhan, 2013
345	*Murraya koenigii* (L.) Spreng.	Leaves	Worm infestation	Nath et al., 2013

TABLE 5.1   (Continued)

S. No.	Name of the plant species	Parts Used	Purpose	Reference(s)
346	*Musa balbisiana* Colla	Inflorescence	Jaundice	Singh et al., 2011
347	*Musa paradisiaca* L.	Leaves, fruit, roots, inflorescence, leaves, petiole	Indigestion, insanity, backache, fever, vomiting, malaria, jaundice, diarrhea	Choudhury et al., 2008; Khongsai et al., 2011; Salam et al., 2011
348	*Mussaenda roxburghii* Hook. f.	Leaves	Fever, cuts and wounds, appendix	Jamir et al., 2011; Ringmichon et al., 2011; Kichu et al., 2015
349	*Myrica esculenta* Buch.-Ham. ex. D. Don.	Stem bark, fruit, leaf	Indigestion, asthma, fever, cuts and wounds, indigestion	Jamir et al., 2008, 2011; Ringmichon et al., 2011; Kichu et al., 2015
350	*Nardostachys jatamansi* DC.	Root	Anti-diabetic	Chhetri et al., 2005
351	*Nasturtium officinale* R.Br.	Shoot	Back pain	Badola and Pradhan, 2013
352	*Natsiatum herpaticum* Buch.-Ham. ex Arn.	Leaves	Backache	Nath et al., 2011
353	*Nelumbo nucifera* (L.) Gaertn.	Rhizome	Fever	Ringmichon et al., 2011
354	*Nephrolepis cordifolia* (L.) Presl.	Rhizome	Scabies	Das, 1997
355	*Nerium indicum* Mill.	Flower	Anti-lice	Kichu et al., 2015
356	*Nicotiana tabacum* L.	Leaves	Cancerous growth	Choudhury et al., 2008
357	*Nicotiana plumbaginifolia* Viv.	Fruits, leaves	Sinusitis	Jamir et al., 2011
358	*Nyctanthes arbor-tristis* L.	Leaves	Cough, gastritis, fever, anthelmintic	Saikia et al., 2010; Badola and Pradhan, 2013; Nath et al., 2013

TABLE 5.1   (Continued)

S. No.	Name of the plant species	Parts Used	Purpose	Reference(s)
359	*Ocimum americanum* L.	Young shoots, seeds, leaves	Sore throat, diabetes, bleeding piles, constipation, cough, stomachache, indigestion, diabetes	Khomdram et al., 2011; Salam et al., 2011
360	*Ocimum basilicum* L.	Shoots, leaves	Fever, stomach troubles, cholera, dysentery, ulcers, food poisoning, cough, bronchitis, gastritis, inflammation, constipation, throat infections	Jamir et al., 2008, 2011; Khomdram et al., 2011; Choudhury et al., 2012; Nath et al., 2013
361	*Ocimum canum* Sims	Leaves, shoot	Fever	Ringmichon et al., 2011;
362	*Ocimum gratissimum* L.	Leaves	Cough, colic, typhoid, fever, expectorant, toothache, leprosy, flatulence, piles	Khomdram et al., 2011
363	*Ocimum kilimandscharicum* Baker ex Garke	Leaves	Cough, fever	Khomdram et al., 2011
364	*Ocimum tenuiflorum* (Syn.: *Ocimum sanctum* L.)	Leaves, seed	Gastric problems, cough, bronchitis, flu, cold, headache, fever, earache, mouth ulcer, skin diseases, malaria, rheumatism, arthritis	Choudhury et al., 2008; Khomdram et al., 2011; Khongsai et al., 2011; Deb et al., 2012; Badola and Pradhan, 2013
365	*Olax acuminata* Wall.	Leaves	Cancer	Choudhury et al., 2008
366	*Oldenlandia diffusa* (Willd.) Roxb.	Young twigs	For lactation	Saikia et al., 2010
367	*Ophioglossum reticulatum* L.	Fronds	Wounds, inflammation	Sen and Ghosh, 2011
368	*Opuntia dillenii* (Ker.-Gawl.) Haw.	Flowers	Anti dandruff	Jamir et al., 2011

TABLE 5.1 (Continued)

S. No.	Name of the plant species	Parts Used	Purpose	Reference(s)
369	*Oroxylum indicum* (L.) Kurz.	Fruit, bark, leaves, pods seed, root, stem and root	Bone fracture, cancer, liver problems, stomachache, cough, fever, malaria, diabetes, tuberculosis, diarrhea, rheumatism, loss of appetite, vomiting sensation, throat pain, menstrual pain, jaundice	Jamir et al., 2011; Khongsai et al., 2011; Ringmichon et al., 2011; Salam et al., 2011; Deb et al., 2012; Badola and Pradhan, 2013
370	*Osbeckia crinata* Benth.	Leaves	Toothache	Chhetri, 2005
371	*Osysris arborea* Salz. ex Dacne	Stem bark	Bone fracture and sprain	Badola and Pradhan, 2013
372	*Oxalis corniculata* L.	Aerial part	Bowel disorder, scurvy, cough, diarrhea, dysentery, wounds of dog and cat bites, stomach complaints, painful urination, colic	Khongsai et al., 2011; Salam et al., 2011; Badola and Pradhan, 2013; Nath et al., 2013
373	*Paedaria foetida* L.	Root, leaves	Gastric problems, kidney problems, body pain; anti-diabetic	Jamir et al., 2011; Khongsai et al., 2011; Chhetri et al., 2005
374	*Paederia scandens* (Lour.) Merr.	Leaves, stem	Stomach pain, vomiting, rheumatism, constipation	Gajurel et al., 2006; Nath et al., 2011; Nath et al., 2013
375	*Pajanelia longifolia* (Willd.) K. Schuman	Leaves and Bark	Nail infection and jaundice	Choudhury et al., 2012
376	*Palhinhaea cernua* (L.) Franco	Plant	Snake bite	Das, 1997
377	*Panax pseudoginseng* Wall.	Roots	Aphrodisiac	Badola and Pradhan, 2013
378	*Papaver somniferum* L.	Leaves	High blood pressure, piles, intestinal problems, sinusitis	Jamir et al., 2008

TABLE 5.1   (Continued)

S. No.	Name of the plant species	Parts Used	Purpose	Reference(s)
379	*Paris polyphylla* Sm.	Root, rhizome	Bronchitis, stomach ulcers	Salam et al., 2011;
380	*Parkia roxburghii* G.Don	Pods, bark, seeds	Stomach disorders, diarrhea, dysentery, cancer, piles	Khumbongmayum et al., 2005; Jamir et al., 2011
381	*Parkia timoriana* (DC.) Merr.	Bark, pods	Diarrhea, dysentery, intestinal disorder, piles	Salam et al., 2011; Singh et al., 2011
382	*Perilla frutescens* Britt.	Leaves, seeds	Boils, cough, nausea, rheumatism, muscular sprain, backache	Khomdram et al., 2011; Badola and Pradhan, 2013
383	*Perilla ocimoides* L.	Seeds	Headache, bodyache, rheumatism	Jamir et al., 2008
384	*Phlogacanthus tubiflorus* Nees	Flowers	Rheumatism	Nath et al., 2011
385	*Phlogacanthus thyrsiflorus* Nees	Leaves, flower	Fever, acute dry cough, flu, dysentery, worm infestation	Ringmichon et al., 2011; Salam et al., 2011; Nath et al., 2013; Ningthoujam et al., 2013
386	*Phyla nodiflora* (L.) Greene	Leaves	Piles	Devi and Singh, 2008
387	*Phyllanthus emblica* L. (Syn.: *Emblica officinalis* L.)	Stem bark, fruit, root	Indigestion, cough, liver trouble, eye disease, diabetes, jaundice, cough, dysentery, diarrhea, stomach problems, irregular menstruation, constipation, antidandruff	Choudhury et al., 2008; Jamir et al., 2008; Khongsai et al., 2011; Salam et al., 2011; Badola and Pradhan, 2013
388	*Phyllanthus fraternus* Webst.	Whole plant	Intestinal disorders	Gajurel et al., 2006
389	*Phytolacca acinosa* Roxb.	Shoot	Body pain, sinusitis	Badola and Pradhan, 2013
390	*Picrorhiza kurroa* Royle ex Benth.	Rhizome,	Cough, cold, fever, stomach ache, throat pain, diarrhea, dysentery, headache	Badola and Pradhan, 2013

TABLE 5.1 (Continued)

S. No.	Name of the plant species	Parts Used	Purpose	Reference(s)
391	*Piper betle* L.	Leaves	Cuts, hemostatic, indigestion, dysentery	Choudhury et al., 2008; Jamir et al., 2008; Nath et al., 2013
392	*Piper brachystachyum* Wall.	Whole plant, leaves	Rheumatism, cough, bronchitis	Khongsai et al., 2011
393	*Piper longum* L.	Roots, fruits	Vermifuge, stomachache, diarrhea, dysentery	Badola and Pradhan, 2013
394	*Piper mullesua* Ham. ex D.Don	Leaves, fruit, seed	Rheumatism, joint pain, cold, cough, bronchitis problems, fever	Jamir and Rao, 1990; Gajurel et al., 2006; Khongsai et al., 2011
395	*Piper nigrum* L.	Seed, fruit	Stimulant, to eradicate lice	Khongsai et al., 2011
396	*Plantago erosa* Wall.	Flower, fruits, root, whole plant	Hemostatic, high blood pressure, cough, cold, indigestion, diarrhea, dysentery, fever, headache, laxative	Jamir et al., 2008, 2011; Ringmichon et al., 2011; Badola and Pradhan, 2013; Kichu et al., 2015
397	*Plantago major* L.	Leaves, whole plant	Boils, muscular pain, stomach ulcers, cuts, wounds	Salam et al., 2011
398	*Plectranthus amboinicus* (Lour.) Spreng.	Plant, leaf	Urinary troubles, calculus, bronchitis, asthma, chronic cough, colic, flatulence	Khomdram et al., 2011
399	*Plumbago zeylanica* L.	Root	Dog bite	Saikia et al., 2010
400	*Pogostemon auricularis* (L.) Hass	Plant	Headache, stomach complaints, abdominal pains, colic, boils	Khomdram et al., 2011
401	*Pogostemon benghalensis* (Burm.f.) O.Kuntze	Leaves	Constipation, piles, wounds	Khomdram et al., 2011

TABLE 5.1   (Continued)

S. No.	Name of the plant species	Parts Used	Purpose	Reference(s)
402	*Pogostemon cablin* (Blanco) Benth.	Leaves	Fever, menstrual problems	Khomdram et al., 2011
403	*Pogostemon elsholtzioides* Benth.	Leaves	Stomach and throat complaints, leucorrhoea	Khomdram et al., 2011
404	*Polygonum capitatum* Ham.	Leaves	Tumorous growth	Choudhury et al., 2008
405	*Polygonum chinense* L.	Young shoot, leaves	Fever	Ringmichon et al., 2011
406	*Polygonum hydropiper* L.	Leaf	Skin infection, fungal infection	Kichu et al., 2015
407	*Polygonum kawagoeanum* Makino	Flowers	Asthma, tuberculosis	Jamir et al., 2011
408	*Pongamia pinnata* (L.) Pierre	Seed oil	Rheumatic pain	Nath et al., 2011
409	*Potentilla fulgens* Wall. ex Hook.	Root	Toothache, diarrhea	Badola and Pradhan, 2013
410	*Pratia nummularia* A.Braun & Asch.	Plant	Urinary tract stones	Salam et al., 2011
411	*Premna bengalensis* C. B.Clarke	Bark	Paralysis	Devi and Singh, 2008
412	*Premna latifolia* Roxb.	Leaves	Dysentery	Choudhury et al., 2012
413	*Pronephrium nudatum* (Rpxb.) Holttum	Pinnae	Pyorrhea	Sen and Ghosh, 2011
414	*Prunus persica* (L.) Stokes	Leaf, root, seed	Typhoid, skin infection, dysentery, diarrhea, skin disease	Kichu et al., 2015
415	*Psidium guajava* L.	Leaves, tender shoots, root	Stomach disorders, fever, cough, sore throat, diarrhea, dysentery, piles, anthelmintic	Choudhury et al., 2008; Ringmichon et al., 2011; Salam et al., 2011; Deb et al., 2012; Badola and Pradhan, 2013; Nath et al., 2013

TABLE 5.1 (Continued)

S. No.	Name of the plant species	Parts Used	Purpose	Reference(s)
416	*Pteris semipinnata* L.	Fronds	Carbuncle	Sen and Ghosh, 2011
417	*Pteris vittata* L.	Fronds, rhizome	Wounds, skin diseases	Sen and Ghosh, 2011; Yumkham and Singh, 2011
418	*Punica granatum* L.	Fruit, leaves	Dysentery, diarrhea, cholera, anthelmintic	Choudhury et al., 2008; Jamir et al., 2011; Kichu et al., 2015
419	*Pyrrosia adnascens* (Sw.) Ching	Rhizome	Cough, cold	Sen and Ghosh, 2011
420	*Quercus lanata* Sm.	Stem Bark	Anti-diabetic	Chhetri et al., 2005
421	*Rauvolfia serpentina* (L.) Benth. ex Kurz.	Root	Blood pressure	Khongsai et al., 2011
422	*Rheum acuminatum* Hook.f. & Thoms.	Root, shoot	Headache, dysentery	Badola and Pradhan, 2013
423	*Rhododendron arboretum* Smith	Petals, young leaves	Fish bones stuck in the throat, diarrhea, blood dysentery, throat pain, headache, for easy delivery	Jamir et al., 2011; Badola and Pradhan, 2013
424	*Rhus griffithii* Hook.f.	Leaves	Skin infections	Jamir et al., 2008
425	*Rhus semialata* Murray	Fruit, leaves	Indigestion, constipation, vomiting, stomachache, blood dysentery, allergy	Jamir et al., 2008; Badola and Pradhan, 2013
426	*Rhus roxburghii* Hook. F.	Whole plant	Dermatitis	Kichu et al., 2015
427	*Rhus semialata* Murr.	Seeds	Stomachache, food poisoning, allergy	Jamir et al., 2011

TABLE 5.1　(Continued)

S. No.	Name of the plant species	Parts Used	Purpose	Reference(s)
428	*Rhynchostylis retusa* (L.) Bl.	Leaves	Otorrhoea	Saikia et al., 2010
429	*Ricinus communis* L.	Leaves, seed oil	Antiseptic, bodyache, sprains, paralysis, rheumatism, inflammation of joints,	Choudhury et al., 2008; Jamir et al., 2008, 2011; Nath et al., 2011
430	*Rosa sericea* Lindl.	Leaves, flower	Wounds, headache	Badola and Pradhan, 2013
431	*Rubia cordifolia* Roxb. ex Fleming	Leaves, root, fruit	Fever, vermifuge, stomachache, cuts, wounds, dysentery, lower body temperature	Badola and Pradhan, 2013
432	*Rubus ellipticus* Smith	Root bark, tender shoots	Malaria, fever, stomachache	Jamir et al., 2008; Ringmichon et al., 2011
433	*Rumex nepalensis* Sreng.	Root, leaf	Body pain, skin diseases, hair loss, cuts, wounds, swellings	Badola and Pradhan, 2013
434	*Saccharum officinarum* L.	Culm	Jaundice, gall bladder disorder	Choudhury et al., 2008; Jamir et al., 2008
435	*Sansevieria roxburghiana* Schult. & Schult.f.	Leaves	Burns, snake bite	Deb et al., 2012
436	*Sapindus mukorossi* Gaertn.	Fruit	Toothache, wounds, dandruff, dysentery, stomachache, fever, anthelmintic	Salam et al., 2011; Badola and Pradhan, 2013
437	*Saraca asoca* (Roxb.) De Wilde	Flower	Anti-diabetic	Chhetri et al., 2005
438	*Sarcandra glabra* (Thunb.) Nakai	Root	Dysentery	Nath et al., 2013
439	*Schefflera hypoleuca* (Kurz) Harms	Root	Tonic to women after child birth	Chhetri, 1994

TABLE 5.1 (Continued)

S. No.	Name of the plant species	Parts Used	Purpose	Reference(s)
440	*Schima wallichii* (DC.) Korth.	Bark	Cuts, wounds	Salam et al., 2011; Badola and Pradhan, 2013
441	*Schrebera swietenioides* Roxb.	Roots	Gout	Nath et al., 2011
442	*Scoparia dulcis* L.	Stem, leaves	Eye trouble, acidity, cuts, wounds	Choudhury et al., 2008; Deb et al., 2012; Nath et al., 2013
443	*Scutellaria assamica* Mukerjee	Leaves	Rheumatic arthritis, muscle pains	Khomdram et al., 2011
444	*Scutellaria discolor* Wall. ex Benth.	Leaves, whole plant	Arthritis, cuts, wounds, injuries, hypertension, fever, colic, cough, painful urination, typhoid, menstrual disorder, stomach upsets	Khomdram et al., 2011; Ringmichon et al., 2011; Salam et al., 2011
445	*Selaginella semicordata* (Wall. ex Hook. & Grev.) Spring.	Whole plant	Wounds, cuts, antiseptic	Yumkham and Singh, 2011
446	*Sesamum orientale* L.	Leaf, fruit, root	Wounds	Saikia et al., 2010
447	*Sesbanbia grandiflora* (L.) Pers.	Leaf	Sprain	Nath et al., 2011
448	*Sigesbeckia orientalis* L.	Leaves	Sores	Badola and Pradhan, 2013
449	*Solanum esculentum* L.	Seeds	High blood pressure, diabetes, appetizer	Jamir et al., 2008
450	*Solanum ferox* L.	Flowers, seeds	Tooth decay	Saikia et al., 2010
451	*Solanum indicum* L.	Fruits	Stimulation, cough, toothache, fever	Khongsai et al., 2011; Salam et al., 2011

TABLE 5.1   (Continued)

S. No.	Name of the plant species	Parts Used	Purpose	Reference(s)
452	*Solanum khasianum* C. B.Clarke	Fruit	Tooth ache, gum problems, tooth decay	Khongsai et al., 2011; Badola and Pradhan, 2013
453	*Solanum nigrum* L.	Fruit, root	Fever, cough, lung congestion, kidney and pancreatic disorders	Salam et al., 2011
454	*Solanum xanthocarpum* Schrad. & Wendl.	Ripe fruits	Fever	Ringmichon et al., 2011
455	*Sonerila aculeata* Roxb.	Leaf	Insect bite, inflammation	Kichu et al., 2015
456	*Solanum ferox* L.	Fruits	Diarrhea	Choudhury et al., 2008
457	*Slanum melongena* L.	Fruit	Boil	Singh et al., 2011
458	*Solanum nigrum* L.	Young fruit; shoots	Cough, rheumatic pain	Gajurel et al., 2006; Nath et al., 2011
459	*Solanum torvum* Sw.	Roots, leaves, fruits	Oral contraceptive, indigestion, itching	Khongsai et al., 2011
460	*Spermacoce poaya* L.	Leaf	Laxative	Kichu et al., 2015
461	*Spermacoce scaberrima* Blume	Leaf	Snake bite	Kichu et al., 2015
462	*Spilanthes acmella* L.	Plant, inflorescence	Baldness, tongue and mouth disease	Gajurel et al., 2006; Choudhury et al., 2008
463	*Spilanthes calva* DC.	Flower	Toothache	Singh et al., 2011
464	*Spilanthes paniculata* Wall. ex DC.	Flowers, stems, leaves	Toothache, bodyache, diarrhea, ascariasis	Khongsai et al., 2011; Deb et al., 2012; Nath et al., 2013
465	*Spondias pinnata* (L. f.) Kurz.	Root, bark, drupes, leaf	Gonorrhea, gastro-intestinal problems, liver tonic	Deb et al., 2012; Nath et al., 2013; Kichu et al., 2015

TABLE 5.1 (Continued)

S. No.	Name of the plant species	Parts Used	Purpose	Reference(s)
466	*Stachytarpheta urticifolia* (Salisb.) Sims	Leaves	Stomach disorders	Devi and Singh, 2008
467	*Stellaria media* (L.) Vill.	Twig juice	Snake bite	Saikia et al., 2010
468	*Sterculia villosa* Roxb.	Stem bark	Lumbago	Nath et al., 2011
469	*Stereospermum personatum* (Hassk.) Chatterjee	Bark	Arthritis, bodyache	Deb et al., 2012
470	*Stephania glabra* (Roxb.) Miers.	Root	Anti-diabetic	Chhetri et al., 2005
471	*Swertia angustifolia* Buch.-Ham. ex. D. Don	Whole plant	Anti-diabetic	Chhetri et al., 2005
472	*Swertia chirata* Ham.	Whole plant	Fever	Ringmichon et al., 2011
473	*Swertia chirayita* (Roxb. ex Flem.) H.Karst.	Whole plant	Fever, cough, cold, stomach pain, gastritis, throat pain, diarrhea, dysentery, headache, backache, diabetes	Badola and Pradhan, 2013
474	*Swertia paniculata* Wall.	Whole plant	Substitute to *Swertia chirayita*	Badola and Pradhan, 2013
475	*Symplocos theifolia* D.Don	Fruit juice	Diarrhea	Badola and Pradhan, 2013
476	*Syzygium cumini* L.	Fruits, twigs	Stomach disorder, diarrhea, dysentery	Khongsai et al., 2011; Nath et al., 2013
477	*Tabernaemontana divaricata* (L.) R.Br.	Root	Toothache	Choudhury et al., 2008
478	*Tagetes erecta* L.	Leaves	Muscular pain	Salam et al., 2011
479	*Tagetes patula* L.	Flowers	Sore throat, cough, mouth ulcers	Badola and Pradhan, 2013

TABLE 5.1　(Continued)

S. No.	Name of the plant species	Parts Used	Purpose	Reference(s)
480	*Tamarindus indica* L.	Fruit, leaves	Constipation, headache, migraine	Choudhury et al., 2012; Deb et al., 2012; Nath et al., 2013
481	*Taxus baccata* L.	Leaves	Cough, fever	Salam et al., 2011
482	*Terminalia arjuna* (Roxb.) Wight & Arn.	Bark	Cough, jaundice, piles, hypertension, poisonous bites	Gogoi and Borthakur, 2001; Sarmah et al., 2006; Choudhury et al., 2012
483	*Terminalia bellirica* Roxb.	Fruit	Fever, stomach trouble	Gajurel et al., 2006
484	*Terminalia chebula* Retz.	Fruit	Dehydration, diarrhea, constipation, cough, sore throat, hiccups, vomiting sensation	Khongsai et al., 2011; Badola and Pradhan, 2013; Nath et al., 2013
485	*Terminalia myriocarpa* Haurck & Mull. Arg.	Bark	Cuts, wounds	Badola and Pradhan, 2013
486	*Thalictrum foliolosum* DC.	Rhizome	Fever	Ringmichon et al., 2011
487	*Thunbergia grandiflora* Roxb.	Watery latex	Cataract, eye infection	Deb et al., 2012
488	*Thysanolaena maxima* (Roxb.) O.Kuntze	Root	Fever, sores, boils	Jamir et al., 2011; Badola and Pradhan, 2013
489	*Tinospora cordifolia* (Willd.) Hook. f. & Thoms.	Leaves, bark, stem	Stomach problems, diabetes; rheumatic pain, skin infections, diarrhea, dysentery, diabetes, chicken pox, measles	Salam et al., 2011; Choudhury et al., 2012; Deb et al., 2012
490	*Tinospora sinensis* (Lour.) Merr.	Bark	Malaria	Choudhury et al., 2012
491	*Toona ciliata* M.Roem.	Stem bark, fruit	Tooth ache, chest pain, fever, measles	Badola and Pradhan, 2013

TABLE 5.1 (Continued)

S. No.	Name of the plant species	Parts Used	Purpose	Reference(s)
492	*Trichosanthes lepiniana* (Naud.) Cogn.	Seed	Skin diseases	Badola and Pradhan, 2013
493	*Trigonella foenum-graecum* L.	Sprouted Seeds	Anti-diabetic	Chhetri et al., 2005
494	*Tupistra nutans* Wall.	Herb	Increases appetite	Badola and Pradhan, 2013
495	*Urtica ardens* Link	Roots	Dog bite	Jamir et al., 2011
496	*Urtica dioica* L.	Leaves	Nose bleeding	Salam et al., 2011
497	*Urtica parviflora* Roxb.	Root	Skin diseases, kidney problems, toothache	Badola and Pradhan, 2013
498	*Viscum articulatum* Burm.f.	Root	Bone fracture, wounds, boils	Badola and Pradhan, 2013
499	*Vitex negundo* L.	Leaves, flowers	Rheumatic pain, bowel complaints	Choudhury et al., 2008; Nath et al., 2011, 2013
500	*Vitex peduncularis* Wall. ex Schaen.	Bark	Gall bladder stone	Deb et al., 2012
501	*Vitex trifolia* L.	Leaves, young shoots	Piles, scabies, toothache, epilepsy	Devi and Singh, 2008
502	*Wedelia chinensis* (Osb.) Merr.	Leaves	Acidity, indigestion	Nath et al., 2013
503	*Xanthium strumarium* (Roxb.) L.	Leaves	Urinary problems	Salam et al., 2011
504	*Zanthoxylum acanthopodium* DC.	Fruit	Bad breath, indigestion, tooth decay, cold, stomachache, anthelmintic	Badola and Pradhan, 2013
505	*Zanthoxylum alatum* Roxb.	Fruit	Similar to *Z. acanthopodium*	Badola and Pradhan, 2013
506	*Zanthoxylum armatum* DC.	Fruits, bark, leaves	Tonic, lice, stomach disorders, cough, bronchitis, throat pain,	Gajurel et al., 2006; Khongsai et al., 2011
507	*Zea mays* L.	Corn	Diuretic, kidney stones	Jamir et al., 2011

TABLE 5.1   (Continued)

S. No.	Name of the plant species	Parts Used	Purpose	Reference(s)
508	*Zingiber cassumunar* Roxb.	Rhizome	Indigestion, gas formation	Saikia et al., 2010;
509	*Zingiber officinale* Roscoe	Rhizome	Cough, bronchitis, throat pain, bone fracture, tuberculosis, fever, influenza, throat problems, expectorant, rheumatic pain, flatulence	Jamir et al., 2008; Khongsai et al., 2011; Ringmichon et al., 2011; Salam et al., 2011; Deb et al., 2012; Badola and Pradhan, 2013; Nath et al., 2013
510	*Zingiber rubens* Roxb.	Leaves	Snake bite precaution	Choudhury et al., 2012
511	*Ziziphus mauritiana* Lam.	Leaves, fruits, bark	Skin infections, constipation, dysentery	Choudhury et al., 2008, 2012; Nath et al., 2013

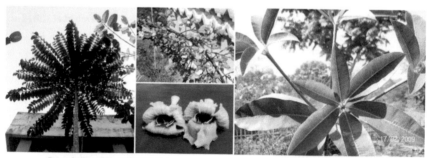

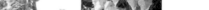

Pajanelia longifolia (Willd.) K. Schuman   *Alstonia scholaris* (L.) R.Br

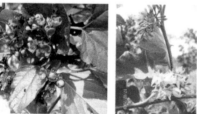

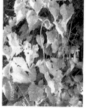

Clerodendrum viscosum Vent.   *Solanum torvum* Sw.   *Mikania micrantha* Kunth.

PLATE 1   *(Photo Courtesy: Dr. Debjyoti Bhattacharyya, Assam University, Silchar).*

KEYWORDS

- **ethnomedicinal plants**
- **North East India**
- **tribal medicine**

REFERENCES

1. Ahmed, A. A., & Borthakur, S. K. (2005). Ethnobotanical wisdom of Khasis (Hynniewtreps) of Meghalaya. Bishen Singh Mahendra Pal Singh, Dehra Dun.
2. Badola, H. K., & Pradhan, B. K. (2013). Plants used in healthcare practices by Limboo tribe in South-West of Khangchendzonga Biosphere reserve, Sikkim, India. *Indian J. Trad. Knowle. 12(3)*, 355–369.
3. Banik, G., Bawari, M., Choudhury, M. D., Choudhury, S., & Sharma, G. D. (2010). Some anti-diabetic plants of Southern Assam. *Assam Univ. J. Sci. & Tech.: Biol. Environ. Sci. 5*, 114–119.
4. Bantawa, P., & Rai, R. (2009). Studies on ethnomedicinal plants used by traditional practitioners, *Jhankri, Bijuwa and Phedangma* in Darjeeling Himalaya. *Nat Prod Radiance 8(5)*, 537–541.
5. Baruah, P., & Sharma, G. C. (1984). Studies of medicinal uses of plants by Bodo tribes of Assam. *J. Econ. Taxon. Bot. 5*, 599–604.
6. Baruah, P., & Sharma, G. C. (1987). Studies on the medicinal uses of plants by the Northeast tribes – III. *J. Econ. Taxon. Bot. 11*, 71–76.
7. Basumatary, N., Teron, R., & Saikia, M. (2014). Ethnomedicinal practices of the Bodo-Kachari tribe of Karbi Anglong district of Assam. *Int. J. Life Sc. Bt. & Pharm. Res. 3(1)*, 161–167.
8. Benniamin, A. (2011). Medicinal ferns of North Eastern India with special reference to Arunachal Pradesh. *Indian J. Trad. Knowl. 10(3)*, 516–522.
9. Bharadwaj, S., & Gakhar, S. K. (2003). Ethnomedicinal plants used by the tribals of Mizoram to cure dysentery. *Ethnobotany 15*, 51–54.
10. Bharadwaj, S., & Gakhar, S. K. (2005). Ethnomedicinal plants used by the tribals of Mizoram for cuts and wounds. *Indian J. Trad. Knowl. 4*, 75–80.
11. Bhattacharjee, S., Tiwari, K. C., Majumder, R., & Mishra, A. K. (1980). Folklore medicine from Kamrup district (Assam). *Bull. Medico. Ethnobot. Res. 1*, 447–460.
12. Bhuyan, M.(2015). Comparative study of ethnomedicine among the tribes of North East India. *Int. J. Soc. Sci. 4(2)*, 27–32.
13. Bhuyan, S. I., Mewiwapangla & Laskar, I. (2014). Indigenous Knowledge and traditional use of medicinal plants by four major tribes of Nagaland, North East India. *Intertl. J Innovative Sci, Engin Technol, 1(6)*, 481–484.

14. Boissya, C. L., & Majumdar, R. (1980). Some folklore claims from Brahmaputra valley (Assam). *Ethnomedicines 6*, 139–145.
15. Bora, A. (2001). Ethnobotany of Morigaon district of Assam. PhD thesis, Gauhati University, Guwahati, India.
16. Bora, A., Devi, P., & Borthakur, S. K. (2012). Phyto-remedies of jaundice, a traditional approach on Majuli, special reference to Satra culture people, Assam. *Asian J. Plant Sci. Res. 2(6)*, 664–669.
17. Bora, P. J. (1999). A study on ethnomedicinal uses of plants among the Bodo tribe of Sonipur district, Assam. *J. Econ. Taxon. Bot. 23*, 609–614.
18. Borborah, E., Dutta, B., & Borthakur, S. K. (2014). Traditional uses of *Allium* L. species from North East India with special reference to their Pharmacological activities. *American J Phytomed Clinical Therapeut. 2(8)*, 1037–1051.
19. Borthakur, S. K. (1976). Less known medicinal uses of plants among tribes of Karibi-Anglong (Mikir Hills), Assam. *Bull. Bot. Surv. Ind. 18*, 166–171.
20. Borthakur, S. K. (1981). Certain plants in folklore and folk life of Karbis (Mikirs) of Assam. In: Jain, S. K. (ed.) Glimpses of Indian Ethnobotany, Scientific Publishers, Jodhpur, pp. 180–190.
21. Borthakur, S. K. (1992). Native phytotherapy for child and women disease from Assam. *Fitoterapia 63*, 483–488.
22. Borthakur, S. K., Choudhury, B. T., & Gogoi, R. (2004). Folklore hepato-protective herbal recipes from Assam in Northeast India. *Ethnobotany 16*, 76–82.
23. Borthakur, S. K., & Goswami, N. (1995). Herbal remedies from Dimasa of Kamrup district of Assam in North-Eastern India. *Fitoterapia 66 (4)*, 333–339.
24. Borthakur, S. K., Nath, K., & Gogoi, P. (1996). Herbal remedies of Nepalese of Assam. *Fitoterapia 67(3)*, 231–237.
25. Buragohain, J. (2011). Ethnomedicinal Plants used by the ethnic communities of Tinsukia district of Assam, India. *J. Rec. Res. Sci. and Technol, 3(9)*, 31–42.
26. Changkija, S., & Kumar, Y. (1996). Ethnobotanical folk practices and beliefs of Ao-Nagas in Nagaland, Inida. *Ethnobotany 8*, 26–30.
27. Chaturvedi, S. K., & Jamir, N. S. (2007). Some ethnomedicinal plants of Nagaland, India. Advances in ethnobotany. pp. 83–93.
28. Chankija, S. (1999). Folk medical Plants of the Nagas in India. *Asian Folk Studies*, 58: 205–230.
29. Chettri, D., Moktan, S., & Das, A. P. (2014). Ethnobotanical studies on the tea garden workers of Darjeeling hills. *Pleione 8(1)*, 124–132.
30. Chhetri, D. R. (2005). Ethnomedicinal plants of the Khangchendzonga National Park, Sikkim, India. *Ethnobotany 17*, 96–103.
31. Chhetri, D. R., Parajuli, P., & Subba, G. C. (2005). Antidiabetic plants used by Sikkim and Darjeeling Himalayan tribes, India. *J. Ethnopharmacol. 99*, 199–202.
32. Chhetri, R. B. (1994). Further observations on Ethnomedicobotany of Khasi hills in Meghalaya, India. *Ethnobotany 6*, 33–36.
33. Choudhury, B. I., Nath, A., Barbhuiya, A. R., Choudhury, S., & Dutta Choudhury, M. (2005). Ethnomedicinal aspects of Rongmai Naga of Cachar district of Assam, India: A study. *Ecobios 3*, 26–34.
34. Choudhury, D., & Neogi, B. (2003). Ethnobotany of Khasi and Chakma tribes of Northeast India. In: J. K. Maheshwari (ed.). Ethnobotany and Medicinal plants of Indian Subcontinent. Scientific Publishers, Jodhpur, pp. 583.

35. Choudhury, M. D (1999). Ethnomedico – botanical aspects of Reang tribe of Assam: a comprehensive study. PhD Thesis Gauhati University (Unpublished).

36. Choudhury, M. D., & Chowdhury, S. (2002). Ethnomedico-botanical aspects of Reangs of Assam: Part II, New ethnomedicinal plants. Bhattacharyya, M. et al. (Eds). Biodiversity and its conservation, Karimganj (India).

37. Choudhury, M. D., Shil, S., & Chakraborty, G. (2008). Ethno-medicobotanical studies on Dimasa Kachari of Cachar district, Assam. *Ethnobotany 20*, 128–132.

38. Choudhary, N., Mahanta, B., & Kalita, J. C. (2011). An ethnobotanical survey on medicinal plants used in reproductive health related disorders in rangeia subdivision, Kamprup district, Assam. *Intern. J. Sci. Advanced Technol. 1 (7)*, 154 – 159.

39. Choudhury, P. R., Choudhury, M. D., Ningthoujam, S. S., Das, D., Nath, D., Talukdar, A. (2015). Ethnomedicinal plants used by traditional healers of North Tripura district, Tripura, North East India. *J. Ethnopharmacol. 166*, 135–148.

40. Choudhury, S. (2012). Ethnomedicinal aspects of Chorei tribe of Southern Assam with special reference to phytochemical screening of some selected plants. M. Phil. dissertation, Assam University, Silchar, India (Unpublished).

41. Choudhury, S., Sharma, P., Choudhury, M. D, Sharma, G. D. (2012). Ethnomedicinal plants used by Chorei tribe of Southern Assam, North East India. *Asian Pac. J. Trop. Disease (Suppl)* 141–147.

42. Dam, D. P., & Hajra, P. K. (1997). Observations on ethnobotany of Monpas of Kameng district, Arunachal Pradesh. In: Jain, S. K. (ed.) Contributions to Indian Ethnobotany, Scientific Publishers, Jodhpur.

43. Das, A. K. (1997). Less known uses of plants among the Adis of Arunachal Pradesh. *Ethnobotany 9*, 90–93.

44. Das, A. K., Dutta, B. K., & Sharma, G. D. (2008). Medicinal plants used by different tribes of Cachar district, Assam. *Indian J. Trad. Knowl. 7(3)*, 446–454.

45. Das, A. K., & Saikia, D. C. (2001). Indigeenous practice of treating human liver disorders in Assam. *Ethnobotany 13*, 87–90.

46. Das, A. K., & Saikia, D. C. (2002). Investigation into the folk belief on anti-fertility and fertility-induced plants. *Ethnobotany 14*, 20–22.

47. Das, A. K., & Sharma, G. D. (2003). Ethnomedicinal plants used by Barman and Manipuri community, Cachar district, Assam. *J. Econ. Taxon. Bot. 27*, 421–429.

48. Das, A. K., & Tag, H., 2005. Ethnomedicinal studies of the Khampti tribe of Arunachal Pradesh. *Indian J. Trad. Knowl. 5*, 317–322.

49. Das, A. P., Ghosh, C., Sarkar, A., & Biswas, R. (2007). Ethnobotanical studies in India with notes on Terai-Duars and Hills of Darjiling and Sikkim. *NBU J. Plant Sci. 1*, 67–83.

50. Das, B., Talukdar, A. D., & Choudhury, M. D. (2014). A few traditional medicinal plants used as antifertility agents by ethnic people of Tripura, India. *Intern J Pharm Pharmaceut Sci. 6(3)*, 47–53.

51. Das, N. J., Devi, K., & Goswami, S. R. (2005). Report on the treatment of dysmenorrhoea by the tribes of Nalbari district, Assam. *Indian J. Trad. Knowl. 4(1)*, 72–74.

52. Das, T., Mishra, S. B., Saha, D., & Agarwal, (2012). Ethnobotanical survey of medicinal plants used by Ethnic and rural people in Eastern Sikkim Himalaya region. *Intern. J. Ayurved. Herbal Med. 2(2)*, 253–259.

53. Deb, D., Darlong, L., Sarkar, A., Roy, M., & Datta, B. K. (2012). Traditional Ethnomedicinal plants used by the Darlong tribes in Tripura, Northeast India. *Intern J Ayurved Herbal Med 2(6)*, 954–966.

54. Deb, L., Singh, K. R., Singh, K. R., Singh, K. B., & Thongam, B. (2011). Some ethno-medicinal plants used by the Native practitioners of Chandel district, Manipur, India. *Intern. Res. J. Pharm. 2(12)*, 199–200.

55. Debnath, B., Debnath, A., Shilsharma, S., & Paul, C. (2014). Ethnomedicinal knowledge of Mog and Reang communities of South district of Tripura, India. *Indian J. Advances plant Res. 1(5)*, 49–54.

56. Devi, A. P. (2011). Plants used by Meitei community of Manipur for the treatment of diabetes. *Assam Univ. J. Sci. & Tech.: Biol. Environ. Sci. 7*, 63–66.

57. Devi, W. I., Devi, G. S., & Singh, C. B. (2011). Traditional herbal medicine used for the treatment of diabetes in Manipur, India. *Res. J. Pharmaceut. Biol. Chem. Sci. 2(4)*, 709–715.

58. Devi, Y. N., & Singh, P. K. (2008). Ethnobotany of Verbenaceae in Manipur. *Ethnobotany 20*, 111–114.

59. Dutta, A. (2000). Ethnobotany of Deories of Upper Assam. PhD thesis, Gauhati University, Guwahati, India

60. Fabricant, D. S., & Farnsworth, N. R. (2001). The value of plants used in traditional medicine for drug discovery. *Env. Health Presp. 109(S1)*, 69–75.

61. Farnsworth, N. R., Akerele, O., Bingel, A. S., Soejarto, D. D., & Guo, Z. (1985). Medicinal plants in therapy. *Bull. WHO 63*, 965–981.

62. Gajurel, P. R., Rethy, P., Singh, B., & Angami, A. (2006). Ethnobotanical studies on Adi tribes in Dehang Debang Biosphere Reserve in Arunachal Pradesh, Eastern Himalayas. *Ethnobotany 18*, 114–118.

63. Gogoi, P., & Boissya, C. L. (1984). Information about few herbal medicines used by people of Assam (India) against jaundice. *Himal. Res. Div. 2*, 41–44.

64. Gogoi, R., & Borthakur, S. K. (2001). Notes on herbal recipes of Bodo tribe in Kamrup district, Assam. *Ethnobotany 13*, 15–23.

65. Gohain, N., Prakash, A., Gogoi, K., Bhattacharya, D. R., Sarmah, N., Dahutia, C., & Kalita, M. C. (2015). An ethnobotanical survey of anti-malarial plants in some highly malaria affected districts of Assam. *Intern. J. Pharm. Pharmaceut. Sci. 7 (9)*, 147–152.

66. Gurumayum, S., & Soram, J. S. (2014). Some Anti-diarrhoeic and anti-dysenteric ethno-medicinal plants of Mao Naga tribe community of Mao, Senapati district, Manipur. *Intern J Pure Applied Biosc. 2(1)*, 147–155.

67. Hajra, P. K. (1977). Some important medicinal plants from Kamang district of Arunachal Pradesh. *Bull. Meghal. Sci. Soc. 2*, 16–20.

68. Hajra, P. K., & Baishya, A. K. (1981). Ethno-botanical notes on Miris (Mishings) of Assam. In: S. K. Jain (ed.) Glimpses of Indian Ethnobotany. Oxford & IBH Publ., New Delhi.

69. Hynniewta, S. R., & Kumar, Y. (2008). Herbal remedies among the Khasi traditional healers and the villager folks in Meghalaya. *Indian J. Trad. Knowl. 7(4)*, 581–586.

70. Idrisi, M. S., Badola, H. K., & Singh, R. (2012). Indigenous knowledge and medicinal use of plants by local communities in Rangit valley, south Sikkim, India. *Ne Bio. 1*, 34–45.

71. Islam, M. (1996). Ethnobotany of certain underground parts of plants of North Eastern Region, India. *J. Econ. Taxon. Bot. Adl. Ser. 12*, 338–343.

72. Jain, S. K., & Borthakur, S. K. (1980). Ethnobotany of Mikirs of India. *Econ. Bot. 34*, 264–272.

73. Jain, S. K., & Dam, N. (1979). Some ethnobotanical notes from north eastern India. *Econ. Bot. 33*, 52–56.

74. Jamir, K. H., Tsurho, K., & Zhimhomi, A. (2015). Some indigenus medicinal plants and its uses in Zuheboto district, Nagaland. *Int. J. Dev. Res. 5(8)*, 5195–5200.

75. Jamir, N. S. (1990). Some interesting medicinal plants used by Nagas. *J. Edu. Indian Med. 9*, 81–87.

76. Jamir, N. S. (1991). Studies on some medico-herbs from North-East India. *Recent Advances in Medicinal Aromatic and Spices crops 1*, 235–239.

77. Jamir, N. S. (1999). Ethnobotanical studies among Naga tribes in Nagaland. In: *Biodiversity North East India Perspective*, B. Kharbuli, D. Syiem & H. Kayang, eds. North Eastern Biodiversity Research Cell, North Eastern Hill University, Shillong. 128–140.

78. Jamir, N. S. (2006). Indigenous knowledge of medicinal plants in the state of Nagaland. In: *Proc. Horticulture for sustainable income and Protection 2*, 677–683.

79. Jamir, N. S. (2012). Traditional knowledge of medicinal plants used by Ao-Naga tribes of Mokokchung district, Nagaland (India). In: G. G. Maiti & S. K. Mukherjee (eds.). International Seminar on "Multidisciplinary approaches in Angiosperm systematics." Universty of Kalyani, Kalyani, India, pp. 602–607.

80. Jamir, N. S., Lanusunep & Konyak, C. H. M. (2011). Some less known ethnomedicinal plants used by Angami-Naga tribes in Kohima district, Nagaland (India). *Ethnobotany 23*, 116–120.

81. Jamir, N. S., Lanusunep & Pongener, N. (2012). Medico- herbal medicine practiced by the Naga tribes in the state of Nagaland (India). *Indian J. Fundamen Applied Life Science. 2(2)*, 328–333.

82. Jamir, N. S., Limasemba & Jamir, N. (2008). Ethnomedcinal plants used by Konyak Naga tribes of Mon district in Nagaland. *Ethnobotany 20*, 48–53.

83. Jamir, N. S., & Rao, R. R. (1990). Fifty new or interesting medicinal plants used by the Zeliangs of Nagaland (India). *Ethnobotany 2*, 11–18.

84. Jamir, N. S., Takatemjen & Limasemba. (2010). Traditional knowledge of Lotha-Naga tribes in Wokha district, Nagaland, *Indian J. Tradit. Knowl. 9(1)*, 45–48.

85. Joseph, J., & Kharkongor, P. (1980). A preliminary ethnobotanical survey in Khasi and Jaintia Hills, Meghalaya. In: Jain, S. K. (Eds). Glimpses of Indian Ethnobotany, pp: 115–123, Oxford & IBH, New Delhi.

86. Kagyung, R., Gajurel, P. R., Rethy, P., & Singh, B. (2010). Ethnomedicinal plants used for gastro-intestinal diseases by Adi tribes of Dehang-Debang Biosphere reserve in Arunachal Pradesh. *Indian J. Trad. Knowl. 9(3)*, 496–501.

87. Kala, C. P. (2005). Ethnomedicinal botany of the Apatani in the Eastern Himalayan region of India. *J. Ethnobiol. Ethnomed. 1*, 11–18.

88. Kalita, D., & Deb, B. (2006). Folk medicines for some diseases prevalent in Lakhimpur district of Brahmaputra valley, Assam. *Nat. Prod. Radiance 5(4)*, 319–322.

89. Kalita, D., Dutta, M., & Islam, N. F. (2005). Few plants and animals based folk medicines from Dibrugarh district, Assam. *Indian J. Trad. Knowl. 4(1)*, 81–85.

90. Kayang, H., Kharbuli, B., Myrboli, B., & Syiem, D. (2005). Medicinal plants of Khasi Hill of Meghalaya, India. *Bioprospecting & Ethnopharmacol 1*, 75–80.

91. Khan, T. U., Agrahari, R. K., Chowdhury, B., & Borthakur, S. K. (2014). Plants used by Hmar, Manipuri and Barman community of Hailakandi district of Assam (India) for the treatment of diabetes. *Pleione 8(2)*, 456–461.

92. Kharkongor, P., & Joseph, J. (1981). Folklore medicobotany of rural Khasi and Jaintia tribes in Meghalaya. In: S. K. Jain (ed.) Glimpses of Indian Ethnobotany. Oxford & IBH, New Delhi, pp. 115, 124–136.

93. Khomdram, S. D, Devi, Y. N., & Singh, P. K. (2011). Ethnobotanical uses of Lamiaceae in Manipur, India. *Ethnobotany 23*, 64–69.

94. Khongsai, M., Saikia, S. P., & Kayang, H. (2011). Ethnomedicinal plants used by different tribes of Arunachal Pradesh. *Indian J. Trad. Knowl. 10(3)*, 541–546.

95. Khumbongmayum, A. D., Khan, M. L., & Tripathi, R. S. (2005). Ethnomedicinal plants in the sacred groves of Manipur. *Indian J. Trad. Knowl. 4*, 21–32.

96. Kichu, M., Malewska, T., Akter, K., Imchen, I., Harrington, D., Kohen, J., Vemulpad, S. R., & Jamie, J. F. (2015). An ethnobotanical study of medicinal plants of Chungtia village, Nagaland, India. *J. Ethnopharmacol. 166*, 5–17.

97. Kumar, Y., Fancy, S., & Rao, R. R. (1987). Further contribution to the ethnobotany of Meghalaya. Plants used by War Jaintia of Jaintia Hills district. *J. Econ. Taxon. Bot. 11(1)*, 65.

98. Kumar, Y., Haridasan, K., & Rao, R. P. (1980). Ethnobotanical notes on medicinal plants among Garo people around Balpahakarh Sanctuary in Meghalaya. *Bull. Bot. Surv. Ind. 22*, 161–165.

99. Lafakzuala, R., Lalramnghinglova, H., & Kayang, H. (2007). Ethnobotanical usage of plants in Western Mizoram. *Indian J. Trad. Knowl. 6(3)*, 486–493.

100. Lalrammnghinglova, H. (2003). Ethno-Medicinal plants of Mizoram. Bishen Singh Mahendra Pal Singh, dehra Dun.

101. Lalmuanpuii, J., Rosangkima, G., & Lamin, H. (2013). Ethno-medicinal practices among the Mizo ethnic group in Lunglei district, Mizoram. *Science Vision 13(1)*, 24–34.

102. Laloo, D., & Hemalatha, S. (2011). Ethnomedicinal plants used for diarrhea by tribals of Mehalaya, Northeast India. *Pharmacognosy Reviews 5(10)*, 147–154.

103. Leishangthem, S., & Sharma, L. D. (2014). Study of some important medicinal plants found in Imphal-East district, Manipur, India. *Intern. J. Scienti. Res. 4 (9)*, 1–5.

104. Lokho, A. (2012). The folk medicinal plants of the Mao Naga in Manipur, North East India. *Int. J. Sci. Res. Pub. 2(6)*, 1–8.

105. Lokho, K., & Narasimhan, D. (2013). Ethnobotany of Mao-Naga tribe of Manipur, India. *Pleione 7(2)*, 314–324.

106. Lunusnep & Jamir, N. S. (2010). Folk medicinal herbs used by the Sumi-Naga tribes of Zunheboto district, Nagaland. *Pleione 4*, 215–220.

107. Maiti, D. C., Chauhan, A. S., & Maiti, G. (2003). Ethnonbotanical notes on some unexploited plants used by Lepchas and Nepalese communities of North Sikkim. In: V. Singh & A. P. Jain (eds.). Ethnobotany and Medicinal Plants of India and Nepal. Vol 1, Pp. 325–332, Scientific Publishers, Jodhpur, India.

108. Majumdar, K., & Datta, B. K. (2007a). A study on ethnomedicinal usage of plants among the Tripura tribes of Tripura state, India. *Nat. Prod. Radiance 6(1)*, 68–72.

109. Majumdar, K., & Datta, B. K. (2007b). Ethnobotanical observation on the traditional usage of medicinal plants among the tribals of Tripura. In: Trivedi, P. C. (ed.) Ethnomedicinal plants of India. Aaviskar publishers, Jaipur, pp. 136–161.

110. Majumdar, K., & Datta, B. K. (2013). Practice pattern of Traditional pharmaceutical formulations by the tribes of Tripura, Northeast India. *Global J. Phmacol. 7(4)*, 442–447.

111. Majumdar, K., Saha, R. Datta, B. K., & Bhakta, T. (2006). Medicinal plants prescribed by different tribal and non-tribal medicine men of Tripura. *Indian J. Trad. Knowl. 5(4)*, 559–562.

112. Majumder, R., Bhattacharjee, S., & Nair, A. R. (1978). Some folklore medicines of Assam and Meghalaya. *Int. J. Crude Drug Res. 16*, p. 4.

113. Mao A. A. (1993). A preliminary report on the folklore Botany of Mao Naga of Manipur (India), *Ethnobotany 5*, 143–147.

114. Mao, A. A. (2013). Ethnobotany of Rhododendrons in North-Eastern India. *Ethnobotany 25*, 124–128.

115. Mao, A. A., Hynniewata, T. M., & Sanjappa, M. (2009). Plant wealth of North-east India with reference to Ethnobotany. *Indian J. Trad. Knowl. 8(1)*, 96–103.

116. Mazumder, R., Tiwary, K. C., Bhattacharya, S., & Nair, R. R. (1978). Some folklore medicine of Assam and Meghalaya. *Quart. J. Crude. Drug Res. 16*, p. 4.

117. Medhi, R. P., & Chakrabarti, S. (2009). Traditional knowledge of NE people on conservation of wild orchids. *Indian J. Trad. Knowl. 8(1)*, 11–16.

118. Megoneitso & Rao, R. R. (1983). Ethnobotanical studies in Nagaland – Sixty-two medicinal plants used by the Agami-Nagas. *J. Econ. Taxon. Bot. 4*, 167–172.

119. Mir, A. H., Krishna Upadhaya, K., & Hiranjit Choudhury, H. (2014). Diversity of Endemic and Threatened Ethnomedicinal Plant Species in Meghalaya, North-East India. *Intern. Res. J. Environment Sci. 3(12)*, 64–78.

120. Moktan, S., & Das, A. P. (2013). Ethnomedicinal approach for diarrheal treatment in Darjiling district (WB), India. *Ethnobotany 25*, 160–163.

121. Namsa, N. D., Mandal, M., Tangjang, S., & Mandal, S. C. (2011). Ethnobotany of the Monpa ethnic group at Arunachal Pradesh, India. *J Ethnobiol Ethnomed* http://www.ethnobiomed.com/content/7/1/31

122. Nath, A., & Maiti, G. G. (2003). Ethnobotany of Barak valley (Southern Assam) with special reference to folk medicine. *J. Econ. Taxon. Bot. 27(4)*, 964-971.

123. Nath, K. K., Deka, P., & Borthakur, S. K. (2007). Ethnomedicinal aspects of some weeds from Darrang district of Assam. *Ethnobotany 19*, 82–87.

124. Nath, K. K., Deka, P., & Borthakur, S. K. (2011). Traditional remedies of joint diseases in Assam. *Indian J. Trad. Knowl. 10(3)*, 568–571.

125. Nath, M., Dutta, R. K., & Hajra, P. K. (2013). Ethnomedicinal plants used in stomach disorders by Dimasa tribe of Barak valley (South Assam). *Ethnobotany 25*, 78–82.

126. Neogi, B., Prasad M. N. V., & Rao R. R. (1989). Ethnobotany of some weeds of Khasi and Garo Hills, Meghalaya, Northeastern India. *Economic Bot. 43(4)*, 471–479.

127. Nima, D. N., Hui, T., Mandal, M., Das, A. K., & Kalita, P. (2009). An ethnobotanical study of traditional anti-inflammatory plants used by the Lohit community of Arunachal Pradesh, India. *J. Ethnopharmacol. 125*, 234–245.

128. Ningombam, D. S., Devi, S. P., Singh, P. K., Pinokiyo, A., & Thongam, B. (2014). Documentation and assessment on knowledge of Ethno-medicinal practitioners; A case study on Local Meetei healers of Manipur. *J. Pharm. Biol. Sci. 9(1)*, 53–70.

129. Panda, A. K. (2012). Medicinal plants used and primary health care in Sikkim. *Intern. J. Ayurved. Herbal Med. 2(2)*, 253–259.

130. Pandey, A., & Mavinkurve, R. G., (2014). Ethno-botanical usage of plants by the Chakma community of Tripura, Northeast India. *Bulletin Environ, Pharmacol Life Sci. 3(6)*, 11–14.

131. Parkash, V., Saikia, A. J., Dutta, R., & Borah, D. (2013). Wild medicinal plants of Umtasoar Range under Nonghkyllem Reserve Forest, Nongpoh, Meghalaya, India and their traditional usage by Khasi tribe I. *The Journal of Ethnobiol, Trad. Med. Photon 118*, 228–237.

132. Pfoze, N. L., & Chhetry, G. K. N. (2004). Traditional folk medicines of the Shepoumaramth Nagas of Senapati district in Manipur. *Proc. Natl. Acad. Sci. India 74B*, 37–57.

133. Pradhan, B. K., & Badola, H. K. (2008). Ethnomedicinal plant use by Lepcha tribe of Dzongu valley bordering Khangchendzonga Biosphere Reserve, in North Sikkim, India, *J. Ethnobiol. Ethnomed., 4(22)*, 1–18.

134. Purkayastha, J., Nath, S. C., & Islam, M. (2005). Ethnobotany of medicinal plants from Dibru-Saikowa Biosphere Reserve of Northeast India. *Fitoterapia 76*, 121–127.

135. Pushpangadan, P. (1995). Ethnobiology in India. A status report, Govt. of India, New Delhi.

136. Rai, P. K., & Lalramnhinglova, H. (2010a). Lesser Known Ethnomedicinal plants of Mizoram, North East India: An Indo-Burma hotspot region. *J. Medicinal Plants Res. 4(13)*, 1301–1307.

137. Rai, P. K., & Lalramnghinglova, H. (2010b). Ethnomedicinal plant resources of Mizoram, India: Implication of traditional knowledge in Health care system. *Ethnobotanical Leaflets 14*, 274–305.

138. Rai, P. K., & Lalramnghinglova, H. (2010c). Ethnomedicinal Plants from Agroforestry Systems and Home gardens of Mizoram, North East India. *Herba Polonica 56 (2)*, 1–13.

139. Rai, P. C., Sarkar, A., Bhujel, R. B., & Das, AP. (1998). Etnobotanical studies in some fringe area of Sikkim and Darjeeling Himalayas. *J. Hill Res. 11*, 12–21.

140. Rao, R. R. (1981). Ethnobotany of Meghalaya, medicinal plants used by Khasi and Garo tribes. *Econ. Bot. 35*, 4–9.

141. Rao, R. R. (1997). Ethnobotanical studies on some Adivasi tribes of North East India with special reference to the Naga people. In: S. K. Jain (ed.) Contribution to Indian Ethnobotany, Scientific Publishers, Jodhpur, pp. 209–223.

142. Rao, R. R., & Jamir, N. S. (1982a). Ethnobotanical studies in Nagaland I: Medicinal Plants. *Econ. Bot. 36*, 176–181.

143. Rao, R. R., & Jamir, N. S. (1982b). Ethnobotanical studies of Nagaland II: 54 medicinal plants used by the Nagas. *J. Econ. Taxon. Bot. 3*, 11–17.

144. Rao, R. R., Neogi, B., & Prasad, M. N. V. (1989). Ethnobotany of som weeds of Khasi and Garo hills of Meghalaya and North-east India. *Econ. Bot. 43(3)*, 471.

145. Rawat, M. S., & Choudhury, S. (1998). Ethnomedicobotany of Arunachal Pradesh (Nishi and Apatani tribes). Bishen Singh Mahendra Pal Singh, Dehra Dun.

146. Rethy, P., Singh, B., Kagyung, R., & Gakurel, P. R. (2010). Ethnobotanical studies of Dehang–Debang biosphere reserve of Arunachal Pradesh with special reference to Memba tribe. *Indian J. Trad. Knowl. 9*, 61–67.

147. Ringmichon, C. L., Shimpi, S. N., & Gopalakrishnana, B. (2011). Some noteworthy antipyretic herbal remedies used by Naga tribes in Manipur. *Ethnobotany 23*, 82–85.

148. Rout, J., Sanjem, A. L., & Nath, M. (2010). Traditional Medicinal Knowledge of the Zeme (Naga) tribe of North Cachar Hills District, Assam on the treatment of Diarrhoea. *Assam Univ. J. Sci. and Tech. Biol. and Environ. Sci. 5(1)*, 63–69.

149. Rout, J., Sajem, A. L., & Nath, M. (2012). Medicinal plants of North Cachar hills district of Assam used by Dimasa tribe. *Indian J. Trad. Knowl. 11 (3)*, 520–527.

150. Saikia, B. (2006). Ethnomedicinal plants from Gohpur of Sonitpur district, Assam. *Indian J. Trad. Knowl. 5(4)*, 529–530.

151. Saikia, B., Borthakur, S. K., & Saikia, N. (2010). Medico-ethnobotany of Bodo tribals in Gohpur of Sonitpur district, Assam. *Indian J. Trad. Knowl. 9(1)*, 52–54.

152. Sajem, A. L., & Gosai, K. (2006). Traditional use of medicinal plants by the Jaintia tribes in North Cachar Hills district of Assam, northeast India. *J. Ethnobiol. Ethnomed. 2*, 33. Doi: 10.1186/1746-4269-2-33.

153. Sanjem, A. L., Rout, J., & Nath, Minaram, (2008). Traditional tribal knowledge and status of some rare and endemic medicinal plants of north Cachar Hills district of Assam, Northeast India, *J. Ethnobotanical Leaflets. 12*, 261–275.

154. Salam, S., Jamir, N. S., & Singh, P. K. (2011). Ethnomedicinal studies on Tangkhul-Naga tribe in Ukhrul district, Manipur. *Ethnobotany 23*, 129–134.

155. Sarmah, R., Arunachalam, A., Melkania, U., Majumder & Adhikari, D. (2006). Ethno-Medico-Botany of Chakmas in Arunachal Pradesh, India. *Indian Forester 132(4)*, 474–484.

156. Schipmann, U., Leaman, D. J., & Cunningham, A. B. (2002). Impact of cultivation and gathering of medicinal plants on biodiversity: Global trends and issues. In: (FAO), Biodiversity and ecosystem approach in agriculture, forestry and fisheries. Satellite event on the occasion of 9th regular session of the commission of genetic resource for food and agriculture, Rome, 12–13 October 2002.

157. Sen, S., Chakraborty, R., De, B., & Devanna, N. (2011). An ethnobotanical survey of medicinal plants used by ethnic people in west and South of Tripura, India. *J. Forestry Res. 22(3)*, 417–426.

158. Sen, A., & Ghosh, P. D. (2011). A note on the ethnobotanical studies of some pteridophyte in Assam. *Indian J. Trad. Knowl. 10(2)*, 292–295.

159. Shanker, R., Lavekar, G. S. Deb, S., & Sharma, B. K. (2012). Traditional healing practice and folk medicines used by Mishing community of Northeast India. *J. Ayurved Integr. Med. 3(3)*, 124–129.

160. Shankar, R., & Rawat, M. S. (2013). Medicinal Plants Used in Traditional Medicine in Aizawl and Mamit Districts of Mizoram. *J. Biol. Life Sci. 4(2)*, 95–102.

161. Shankar, R., Rawat, M. S., Majumdar, R., Baruah, D., & Bharali, B. K. (2012). Medicinal plants used in traditional medicine in Mizoram. *World J. Sci. Technol. 2(12)*, 42–45.

162. Sharma, B. C. (2013). Ethnomedicinal plants used against skin diseases by indigenous population of Darjeeling Himalayas, India. *Indian J Fundamen Applied Life Sci. 3(3)*, 299–303.

163. Sharma, M., Sharma, C. L., & Marak, P. N. (2014). Indigenous uses of medicinal plants in north Garo hills, Meghalaya, NE India. *Res. J. Recent Sci. 3*, 137–146.

164. Sharma, U. K., Pegu, S., Hazarika, D., & Das, A. (2012). Medico-religious plants used by the Hajong community of Assam, India. *J. Ethnopharmacol. 143*, 787–800.

165. Shil, S., & Choudhury, M. D. (2009). Ethnomedicinal Importance of Pteridophytes used by Reang tribe of Tripura, North East India. *J. Ethnobotanical Leaflets. 13*, 634–643.

166. Shil., S., Choudhury, M. D., & Das, S. (2014). Indigenous knowledge of medicinal plants used by the Reang tribe of Tripura state of India. *J. Ethnopharmacol. 152*, 135–141.

167. Singh, H. B., Hynniewata, T. M., & Bora, P. J. (1997). Ethnomedico botanical studies in Tripura, India. *Ethnobotany 9*, 56–58.

168. Singh, H. B., Prasad, P., & Rai L. K. (2002). Folk Medicinal Plants in the Sikkim Himalayas of India. *Asian Folklore studies 61*, 295–310.

169. Singh, J., Bhuyan, T. C., & Ahmed, A. (1996). Ethnobotanical studies on the Mishing tribes of Assam with special reference to food and medicinal plants. *J. Econ. Tax. Bot. Addl. Ser. 12*, 350–356.

170. Singh, K. J., & Huidrom, D. (2013). Ethnobotanical uses of medicinal plant, *Justicia adhatoda* L. by Meitei community of Manipur, India. *J Coastal Life Med* 1(4): 322–325.

171. Singh, L. S., Singh, P. K., & Singh, E. J. (2001). Ethnobotanical uses of some pteridophytic species in Manipur. *Indian Fern. J. 18*, 14–17.

172. Singh, N. P., Gajurel, P. R., Panmei, R., & Rethy, P. (2015). Indigenous healing practices and ethnomedicinal plants used against jaundice by some Naga tribes in Nagaland, India. *Pleione 9(1)*, 40–48.

173. Singh, T. T., Sharma, H. M., Devi, A. R., & Sharma, H. R. (2014). Plants used in the treatment of piles by the Scheduled caste community of Andro village in Imphal East District, Manipur (India). *J. Plant Sci. 2(3)*, 113–119.

174. Singh, V. N., Chanu, L. I., Chiru Community & Baruah, M. K. (2011). An ethnobotanical study of Chirus – A less known tribe of Assam. *Indian J. Trad. Knowl. 10(3)*, 572–574.

175. Sinha, S. C. (1987). Ethnobotany of Manipur Medicinal plants. *Front. Bot. 1*, 123–152.

176. Solecki, R., & Shanidar, I. V. (1975). A Neanderthal flower buried in northern Iraq. *Science 190*, 880–881.

177. Sonowal, R., & Barua, I. (2011). Ethnomedical Practices among the Tai-Khamyangs of Asssam, India. *J. Ethno. Med. 5(1)*, 41–50.

178. Sumitra, S., & Jamir, N. S. (2009). Traditional uses of medicinal plants used by Tangkhl-Naga tribe in Manipur, India. *Pleione 3*, 157–162.

179. Tag, H., Kalita, P., Dwivedi, P., Das, A. K., & Nima, N. D. (2012). Herbal medicines used in the treatment of diabetes mellitus in Arunachal Himalaya, northeast, India. *J. Ethnopharmacol. 141*, 786–795.

180. Tamuli, P., & Saikia, R. (2004). Ethno-medico-botany of the Zeme tribe of North Cachar Hills district of Assam. *Indian J. Trad. Knowl. 3(4)*, 430–436.

181. Tangjang, S., Nima, D. N., Aran, C., & Litin, A. (2011). An ethnobotanical survey of medicinal plants in the Eastern Himalayan zone of Arunachal Pradesh, India. *J. Ethnopharmacol. 134*, 18–25.

182. Tarafdar, R. G., Nath, S., Talukdar, A. D., & Choudhury, M. D. (2015). Antidiabetic plants used among the ethnic communities of Unakoti district of Tripura, India. *J. Ethnopharmacol. 160*, 219–226.

183. Tiwari, U. L., Kotia, A., & Rawat, G. S. (2009). Medico-ethnobotany of Monpas in Tawang and West Kaming districts of Arunachal Pradesh, India. *Pleione 3*, 1–8.

184. Tiwary, K. C., Mazumder, R., & Bhattacharya, S. (1978). Some medicinal plants from district Tirap of Arunachal Pradesh. *Indian J. Pharm. Sci. 40*, 206–208.

185. Tiwary, K. C., Mazumder, R., & Bhattacharya, S. (1979). Floklore medicine from Assam and Arunachal Pradesh. *Int. Crud. Drug Res. 17*, 61–67.

186. Tripathi, S., & Goel, A. K. (2001). Ethnobotanical diversity of Zingiberaceae in North-Eastern India. *Ethnobotany 13*, 67–79.

187. Tushar, Basak, S., Sarma, G. C., & Rangan, L. (2010). Ethnomedical uses of Zingiberaceous plants of Northeast India. *J. Ethnopharmacol. 132(1)*, 286–296.

188. Yumkham, S. D., & Singh, P. K. (2011). Less known ferns and fern allies of Manipur with ethnobotanical uses. *Indian J. Trad. Knowl. 10(2)*, 287–291.

189. Yumnam, R. S., Devi, C. O., Abujam, S. K., & Chetia, D. (2012). Study on the Ethno-medicinal System of Manipur. *Intern J. Pharmaceut. Biol. Archives. 3(3)*, 587–591.

190. Zhasa, N. N., Hazarika, P., & Tripathi, Y. C. (2015). Indigenous Knowledge on utilization of plant biodiversity for treatment and cure of diseases of Human beings in Nagaland, India: A case study. *Intern Res J Biol Sci 4(4)*, 89–106.

CHAPTER 6

ETHNOBOTANY OF OTHER USEFUL PLANTS IN NORTH-EAST INDIA: AN INDO-BURMA HOT SPOT REGION

PRABHAT KUMAR RAI

Department of Environmental Science, School of Earth Science and Natural Resource Management, Mizoram University, Aizawl–796004, Mizoram, India, E-mail: prabhatrai24@gmail.com

CONTENTS

Abstract 164

6.1   Introduction 164

6.2   Bamboo: A Prominent Non-Timber Forest Product
      Linked with Ethnicity of North East India 165

6.3   Rattans (Cane) 167

6.4   Dye Yielding Plants 168

6.5   Wood Crafts 170

6.6   Incense 171

6.7   Insecticide/Insect Repellent 171

6.8   Ichthyotoxic and Fish Feed Plants 171

6.9   Conclusion 172

Acknowledgement 172

Keywords 173

References 173

ABSTRACT

In the present chapter ethnobotany of other useful plants has been described which may be inextricably and intimately linked with rural livelihood of diverse tribes existing in North East India. Initially, in this chapter ethnobotany of Bamboos and Canes (Rattans) is described and overviewed. Further, ethnobotany of useful plants serving multifaceted purposes apart from ethnomedicine and food are described. These include dye-producing plants, fiber yielding plants and plants used for preparation of wine and pickles have been described. Use of under-utilized plants or less exploited plants to be used for diverse economic benefits for the livelihood improvement is intimately linked with socio-economy of North East India, an Indo Burma hot spot region.

6.1   INTRODUCTION

Biodiversity at local, regional and global level is intimately as well as inextricably linked with environment as well as economy. Plant diversity boosts the economy by providing food, fiber, timber and non-timber forest produce (NTFP), for example, botano-chemicals while it maintains a healthy environment by efficiently regulating the gaseous and nutrient cycling. Forest resources thriving immense biodiversity may be inextricably connected with socio-economic livelihood and hence Sustainable Development of North East India (NE, India) (Rai, 2015).

The Indian Subcontinent is one of the seventeen mega-biodiversity centers of the world particularly rich in plant resources linked with the human health and welfare (Rai and Lalramnghinglova, 2010a,b,c; 2011a,b). North East India encompasses a significant portion of Indo-Burma biodiversity hotspot (Myers et al., 2000; Rai, 2009).

The North East Region (NER) of India is perhaps one of the most vibrant and complex areas to administer, of the 600 odd ethnic communities that inhabit India, well over 200 ethnic groups are found in this region (Rocky, 2013).

World over, the tribal population still stores a vast knowledge on utilization of local plants as food and other specific uses (Sundriyal et al., 1998; Pfoze et al., 2014). In an ethnobotanical exploration of Nagaland

(Pfoze et al., 2014) a total of 628 number of species recorded in the study, 73.88% (464) of the species are used as ethnomedicine, 27.23% (171) as edible plants, 13.69% (86) as edible fruits, 5.73% (36) as dyes, 4.30% (27) as fish poison, 1.60% (10) as fermented food and beverage, 1.75% (11) as fodder and pasture grass and about 7.96% (50) for other uses such as fibers, furniture, jams and pickles, oil and gum, masticatory, plants use as seasonal indicator, etc. (Pfoze et al., 2014). Similarly, about 318 genera of ethnomedicinal plants, 124 genera of edible plants and 53 genera of edible fruits. Hazarika et al. (2015) investigated ethnobotany of other useful plants used for purposes other than ethnomedicine (See Tables 6.1 - 6.3). Devi (1980) has given the details of museological aspects of ethnic tribes of Manipur valley.

Albizzia odoratissima and *Albizzia procera* are the two main sources of fodder tree species in the Mizoram (Sahoo et al., 2010).

6.2 BAMBOO: A PROMINENT NON-TIMBER FOREST PRODUCT LINKED WITH ETHNICITY OF NORTH EAST INDIA

Bamboo is a predominant under-story species in forest ecosystems of NE India. Out of the 150 species of bamboo available in India, 58 species are present in NE India (Rai, 2009). Bamboo is an important commercial source for a variety of purposes, such as manufacture of paper, construction of houses, bridges, furniture, bags and baskets, and is also utilized, although to a limited extent, as fuel and fodder (Rai, 2009). Bhatt et al. (2003) also mentioned the various economic importance of bamboo in the form of food (young shoot), timber, and as agricultural implements (culms and branches) in three states (Mizoram, Meghalaya and Sikkim) of NE India. Bamboo is also inextricably linked with the traditional culture as

TABLE 6.1 Underutilized and Unexploited Fruits from Ethnobotanical Plants Used for Making Oil

S. No.	Plant species	Part Used
1	*Terminalia bellerica* (Combretaceae)	Seed
2	*Phoenix dactylifera* (Arecaceae)	Seed
3	*Emblica officinalis* (Euphorbiaceae)	Fruit

TABLE 6.2 Ethnobotanical Plants Used to Prepare Pickle and Wine of Commercial Importance

S. no.	Food/beverage	Plant species	Preparation
1	Food Pickle	*Emblica officinalis*	Fresh fruits are mixed with spices along with oil and vinegar
2	Pickle	*Ziziphus mauritiana*	Ripe fruits are mixed with spices along with oil and vinegar
3	Pickle	*Tamarindus indica*	Fruits are mixed with spices, oil and vinegar
4	Pickle	*Elaeocarpus floribundus*	Boiled fruits are dried and mixed with spices along with oil and vinegar
5	Pickle	*Artocarpus heterophyllus*	Unripe fruits are slice into pieces and mixed with spices, oil and vinegar
6	Beverages Wine	*Averrhoa carambola*	Squeezed the juice from the fruits, pour in the bottle and fermented for 2 weeks
7	Wine	*Emblica officinalis*	Freshly fruits are mixed with sugar and pour in the bottle and fermented for 3 months
8	Wine	*Citrus grandis*	Crushed and squeezed the juice from the fruits, mixed with sugar and fermented for 2 months
9	Wine	*Elaeagnus latifolia*	Freshly fruits are mixed with sugar and fermented for 5 months

(Reprinted from Hazarika, T. K., Marak, S., Mandal, D., Upadhyay, K., Nautiyal, B. P., & Shukla, A. O. (2015). Underutilized and unexploited fruits of Indo-Burma hot spot, Meghalaya, north-east India: ethno-medicinal evaluation, socio-economic importance and conservation strategies. Genet. Resour. Crop. Evol. 63(2), 289–304. With permission of Springer.)

TABLE 6.3   Other Ethnobotanical Plants of Miscellaneous Use

S. No.	Plant species	Family	Uses
1.	*Dillenia pentagyna*	Dilleniaceae	Leaves for packing material
2.	*Sterculia villosa*	Malvaceae	Bark for making ropes
3.	*Artocarpus heterophyllus*	Moraceae	Wood for making furniture
4.	*Ficus glomerata*	Moraceae	Wood containers
5.	*Ficus lamponga*	Moraceae	Wood containers

well as ethnicity of peoples of NE states, and various festivals are based on it with the performance of bamboo dance (Rai, 2009). Therefore, in real sense, bamboo is poor man's timber in NE states of India.

Bamboo shows a characteristic simultaneous mass flowering after long intervals of several decades. Bamboo species flower suddenly and simultaneously then all the flower clumps die, leading to drastic changes in forest dynamics and environmental conditions, for example, light intensity, seedling survival, organic matter decomposition, and nutrient cycling, although complete destruction of bamboo clumps requires another few years. Bamboo communities follow active nutrient cycling and their vigorous growth and litter production ameliorates nutrient impoverished coal mine spoil and tropical soil fertility (Rao and Ramakrishnan, 1989; Singh and Singh, 1999; Mailly et al., 2007; Takahashi et al., 2007; Rai, 2009). However, after mass flowering and death, nutrient uptake by the bamboo ceases and large amounts of dead organic matter are deposited (Rai, 2012).

Ethnopedology is the documentation and understanding of local approaches to soil perception, classification, appraisal, use and management (WinklerPrins and Sandor, 2003; Nath et al., 2015). It is widely recognized that farmers' hold important knowledge of folk soil classification for agricultural land for its uses, yet little has been studied for traditional agroforestry systems (Nath et al., 2015). Nath et al. (2015) explored the ethnopedology of bamboo (*Bambusa* sp.) based agroforestry system in North East India, and establishes the relationship of soil quality index (SQI) with bamboo productivity.

6.3   RATTANS (CANE)

The name 'cane' (rattan) stands collectively for the climbing members of a big group of palms known as Lepidocaryoideae. Rattans/canes are prickly climbing palms with solid stems, belonging to the family Arecaceae and the sub-family Calamoideae. They are scaly-fruited palms. The rattans/canes comprise more than fifty per cent of the total palm taxa found in India (Basu, 1985; Lalnuntluanga et al., 2010). Rattan forms one of the major biotic components in tropical and sub-tropical forest ecosystem (Lalnuntluanga et al., 2010). The flora of Assam is still regarded as a major floristic account of the North East region (Kanjilal et al., 1940; Lalnuntluanga et al., 2010). Anderson (1871) enumerated 7 species of rattans of Sikkim (viz., *Calamus erectus*, *C. flagellum*, *C. leptospadix*, *C. tenuis*, *C. acanthospathus*, *C. guruba* and *C. latifolius*). In-depth studies on rattans have been started recently in the region. Thomas and Haridasan (1999) reported 24 species of rattans under 4 genera (*Calamus*, *Daemonorops*, *Plectocomia* and *Zalacca*) from Arunachal Pradesh (Lalnuntluanga et al., 2010). Singh et al. (2004) reported 13 species, viz., *C. acanthospathus*, *C. arborescens*, *C. collina*, *C. erectus*, *C. flagellum*, *C. floribundus*, *C. guruba*, *C. inermis*, *C. latifolius*, *C. leptospadix*, *C. tenuis*, *Daemonorops jenkinsianus* and *Plectocomia bractealis*, under 3 genera (*Calamus*, *Daemonorops* and *Plectocomia*) from Manipur. Deb (1983) reported 6 species, viz., *C. viminalis*, *C. floribundus*, *C. tenuis*, *C. leptospadix*, *C. guruba* and *C. erectus*, belonging to the genus *Calamus* from Tripura. Haridasan et al. (2000) reported the presence of 3 species of *Calamus* (viz., *C. leptospadix*, *C. tenuis* and *C. erectus*) from Meghalaya, 1 species of *Daemonorops* (viz., *D. jenkinsianus*) from Nagaland and 6 species of *Calamus* (viz., *C. leptospadix*, *C. inermis*, *C. latifolius*, *C. flagellum*, *C. erectus* and *C. acanthospathus*); 1 species each of *Daemonorops* (viz., *D. jenkinsianus*) and *Plectocomia* (viz., *P. himalayana*) from Sikkim (Lalnuntluanga et al., 2010).

6.4   DYE YIELDING PLANTS

Borthakur (1981), Akimpou et al. (2005), Singh et al. (2009), Teron and Borthakur (2012), Pfoze et al. (2014), and Hazarika et al. (2015) gave an account of dye yielding plants and dyeing system of Manipur and North-East India, details of which are given below.

- *Bixa orellana* L.: The plant imparts reddish color to clothes or yarn threads. Seeds are taken in clean and thin clothes and rubbed into the water with hand. The liquid thus obtained is used for dyeing clothes or yarn threads

- *Carthamus tinctorius* L.: The petals yield a pink dye. The petals are collected and kept until they become decayed. The decayed petals are rolled in the palm making into balls of thumb size. Two or three balls are enough to dye the yarn threads for one phanek (skirt).

- *Clerodendron odoratum* D. Don: This dye gives pale green color to the clothes. Leaves are collected and crushed into the tub containing water. The water turns light green in color. Then the thread or cloth is soaked overnight and slightly squeezed and spread in shade. The process is repeated 6 to 7 times until the desired color is obtained.

- *Croton caudatus* Gelseler: Sap of twigs is used for black dye of crafts.

- *Curcuma domestica* Valenton (Syn.: *C. longa* L.): The plant gives yellowish color. Fresh rhizomes are crushed into pieces and allowed to soak in water. Clothes or threads are soaked overnight and dried.

- *Garcinia xanthochymus* Hook.f. & T. Anderson – Yellow, pale rose and maroon red dye is extracted from the plant used for dyeing the garments.

- *Indigofera tinctoria* L. – Leaves and flower buds are used to extract indigo/blue dye for dyeing garments.

- *Justicia comata* (L.) Lam. – Leaves and shoots used to extract pink dye used for crafts.

- *Machilus gamblei* King ex Hook.f. Bark is used to extract red dye used for garments.

- *Marsdenia tinctoria* R. Br. Leaves are used to extract indigo/blue dye used for tattoos.

- *Morinda angustifolia* Roxb. – Roots are used to extract yellow dye used for dyeing garments.

- *Pasania pachyphylla* (Kurz) Schottky: Stem bark is cut into pieces and soaked in a pitcher containing water for 6 to 7 days. It is used to obtain black color and dark brown color. For pure black, the thread or cloth is alternately soaked in *Strobilanthes cusia* (Nees) Imlay liquid and *Pasania pachyphylla* liquid until the desired color is obtained. And for dark brown color it is soaked in *Quercus* spp. prepared liquid.

- *Plumbago indica* L.: Flowers are collected in large amount and its petals are crushed and soaked in water. Clothes or yarn threads dipped into the liquid acquire red color.
- *Quercus dealbata* Hook.f. & Thoms. The plant gives dark brown color (of less color intensity) to the clothes/yarn threads. The bark is cut into pieces and soaked in a pitcher containing water.
- *Shorea robusta* Gaertn. – Red dye is extracted from tender leaves for dyeing crafts.
- *Strobilanthes cusia* (Nees) Imlay: Mature leaves are collected and soaked in a pitcher containing water. The pitcher is kept undisturbed until the leaves are completely decayed. The pitcher is stirred with a multipronged stick. Solid things are removed while stirring. Ashes taken from burning oyster is added and stirred continuously. Now liquid is ready for dyeing clothes. It is mainly used to dye black color.
- *Strobilanthes flaccidifolia* Nees – Kum dye is prepared from the plant.
- *Tectona grandis* L.f.: Leaves or barks are cut into pieces and soaked for 2–3 days in water. Clothes or yarn threads which are dipped into this dye give somewhat reddish color.
- *Terminali bellirica* (Gaertn.) Roxb. – Black dye is extracted from fruits for dyeing cordage.

6.5   WOOD CRAFTS

The close and even grained wood of many *Rhododendron* species such as *R. arboreum, R. hodgsonii, R. falconeri*, etc. are used for the 'Khukri' handles, pack-saddle, cups, spoons, ladles, gift boxes, gun-stocks, and posts by Bhutias, Lepchas and Nepalese.

The yak pastoralists, known as Brokpas, of Arunachal Pradesh are expert craftsmen making all the items of their daily utility for processing and storing yak products by themselves. The wood of *Quercus wallichiana* and Bamboo species, *Dendrocalamus hamiltonii, Bambusa tulda* and *B. pallida* are used for these purposes (Bora et al., 2013).

The wood of *Hibiscus tiliaceus* is used by the Great Andamanese to make buoys (phota) for fishnets. Bark from the trunk is removed, sun dried, and scraped to extract fibers used to weave items such as harpoon lines and nets; the fiber is also used to make bracelet.

6.6   INCENSE

The leaves of *Rhododendron anthopogon* are mixed with those of junipers to provide incense that is widely used in Buddhist monasteries in Sikkim and Arunachal Pradesh.

6.7   INSECTICIDE/INSECT REPELLENT

It is reported that the vegetative parts of *Rhododendron thomsonii* is boiled and the highly poisonous extract is used as natural insecticide in Lachen and Lachung villages of north-east Sikkim (Pradhan and Lachungpa, 1990). Similarly the leaves extract of *Rhododendron dalhousiae* var. *rhabdotu* is used as insect repellent by the Monpas of Arunachal Pradesh (Paul et al., 2010).

6.8   ICHTHYOTOXIC AND FISH FEED PLANTS

Community seasonal fishing and hunting are of great economic activities of many tribal people including Monpa ethnic group in addition to agriculture. Chetri et al. (1992) also gave an account of ethnobotany of ichthyotoxic plants in Meghalaya. Tag et al. (2005) reported that the following plants are used as fish poison by the hill Miri tribe of Arunachal Pradesh: *Aesculus pavia* (bark, leaves), *Cyclosorus extensus* (whole plant), *Acacia pennata* (whole plant), *Ageratum conyzoides* (whole plant), *Anamirta cocculus* (fruits), *Croton tiglium* (bark, leaves), *Gynocardia odorata* (pulp of fruits), *Polygonum hydropiper* (whole plant), *Spiranthes oleracea* (whole plant), *Tephrosia candida* (leaves, seeds) and *Zanthoxylum nitidum* (bark, fruits). Namsa et al. (2011) documented the use of the following plants for stupefying and poisoning the fish. The study revealed a wealth of indigenous knowledge and procedures related to poison fishing with the aid of poisonous plants. This easy and simple method of fishing are forbidden in urban areas but still practiced in remote tribal areas. The active ingredients were released by macerating the appropriated plant parts with the help of wooden stick or hammer, which were then introduced into the water environment. Depending upon time and conditions, the fish begin to float to the surface where they can easily be collected with bare hand. A total of seven plant species, namely *Castanopsis indica*, *Derris scandens*, *Aesculus assamica*, *Polygonum hydropiper*, *Spilanthes acmella*, *Ageratum conyzoides*, and *Cyclosorus extensus* were used to poison fish during the month of June-July every year and leaves of three species like *Ipomoea batatas*, *Mannihot esculenta*, and *Zea mays* were used as common fish foodstuffs. The two main molecular groups of fish poisons in plants (the rotenones and the saponins) as well as a third group of plants which liberate cyanide in the water account for nearly all varieties of fish poisons. The underground tuber of *Aconitum ferrox* was widely used in arrow poisoning to kill ferocious animals like bear, wild pigs, gaur and deer. The killing of Himalayan bear was very common practice among the tribal people and the gall bladders are highly priced in the local market. The dried gall bladders of bear are given orally in low doses to cure malaria since ancestral times. Fresh bark of *Aesculus assamica* Griffith collected and pounded with wooden stick used as fish poison. Juice and paste of *Ageratum conyzoides* L. used as fish poison. Whole plant extract of *Castanopsis indica* Roxb. is used to poison fish. *Derris scandens* (Roxb.) Benth. roots are pounded with wooden stick and thrown into the river to poison fishes. *Polygonum hydropiper* L. whole plant extract is used to poison fish. Paste or boiled leaves and young twigs of *Spilanthes oleracea* Murr. are used as fish poison.

6.9   CONCLUSION

The present review emphasizes the use of under-utilized plants or less exploited plants to be used for diverse economic benefits for the livelihood improvement intimately linked with socio-economy of North-East India, an Indo Burma hot spot region. The development of traditional knowledge to suit new lifestyle would result huge benefit upon livings. The global consumers were aware on the benefits of the natural products.

ACKNOWLEDGEMENT

The author is thankful to Professor Amar Nath Rai, Former Director, NAAC, Vice chancellor Mizoram and North Eastern Hill University, India. The author is further thankful to Prof. Lalramghinghlova, Prof. Lanuntluanga, Prof. U. K. Sahoo and Dr. T. K. Hazarika for their kind cooperation and literature provided.

KEYWORDS

- **bamboo**
- **beverages**
- **canes**
- **dye yielding plants**
- **livelihood**

REFERENCES

1. Akimpou, G., Rongmei, K., & Yadava, P. S. (2005). Traditional dye yielding plants of Manipur, Northeast India. *Indian J. Trad. Knowl. 4(1)*, 33–38.
2. Anderson, T. (1871). An enumeration of the palms of Sikkim. *J Linn Soc (Botany), 11*, 4–14.
3. Basu, S. K. (1985). The present status of Rattans Palms in India: An overview. In: Wong & Manokaran (eds.). Proceedings Rattan Seminar, Kuala Lumpur, pp. 77–94.
4. Bhatt, B. P., Singha, L. B., Singh, K., & Sachan, M. S. (2003). Commercial edible bamboo species and their market potential in three Indian tribal states of North Eastern Himalayan Region. *J. Bamboo and Rattan 2(2)*, 111–133.
5. Bora, L., Paul, V., Bam, J., Saikia, A., & Hazarika, D. (2013). Handicraft skills of Yak pastoralists in Arunachal Pradesh. *Indian J. Trad. Knnowl. 12(4)*, 718–724.
6. Borthakur, S. K. (1981). Studies on ethnobotany of Karbis (Mikirs): Plants mastigatories and dyestuffs. In: Jain, S. K. (ed.) Glimpses of Indian Ethnobotany, Scientific Publishers, Jodhpur, pp. 180–190.
7. Chetri, R. B., Kataki, S. K., & Boissya, C. L. (1992). Ethnobotany of some ichthyotoxic plants in Meghalayas, North-eastern India. *J. Econ. Taxon. Bot. Addl. Ser. 10*, 285–288.
8. Devi, D. L. (1980). Ethnobiological studies of Manipiur valley with reference to Museological aspects. PhD thesis, Manipur university.

9. Deb, D. B. (1983). The Flora of Tripura State, Volume-II. Today & Tomorrow's Printers and Publishers, pp. 428–430.

10. Haridasan, K., Thomas, S., & Sharma, A. (2000). Bamboo and rattan (cane) in North-East India with special reference to Arunachal Pradesh. In: S. C. Tiwari & P. P. Dabral, eds. International Book Distributor, 9/3 Rajpur Road, Dehra Dun, pp. 39–58.

11. Hazarika, T. K., Marak, S., Mandal, D., Upadhyay, K., Nautiyal, B. P., & Shukla, A. O. (2015). Underutilized and unexploited fruits of Indo-Burma hot spot, Meghalaya, north-east India: ethno-medicinal evaluation, socio-economic importance and conservation strategies. *Genet. Resour. Crop. Evol.* 63(2), 289–304.

12. Kanjilal, U. N., Kanjilal, P. C., Das, A., De, R. N., & Bor, N. L. (1940). Flora of Assam. Vols. 1–5. Shillong.

13. Mailly, D., Christanty, L., & Kinunins, J. P. (1997). 'Without bamboo, the land dies': nutrient cycling and biogeochemistry of a Javanese bamboo *tahn-kebun* system. *Forest Ecol Manage 91*, 155–173

14. Myers, N., Mittermeier, R. A., Mittermeier, C. G., da Fonseca, G. A. B., & Kent J. (2000) Biodiversity hotspots for conservation priorities. *Nature 203*, 853–858.

15. Namsa, N. D., Mandal, M., Tangjang, S., & Mandal, S. C. (2011). Ethnobotany of the Monpa ethnic group at Arunachal Pradesh, India. *J Ethnobiol Ethnomed* http://www.ethnobiomed.com/content/7/1/31

16. Nath, A. J., Lal. R., & Das, A. K. (2015). Ethnopedology and soil quality of bamboo (*Bambusa* sp.) based agroforestry system. *Science of the Total Environment 521–522*, 372–379.

17. Paul, A., Khan, M. L., & Das, A. K. (2010). Utilization of Rhododendrons by Monpas in Western Arunachal Pradesh, India. *J. Amer. Rhododendron Soc.* 81–84.

18. Pfoze, N. L., Kehie, M., Kayang, H., & A Mao, A. (2014). Estimation of Ethnobotanical Plants of the Naga of North East India. *J. Medicinal Plants Studies. 2 (3)*, 92–104.

19. Pradhan, U. C., & Lachungpa, S. T. (1990). Sikkim-Himalayan Rhododendrons. Primulaceae books, Kalingpong.

20. Rai, P. K. (2009). Comparative Assessment of soil properties after Bamboo flowering and death in a Tropical forest of Indo-Burma Hot spot. *Ambio 38(2)*, 118–120.

21. Rai, P. K. (2015). Environmental Issues and Sustainable Development of North East India. Lambert Publisher, Germany.

22. Rao, K. S., & Ramakrishnan, P. S. (1989). Role of bamboos in nutrient conservation during secondary succession following slash and burn agriculture (jhum) in north-east India. *J Appl Ecol 26*, 625–633

23. Rocky, R. L. (2013). Tribes and Tribal Studies in North East: Deconstructing the Philosophy of Colonial Methodology. *J. Tribal Intellectual Collective India. 1(2)*, 25–37.

24. Sahoo, U. K., Lalremruata, J., Jeeceelee, L., Lalremruati, J. H., Lalliankhuma, C., & Lalramnghinglova, H. (2010). Utilization of Non timber forest products by the tribal around Dampa tiger reserve in Mizoram. *The Bioscan 3*, 721–729.

25. Singh, A. N., & Singh, J. S. (1999). Biomass, net primary production and impact of bamboo plantation on soil redevelopment in a dry tropical region. *For Ecol Manage 119*, 195–207

26. Singh, H. B., Puni, L., Jain, A., Singh, R. S., & Rao, P. G. (2004). Status, utility, threats and conservation options for rattan resources in Manipur. *Current Sci. 87(1)*, 90–94.

27. Singh, N. R., Yaipabha, N., David, T., Babita, R. K., Devi, C. B., & Singh, N. R. (2009). Traditional knowledge and natural dyeing system of Manipur – with special reference to Kum dye. *Indian J. Trad. Knowl. 8(1)*, 84–88.

28. Sundriyal, M., Sundriyal, R. C., Sharma, E., & Purohit, A. N. (1998). Wild edible and other usefulplants from the Sikkim Himalaya, India. *Oecologia Montana 7*, 43–54.

29. Tag, H., Das, A. K., & Kalita, P. (2005). Plants used by the Hill Miri tribe of Arunachal Pradesh in ethnofisheries. *Indian J. Trad. Knowl 4*, 57–64.

30. Takahashi, M., Furusawa, H., Limtong, P., Sunanthapongsuk, V., Marod, D., & Panuthai, S. (2007). Soil nutrient status after bamboo flowering and death in a seasonal tropical forest in western Thailand. *Ecol Res 22*, 160–164.

31. Teron, R., & Borthakur, S. K. (2010). Traditional knowledge of herbal dyes and cultural significance of colors among the Krbis ethnic tribe in Northeast India. *Ethnobotany Research& Applications 10*, 593–603.

32. Thomas, S., & Haridasan, K. (1999). Rattans – the prickly palms. *Arunachal Forest News, 17*, 26–28.

33. WinklerPrins, A., & Sandor, J. A., 2003. Local soil knowledge: insights, applications, and challenges. *Geoderma 111*, 165–170.

CHAPTER 7

ETHNOVETERINARY PRACTICES IN NORTHEAST INDIA AND ANDAMANS

BIPUL SAIKIA

Department of Botany, Chaiduar College, Gohpur – 784168, Sonitpur, Assam, E-mail: bipul_sai@yahoo.com

CONTENTS

Abstract 177

7.1 Introduction 178

7.2 Ancient India 180

7.3 Ethnoveterinary Medicine 181

7.4 Prospects of Ethnoveterinary Medicine 184

7.5 Plants 185

7.6 Conclusion 186

Keywords 203

References 203

ABSTRACT

The relationship of plant and man is as old as humanity. Traditional herbal drugs used for controlling diseases of human is more practiced since long time probably dating back to 4000–5000 B.C. of Rig Veda. Man has utilized plants and animals to produce drugs for treating illnesses and injuries since ancient times. Domestication of wild species has gradually changed the way of livelihood of human beings. It leads to the development of agriculture, transport and food systems together with construct the traditional folk knowledge which was later transformed to the integral part of social tradition and culture. Ethnoveterinary practices concern to animal healthcare is as old as the domestication of various livestock species. According to the World Health Organization, at least 80% of people in developing countries depend largely on traditional practices of various diseases of both animals and humans. These traditional healing practices of animal health care are called 'ethnoveterinary medicine'. The age old practice of shifting cultivation particularly in northern region and the north east helped people to learn more about the plant species especially among tribals. The systems consist of myth, faith, belief, knowledge, practices and skills pertaining to healthcare and management of livestock. The ethnoveterinary health practice in India is a old system and acquired knowledge of the products for centuries of experiences. Presently domestic traditional cattle nurture practices are drastically cut down in rural areas because of lack of livestock keepers and mind changes of younger generations due to their modern life style. In spite of the uses of allopathic medicine in larger extent, all the traditional healers of remote areas are aware about the use of traditional medicines for different purposes.

The aim of this review article is to emphasize the ethno-veterinary health management practices found amongst livestock producers in northeast India and Andaman. The present review pooled information on uses of ethno-veterinary medicine in animal health care and will provide useful information regarding diverse uses and practices. The present review will help to understand the knowledge on EVM uses, promote awareness, provide information for researchers, conservation of sociocultural practices and species and help to find out active biological compounds.

7.1   INTRODUCTION

The study of ethnosciences started in the middle of the last century and workers in several areas began to incorporate the term "ethno" (indicate race, people or culture) into their scientific repertoire, such as in ethno-botany, ethnozoology, ethnoveterinary, etc. Mathias (2001) emphasized that this knowledge is acquired by communities over many years on the basis of exhaustive trial and error and deliberate experimentation. It is a part of a community- based approach and provides basic veterinary treatment for domestic animals in the rural area. Ethnoveterinary medicine was practiced as early as 1800 B.C. at the time of King Hamurabi of Babylon who formulated laws on veterinary fees and charged for treating cattle and donkeys (Schillhorn Van Veen, 1996).

India has one of the sophisticated medical cultures with a tradition of over 5000 years. The livestock owners in India have been using traditional medication based on plant formulations since time immemorial. Livestock raisers and healers everywhere have traditional ways of classifying, diagnosing, preventing and treating common animal diseases. The ethnoveterinary systems differ among ethnic communities because of religion, tribes and types of animals they rear and ecological factors. Due to gradual disappearing of information, the extensive documenting on ethnoveterinary medicines arose in the early 1980s. Later on numerous works have been done and presented in various seminars, conferences and workshops. India is a country rich in biological diversity. According to Misra and Kumar (2004), EVM is the community-based local or indigenous knowledge and methods of caring for healing and managing livestock. This also includes social practices and the ways in which livestock are incorporated into farming systems. Verma and Singh (2009) reported that medicinal herbs as potential sources of therapeutics aids have attained a significant role in health system all over the world for both humans and animals not only in the diseased condition but also as potential material for maintaining proper health. Balaji and Chakravarthi (2010) stated that Ethnoveterinary information is facing extinction because of the current rapid changes in communities across the world and around 75% world population depends on medicine obtained from plants. So far, more than 100,000 biologically active compounds (phenols, flavonoids, quinines, etc.) have been isolated from higher plants.

In spite of various work progress in the use of EVM, knowledge is still kept in documentation records and more work has to be done in future for popularization among younger generation, maintaining proper health system and scientific publications.

7.2 ANCIENT INDIA

Ancient Indian culture stands for treasure of documents of ethnobiological uses. "Domestication of dogs, buffaloes, elephants and fowls occurred in India between 6000 and 4500 B.C. Strong archaeological evidence is available for existence of an advanced civilization in Mohenjo-daro, Harappa (now in Pakistan) and certain other places in northeastern India around 2500 B.C. The people of these civilizations had humped and hump less cows, buffaloes, elephants, goats, fowl, etc. Cattle husbandry was well developed during the Rigvedic period 1500–1000 B.C. (Somvanshi, 2006).

The old great literature like Vedas (*Rigveda, Yajuraveda, Samveda* and *Atharvaveda) Upanishads, Puranas, Brahamanas* and epics like *Ramayana* and *Mahabharata,* etc. had some indications of plants and its uses for both man and animal. According to the study of D. N. Sharma, Emeritus scientists, HP, "there had been evidence on the existence of literature on veterinary science in Rigveda (2000–4000 B.C.), when the physician attended upon humans and animals indiscriminately. Asvini Kumars (Pashu-Chikitsa) are considered to be the physicians of the Gods. There are mentions about the surgical and therapeutic skills of the Asvini Kumars and they did miracles and could replace the head of a man with that horse. Dadhichi has acquired this knowledge from Lord Indra. The nucleus of veterinary science *(Pashu Ayurveda)* existed in *Atharvaveda* it is a repository of therapeutic hints and prescriptions to attain the longevity of man's life up to hundred years, i.e., *Jigivisheth Shatum Samaha* (Yayurveveda, XL, 2)." The earliest available works on elephantology were *Hasti-Ayurveda* and the *Gajasastra.* The four ways were mentioned in *Atharvaveda* are: the drugs of angirasas (juices of plants and herbs), the drugs of the *Atharvans* (a part of the mantra therapy) and the divine drugs in the form of prayers and mental yoga.

The veterinary science has been mentioned in *Charaka, Sushruta, Harita samhita, Gau-Ayurveda, Brahmananda Purana, Skanda Purana,*

Devi Purana, Matsya Purana, Agni Purana, Garuda Purana, Linga Purana, Vayu Purana, Haya-Ayurveda, Asva-Chikitsa, Nakul Samhita, etc. Salihotra the oldest and the greatest veterinarians we ever had composed three texts in Sanskrit. He was the father of veterinary science followed by Palkapya and Atreya. During Vedic (1000–600 B.C.), Buddhist (600 B.C.), Magadha (400 B.C.), Gupta dynasty (300–550 A.D.), *Skandagupta* (455–467 A.D.), *Kannauj* empire (606–647 A.D.), *Mauryan* age (322–232 B.C.), King Ashoka (established veterinary hospitals probably the first ever in the world in 300 B.C.) animal husbandry work was done for different purposes.

"Hindus were pioneers in the use of snake venom in medicine were mentioned in *Rasa Granthas* (mercury and snake venom), Somvanshi (2006). It is known from the report of Indian history of ethnoveterinary practices that Panchgavya or cow therapy is a holistic approach of treatment mentioned in the holy Vedas. It means five products from cows including milk, curd, ghee, urine and dung. They are known for remedial values when consumed or applied externally or sprayed in the environment. Scientific evaluation of these elements revealed individually or collectively that they enhance the immune responses of the body when used. The Kamdhenu Ark prepared from cow urine is effective in treatment of kidney disorders and diabetes mellitus. It has also been found to increase phagocytosis by macrophages and thus helpful in prevention and control of bacterial infections. The cow urine has antioxidant property and protects DNA damage due to mitomycin-C induced chromosomal aberrations. In Ayurveda, the cow urine is also termed as 'Sanjivani'.

7.3 ETHNOVETERINARY MEDICINE

The northeastern region of India is a treasure of indigenous knowledge systems pertaining to agriculture, food, medicine and natural resources management (Mathias). The region has over 100 tribes and communities, each having their unique ethnic foods developed through the ages. Kanjilal et al. (1938) recorded some ethnomedicinal and ethnoveterinary uses of plants from Assam in their book "Flora of Assam." Borthakur and Sharma (1996) studied ethnoveterinary medicine with special reference to prevalent among the Nepalese of Assam. The most important contribution to Indian ethnoveterinary medicine was done by Jain (1999) in his book "Dictionary of Ethnoveterinary plants of India." This book includes 783 plant species for different ailments. He recorded about 92 species belongs to Fabaceae followed by 37 in Asteraceae and 32 in Euphorbiaceae. Sapkota and Sharma (2000) studied ethnoveterinary practices among the Nepalese dwellers of Assam. Jain and Srivastava (2001) presented paper on prospects of herbal drugs for ethnoveterinary practices (EVP) in northeast India. Sapkota and Sharma (2003) studied 35 numbers of herbal medicines that are used to treat various diseases by different ethnic groups of people of Dhemaji and Jonai Sub-Division and confirm the dosage of the herbs before these are commercially exploited. Pradhan and Badola (2008) recorded ethnomedicinal plants used for man and animals by Lepcha tribe of Dzongu valley bordering Khangchendzonga Biosphere Reserve, in North Sikkim. Saikia et al. (2010) presented a paper on utilization of plants with reference to ethno-veterinary herbal medicines of Sonitpur district which included 25 plant species of the district. Saikia and Borthakur (2010) studied the use of medicinal plants in animal healthcare from Gohpur, Assam which included 20 plant species of this region. Lalramnghinglova (2011) studied 45 plant species used in veterinary diseases from Mizoram. In the book "Ethnoveterinary Plants of North East India" (Sharma, 2012), about 300 veterinary medicinal plant species under 80 families have been described. Fifty one different animal ailments have been identified and described. These diseases are treated by different medicinal plants based on the traditional knowledge of different tribes in this remote part of the country. Salam et al. (2013) reported 32 plant species used in veterinary diseases from Manipur.

Khatoon et al. (2013) studied ethnoveterinary plants used by Kom tribe of Manipur. Bharati and Sharma (2013) studied the use of 37 medicinal plants from Sikkim to treat ailments in animals such as diarrhea, dysentery, digestive disorders, injury, wound, fever, maternity complications, skin disease, urinary problems, cough and cold, skeleto-muscular disorders, inflammation, scorpion sting, snake and insect bite, weakness, parasite, ulcer and bleeding. Twelve medicinal plants being used in Sikkim Himalayas have not been documented in ethnoveterinary medicine elsewhere in the world. Fifteen plant species were found to contain previously unreported medicinal properties. Maiti et al. (2013) studied the ethnoveterinary medicine of Monpa tribe of Arunachal Pradesh, who used different ethno-veterinary practices applicable against the ephemeral fever of high altitude yak (*Poephagus grunniens* L.). It is found that the Monpas are using seven ethnoveterinary practices against ephemeral fever, of which *Thalictrum foliolosum* is found to be most significant. Rajkumari et al. (2014) studied the ethnoveterinary plants associated with this particular tribe by collecting 36 plant species and genera belonging to 29 families used for treating as many as 17 ailments of domestic animals (cows, dogs, buffaloes, pigs, etc.). These have been documented based on ethnoveterinary surveys (PRA and interview-questionnaire methods). Laskar et al. (2015) studied the ethnoveterinary uses of plants by the Halam tribe of Hailakandi district of Southern Assam. Thirty ethnoveterinary important medicinal plants belonging to 23 families were recorded in the study area with the help of ethnoveterinary traditional healers. Among the plant parts used by the selected tribe, leaves, flower, fruit, bark, bulb, rhizome, roots are most commonly used for the preparation of medicine for the treatment of domestic animals. The Asteraceae family is found to be the most often used.

People of Andaman villages are depending on farming and animal husbandry. Pigs are the sign of wealth and status among Nicobarese and hence lot of care is taken for its rearing and they are fed with the coconut regularly and almost one third of the total produce is reserved for feeding their pigs (Prasad, 2014). He also highlighted the traditional ethnoveterinary practices of the Nicobarese of Katchal Island and with the socio- cultural practices for the well being of livestock. Sunder et al. (2014) studied and document 41 ethnoveterinary medicinal plants of 27 families from the different villages of South and North Andaman districts of Andaman & Nicobar Islands. Raikwar and Prabhakar (2015) stressed the importance of ethnoveterinary medicinal plants in India and listed 32 ethnoveterinary medicinal plants.

Namsa et al. (2011) reported that a few plants were used to improve the health state and growth of livestocks. The leaves of *Cannabis sativa* were given to the cattle and goat to cure dysentery and diarrhea (These diseases were identified by the presence of watery stool and blood). The stem of wild *Musa paradisiaca* L., was regularly given to cattle particularly during pregnancy to enhance the yield of milk. A paste powder obtained from the whole plant of *Plantago major* and *Ageratum conyzoides* are commonly tied to the affected portions of cattle and goat to relieve from severe pain and inflammations. *Gymnocladus assamicus* ripe pods are soaked in water and used as disinfectant for cleaning wounds and parasites like leeches and lice on the skin of livestocks. The fully ripe pods soaked in water are used as soap for bathing because it does not cause harm to soft skin and burning sensation to eyes. Leaves are used as green manure in agricultural field crops. *Gymnocladus assamicus* is a critically rare and endangered plant species and also endemic to the north-eastern region of India.

The EVM knowledge has been developed through trial and error and deliberate experimentation. In India, ethnoveterinary medicine has seen increasing recognition as a distinct area of study since the publication of books and research articles.

7.4   PROSPECTS OF ETHNOVETERINARY MEDICINE

According to the World Health Organization, at least 80% of people in developing countries depend largely on indigenous practices for the control and treatment of various diseases affecting both human beings and their animals (Balaji and Chakravarthi, 2010). These traditional healing practices are called 'ethnoveterinary medicine'. Ethnoveterinary medicine is cost effective and also dynamic (Warren, 1991). Mathias (2010) stated that the application of ethnoveterinary medicines are accepted by the people due to increasing resistance of microorganisms to antibiotics and other chemical drugs. Ethnoveterinary medicines are easily available, easy to prepare and to administer. These age-old customs cover all parts of the world, especially on domestic animal species. The World Health Organization (WHO) defines traditional medicine (herbal medicine) as "the sum total of the knowledge, skills, and practices based on the theories, beliefs, and experiences indigenous to different cultures, whether explicable or not, used in the maintenance of health as well as in the prevention, diagnosis, improvement or treatment of physical and mental illness." Indian Pharmacopoeia (IP) is an official regulatory document meant for overall quality control and assurance of pharmaceutical products marketed in India and thus, contributing to the safety, efficacy, and affordability of medicines (Rastogi et al., 2015). They also stated that the medicinal plants for various animal diseases in different parts of India are compiled in IP 2014 also, the official statuses of the herbs in the British Pharmacopoeia (BP) 2014 and the United States Pharmacopoeia (USP).

Though, ethnoveterinary medicine is now in threat of extinction due to modern development and changes of people mind-sets, various efforts have been taken to standardized the system in every part of the world to continue and conserve the social and commercial ethics of the society. Encouraging the conservation and use of ethnoveterinary medicine does not mean declining the value of modern system of medicine. Hence, the ethnoveterinary medicine has sustainable profit by means of conservation of species, practices and detection of bioactive compounds towards the benefits of society and environment.

7.5 PLANTS

Plants are the most commonly used ingredients in the preparation of EVM. Leaves, bark, fruits, flowers, seeds, roots are used in medicinal preparations. It is known that at present over 35,000 plants are known to have medicinal values. At least 1,00,000 species of plants are used by humans for as food, medicine, fiber, fuel, oils, shelter, poisons, intoxicants, ornamentals and other purposes. By virtue of specialized biochemical capabilities, plants synthesize and accumulate a vast array of primary and secondary metabolites/chemicals. Thirty five percent veterinary western medicines are phytic in origin (Balaji and Chakravarthi, 2010). Besides secondary metabolites "certain organic acids and polyacetylenes are also known to exist" (Cotton, 1996).

EVM is easily assessable, cost effective effortlessly manage and generally administered topically or orally. But the people are conservative for sharing their knowledge. Hence the scope of further dissemination is inadequate. The effective dosages, symptoms, success depends on experience but not always perfect. Technically all preparations are not totally effective. EVM has little or nothing to offer against the acute viral diseases of animals. New generations are not fully alert for uses of EVM. Deforestation and exploitation are the other causes of habitat loss and decrease of important EVM species.

7.6   CONCLUSION

North Eastern region of India is a rich center of bioresources. Tribals are the dominant groups related with the uses of species for medicinal practices. Traditional knowledge of practice itself is an old-age system and mostly dominated by plant species for its medicinal values. From Kashmir to Kanyakumari and from Rajasthan to Sikkim and northeast, there is no state which does not have its own traditional medicinal practices. Besides maximum application of modern allopathic medicines, the traditional herbal practices are still alive among the tribal and rural people and needs special attention to safeguard the traditional knowledge. Ayurveda, Unani, Siddha, etc. are the earliest medical systems known in India. The Mishing, Bodo, Karbi, Assamese, Nepali, etc., are the communities of Assam have a unique medicinal system of their own. The Lotha-Naga tribes inhabited the hilly tracts of Nagaland are known for curing many ailments using locally grown herbs. The "lekok" plant found in Nagaland is known for its astringent and digestive properties. The Khasis make a herbal concoction called "Ka Dawai Niangsohpetto" eliminate the germs from the body. The people of Meghalaya and Arunachal Pradesh have exceptional medicinal system. In Andaman pig "*Ha-un*" is mostly raring by people. Some species like *Bambusa spinosa*, *Cissus quadrangularis*, *Lagenaria leucantha*, *Nicotiana tabacum* are reported for various ethnoveterinary uses. The knowledge of medicinal plants has true value for research and the discovery of new drugs to cure the diseases of animals. The scientific study for phytochemical screening is considered as much needed effort to protect and conserve under IPR rule.

Ethnoveterinary medicinal plants of Northeast India and Andaman and Nicobar Islands are listed in Table 7.1.

TABLE 7.1 Some Ethnoveterinary Plants of Northeast and Andamans

Scientific name	Disease and plant parts	References
Abelmoschus moschatus (L.) Medic.	Diuretic – seeds, roots	Sharma and Sapcota, 2003
Abies densa Griff.	Appetizer – leaves	Bharati and Sharma, 2012
Abrus fruticulous Wall. ex Wt. & Arn.	Cough – roots	Sharma and Sapcota, 2003
Acacia catechu (L. f.) Willd.	Dysentery – leaves; foot diseases – leaves	Sharma and Sapcota, 2003; Sunder et al., 2014
Achras sapota L.	Diarrhea in cattle – fruits	Sunder et al., 2014
Achyranthes aspera L.	Galactagogue – young shoots/ worm (pig & goat) – leaves	Rajkumari et al., 2014; Lalramnghinglova, 2011
Acorus calamas L.	Dyspepsia/indigestion/appetizer, indigestion and wound – rhizome/diarrhea in cattle – rhizome	Sharma and Sapcota, 2003; Saikia et al., 2010; Jain and Srivastava, 1999; Bharati and Sharma, 2012; Sunder et al., 2014
Adhatoda vasica (L.) Nees.	Diarrhea – leaves	Sunder et al., 2014
Adiantum philippense L.	Delivery – Rhizome	Laskar et al., 2015
Aegle marmelos (L.) Correa	Dysentery/injury/to cure diarrhea, increase the body weight and milk production – fruit	Sharma and Sapcota, 2003; Borthakur and Sarma, 1996; Sunder et al., 2014
Agave americana L.	Bone fracture	Rajkumari et al., 2014
Ageratum conyzoides L.	Sore on legs and toes – leaves	Lalramnghinglova, 2011
Alangium chinense (Lour.) Harms.	Dog – or jackal – bite – roots	Sharma and Sapcota, 2003
Allium cepa L.	Cough/insect bite – bulbs	Sharma and Sapcota, 2003; Borthakur and Sarma, 1996; Saikia and Borthakur, 2010
Allium sativum L.	Foot diseases/Indigestion – rhizome with ginger	Saikia et al., 2010; Saikia and Borthakur, 2010
Allium tuberosum Roxb.	Whopping cough – bulbs	Sharma and Sapcota, 2003
Aloe barbadensis Mill.	Chronic diarrhea and dysentery/ burn – leaves/maggot – leaves	Sharma and Sapcota, 2003; Borthakur and Sarma, 1996; Salam et al., 2013

TABLE 7.1   (Continued)

Scientific name	Disease and plant parts	References
Aloe vera (L.) Burm. f.	Burns on skin – leaves	Rajkumari et al., 2014
Alstonia scholaris (L.) R. Br.	Skin/Restorative – bark/wound and sores of pig – bark	Laskar et al., 2015; Borthakur and Sarma, 1996; Lalramnghinglova, 2011
Alternanthera ficoidea R. Br.	Inflamed lymph nodes	Sharma and Sapcota, 2003
Alternanthera sessilis (L.) R. Br. ex DC.	Ulcer – whole plants	Borthakur and Sarma, 1996
Amaranthus gangeticus L.	Health tonic – whole plants/ roots	Sharma and Sapcota, 2003
Amomum subulatum Roxb.	Inflammation of the eye and insect bites – seed/urinary infection in cattle – roots	Bharati and Sharma, 2012
Ampelocissus sikkimensis (Laws.) Planch.	Sores in mouth and tongue and treats foot and mouth disease in cattle	Pradhan and Kodla, 2008
Andrograpis paniculata Nees.	Fever – leaves	Laskar et al., 2015
Annona squamosa L.	Ectoparasite – leaves	Saikia and Borthakur, 2010
Antidesma acidum Retz.	Dysentery – root and leaves	Sharma and Sapcota, 2003
Aralia species	Bodyache and joints pain – roots	Maiti et al., 2013
Arachis hypogaea L.	To increase the milk production and body weight – leaves	Sunder et al., 2014
Areca catechu L.	Endoparasite	Rajkumari et al., 2014
Aristolochia indica L.	Fever – leaves	Saikia et al., 2010
Artemisia maritima L.	Diarrhea – leaves	Salam et al., 2013
Artemisia nilagirica C. B. Clarke.	Dermatitis	Rajkumari et al., 2014
Artemisia vulgaris L.	Treat itching and stop nose bleeding – leaves/sore, worm and internal bleeding – leaves	Bharati and Sharma, 2012; Lalramnghinglova, 2011
Artocarpus heterophyllus Lam.	Diarrhea – roots part	Sharma and Sapcota, 2003

TABLE 7.1 (Continued)

Scientific name	Disease and plant parts	References
Arundinaria maling Gamble	Ringworm –root paste; dysentery – leaves	Bharati and Sharma, 2012
Asparagus racemosus Willd.	Increase milk mixed with hay or grain – roots	Bharati and Sharma, 2012
Asparagus officinalis L.	Cough and cold – rhizome	Salam et al., 2013
Azadirachta indica A. Juss.	Constipation – leaf and fruit/ removal of insects/To cure stomachache, cure in cut and wounds, abscess and broken horn, remove insects from the eyes and to control flies nuisance – leaves/cough – leaves	Sharma and Sapcota, 2003; Borthakur and Sarma, 1996; Rajkumari et al., 2014; Sunder et al., 2014; Salam et al., 2013
Bambusa balcooa Roxb.	Stop bleeding – rhizome	Saikia et al., 2010
Bambusa tulda Roxb.	Removal placenta – leaves	Borthakur and Sarma, 1996; Rajkumari et al., 2014
Bambusa spinosa Roxb.	To kill ectoparasites, diarrhea, retention of placenta, tongue sore, appetizer, digestion, cure the stomach problem and fever – leaves	Sunder et al., 2014
Basella alba L.	Cuts and wounds	Rajkumari et al., 2014
Bauhinia racemosa Lamk.	Heal redness of eye – leaf juice	Sunder et al., 2014
Bauhinia variegata L.	Diarrhea and dysentery – fresh flowers and bark/to treat blindness, to wash and cure wounds in foot and mouth, expel the placenta – bark and root	Bharati and Sharma, 2012; Sunder et al., 2014
Bergenia ciliata Sternb.	Dysentery – roots	Bharati and Sharma, 2012
Bixa orellana L.	Intermittent fever – seeds	Sharma and Sapcota, 2003
Blumea lanceolaria (Roxb.) Druce	Sore and wound for dog and worm – leaves	Lalramnghinglova, 2011
Butea superba Roxb.	Snakebites – root	Lalramnghinglova, 2011
Bombax ceiba (L.) Sw.	Dog – bite/parturition – bark	Laskar et al., 2015; Sharma and Sapcota, 2003; Borthakur and Sarma, 1996

TABLE 7.1 (Continued)

Scientific name	Disease and plant parts	References
Brassica campestris L.	Yoke gall – leaves	Rajkumari et al., 2014
Brassica nigra L.& turmeric	Mischief – rhizome	Saikia and Borthakur, 2010
Bryophylum pinnatum (Lam.) Oken	Indigestion in goat – leaves	Sunder et al., 2014
Cajanus cajan (L.) Millsp.	Appetite – leaves	Salam et al., 2013
Calotropis gigantea (L.) R. Br.	Fracture – leaves/treat hump sore – latex/Sprain – leaves/ sickness – latex/skin – leaves	Laskar et al., 2015; Sharma and Sapcota, 2003; Borthakur and Sarma, 1996; Sunder et al., 2014; Lalramnghinglova, 2011
Cannabis sativa L.	Carminative – leaves and seeds/ tonic and inflammation – stem/ diarrhea – leaves/leaves given to cattle in flatulence/strengthens animals and worm – leaves/ fever – leaves	Sharma and Sapcota, 2003; Bharati and Sharma, 2012; Rajkumari et al., 2014; Lalramnghinglova, 2011; Salam et al., 2013
Canavalia gladiata (Jacq.) DC.	Anthrax –fruits	Sharma and Sapcota, 2003
Capsicum frutescens L.	Boils – fruits	Saikia and Borthakur, 2010
Carica papaya L.	Cure fever in goat – fruit, seeds and roots	Sunder et al., 2014
Cassia alata L.	Asthma – flower	Laskar et al., 2015
Cassia fistula L.	Anthrax – fruit/constipation/ dysentery – leaves	Sharma and Sapcota, 2003; Rajkumari et al., 2014; Salam et al., 2013
Cassia hirsuta L.	Snakebites of animal and human – leaves and roots	Lalramnghinglova, 2011
Cassia occidentalis L.	Skin infection – leaves	Laskar et al., 2015
Centella asiatica (L.) Urb.	Ulcer/diarrhea and dysentery – whole plants	Borthakur and Sarma, 1996; Rajkumari et al., 2014; Sunder et al., 2014
Celastrus paniculatus Willd.	Urinary disorders – whole plants	Bharati and Sharma, 2012
Chenopodium album L.	Dysentery – whole plants	Salam et al., 2013

TABLE 7.1 (Continued)

Scientific name	Disease and plant parts	References
Christella parasitica (L.) H.Lev.	Snake bite/pain –fronds	Saikia et al., 2010; Saikia and Borthakur, 2010
Chromolaena odorata (Linn.) R. M. King & H. Robinson	Injured part – leaves	Prasad, 2014
Cinnamomum tamala L.	Diarrhea – leaves	Laskar et al., 2015
Cissampelos pareira L.	Insect bite and scorpion sting and blood in urine – root	Bharati and Sharma, 2012
Cissus adnata Roxb.	Bone fracture – stem	Rajkumari et al., 2014
Cissus quadrangularis L.	Fracture/bone fracture, increase the body weight and milk production and as dewormer – stem	Laskar et al., 2015; Sunder et al., 2014
Citrus aurintifolia (Christm.) Swingle	Dysentery – fruit/mucus in the feces/relive stomachache in cattle – fruits	Saikia et al., 2010; Saikia and Borthakur, 2010
Citrus limon (L.) Burm. f.	Bloat – fruit	Rajkumari et al., 2014
Clerodendrum infortunatum L.	Wounds of pig – leaves	Lalramnghinglova, 2011
Clerodendrum serratum (L.). Moon.	Vitiated – roots	Sharma and Sapcota, 2003
Cocos nucifera L.	To increase the milk production and body weight, cure wound – fruit oil	Sunder et al., 2014
Congea tomentosa Roxb,	Worm, wounds and sores – leaves	Lalramnghinglova, 2011
Colocasia antiquorum var. *esculenta* L.	Rhizomes are used to stimulate lactation in cows/sore, hardening and diarrhea – stem	Sunder et al., 2014
Costus specious (J. Koing) Sm.	Foot mouth diseases – rhizome/inflammation – rhizome	Saikia et al., 2010; Bharati and Sharma, 2012
Crinum asiaticum L.	Diuretic/indigestion – bulb	Sharma and Sapcota, 2003; Saikia et al., 2010
Croton caudatus Geisl.	Worm, sores ulcers – leaves	Lalramnghinglova, 2011

TABLE 7.1   (Continued)

Scientific name	Disease and plant parts	References
Curcuma domestica Val./*Curcuma longa* L.	Stomach pain–rhizome Mastitis–rhizome/wound, ulcers and sores – rhizome/bone fracture – rhizome	Prasad, 2014 Rajkumari et al., 2014; Lalramnghinglova, 2011; Salam et al., 2013
Curcuma minor King	Snakebites–rhizome	Lalramnghinglova, 2011
Cucumis sativus L.	Swallowed leech – fruits/appetite – leaves	Saikia and Borthakur, 2010; Salam et al., 2013
Cucurbita maxima Duchesne	Endoparasite/wounds of dog – fresh fruit	Rajkumari et al., 2014; Salam et al., 2013
Curculigo orchioides Gaertn.	Cough and fever – root	Sharma and Sapcota, 2003
Curculigo crassifolia (Baker) Hook.f.	Wounds, cuts and snake bites – rootstock	Lalramnghinglova, 2011
Curcuma angustifolia Salisbury	Injured by leech – rhizome	Saikia and Borthakur, 2010
Curcuma aromatica Salisbury	Scabies – rhizome	Sharma and Sapcota, 2003
Curcuma caesia Roxb.	Dysentery – rhizome	Saikia and Borthakur, 2010
Cynodon dactylon (L.) Pers.	Dyspepsia, wound – rhizome/hematuria	Borthakur and Sarma, 1996; Sunder et al., 2014; Saikia and Borthakur, 2010
Dalbergia sissoo Roxb.	Diarrhea	Borthakur and Sarma, 1996
Daphne cannabina Wall.	Baby goats during diarrhea and fever – leaves	Pradhan and Kodla, 2008
Datura metel L.	Dysentery – fruit/rabies/skin diseases, insect bite, tick infection and mastitis – twigs	Laskar et al., 2015; Saikia and Borthakur, 2010; Sunder et al., 2014
Datura stramonium L.	Maggot – leaves	Salam et al., 2013
Dillenia indica L.	Diarrhea of dogs – stem bark	Lalramnghinglova, 2011
Dillenia pentagyna Roxb.	Cough and sickness of pig – dried roots	Lalramnghinglova, 2011
Diplazium esculentum (Retz.) Sw.	Cuts & wounds – roots	Laskar et al., 2015
Drymaria cordata (L.) Willd. ex Roem. & Schult.	Fractured bone and mouth ulcer – plant paste/constipation – plant paste	Bharati and Sharma, 2012; Rajkumari et al., 2014

TABLE 7.1   (Continued)

Scientific name	Disease and plant parts	References
Eclipta alba L.	To improve body weight and milk production – whole plants	Sunder et al., 2014
Elatostema ficoides Wedd.	Fever – plant paste	Bharati and Sharma, 2012
Elsholtzia communis (Collett. & Hemsl.) Diels	Foot and mouth disease/snakebites	Rajkumari et al., 2014; Lalramnghinglova, 2011
Embelia ribes Burm. f.	Kill tapeworm – fruits	Bharati and Sharma, 2012
Enhydra fluctuans Lour.	Deworming – leaves	Sunder et al., 2014
Entada phaseoloides L.	Diarrhea, dysentery and appetizer – fruits and seeds	Sunder et al., 2014
Entada pursaetha DC.	Vermicide	Borthakur and Sarma, 1996
Entada scandens auct non Benth.	Dysentery and fever – bark	Salam et al., 2013
Equisetum debile Roxb. ex Vaucher	Stop bleeding – stem	Bharati and Sharma, 2012
Erythrina stricta Roxb.	Sores and worms – wood pieces	Lalramnghinglova, 2011
Erythrina variegata L.	Conjunctivitis – bark	Sharma and Sapcota, 2003
Euphorbia antiquorum L.	Wounds – latex	Salam et al., 2013
Ficus auriculata Lour.	Sores and ulcers – milky juice	Lalramnghinglova, 2011
Ficus cunia Buch.-Ham. ex. Roxb.	Maggot – latex	Salam et al., 2013
Ficus glomerata L., & *Foeniculum vulgare* Mill	Galactagogue – bark	Sharma and Sapcota, 2003
Ficus hispida L.	Rubbed on tongue to cure sore of cow and bullock – leaves	Saikia and Borthakur, 2010
Ficus racemosa L.	Retention of placenta	Rajkumari et al., 2014
Ficus semicordata Buch. Ham.ex Sm.	Snake bites – root	Lalramnghinglova, 2011
Flemingia strobilifera R.Br.	Flowering twigs – beaten to cure disease	Kanjilal et al., 1938

TABLE 7.1   (Continued)

Scientific name	Disease and plant parts	References
Fragaria nubicola (Hook. f.) Lindl. ex Lacaita	Diarrhea and dysentery – leaves and fruits	Bharati and Sharma, 2012
Ficus religiosa Roxb.	Constipation – bark	Sharma and Sapcota, 2003
Garcinia coronaria	Snakebites – roots	Lalramnghinglova, 2011
Garcinia cowa Roxb.	Dysentery – fruits	Saikia et al., 2010
Garcinia sopsopia (Buch.Ham) Mabb.	Wound of snake bites – bark and twigs	Lalramnghinglova, 2011
Gelsemium elegans Benth.	Mange, diarrhea, sickness and cough – root	Lalramnghinglova, 2011
Gynocardata odorata R. Br.	Poisonous to animal and fish poison – fruits, leaves and stem bark	Lalramnghinglova, 2011
Hibiscus rosa-sinensis L.	Scabies – leaves	Borthakur and Sarma, 1996
Hibiscus sabdariffa L.	Dysentery –leaves and fruit/ dysentery – leaves	Saikia and Borthakur, 2010; Salam et al., 2013
Hippeastrum puniceum (Lam.) Voss.	Gripping pain – bulb	Saikia et al., 2010
Holarrhena antidysenterica (L.) Wall. ex A. DC.	Scabies – bark/dysentery – bark	Borthakur and Sarma, 1996; Bharati and Sharma, 2012
Ilex umbrellulata Loes.	Sickness and mange of pig – stem bark	Lalramnghinglova, 2011
Ipomoea batatas (L.) Lam.	Improve milk production and body weight – leaves	Sunder et al., 2014
Jatropa curcus L.	Maggot/to treat constipation in cattle and goats – seeds	Rajkumari et al., 2014; Sunder et al., 2014
Juglans regia L.	Poison for fish, prawn and crab	Lalramnghinglova, 2011
Justicia adhatoda L., and *Curcuma longa* L.	Bronchitis – leaves	Sharma and Sapcota, 2003
Justicia gendarussa Burm. f.	Fever and cold – roots	Laskar et al., 2015
Lagenaria leucantha Rusby	Diarrhea, retention of placenta and hump sore – fruits and leaves	Sunder et al., 2014

TABLE 7.1 (Continued)

Scientific name	Disease and plant parts	References
Lepidagathis incurva F. Ham. ex. D. Don.	Leech bites – leaves	Lalramnghinglova, 2011
Leucas aspera (L.) Link.	Worms – leaves/pain – leaves	Laskar et al., 2015; Saikia et al., 2010
Lecanthus peduncularis (Wall. ex Royle) Wedd.	Cuts and wounds leaf paste	Bharati and Sharma, 2012
Lindernia ruellioides (Colms.) Penn.	Chicken bone setting and contraction of nerve – plant	Lalramnghinglova, 2011
Litchi chinensis Sonner	Animal bite – leaves	Lalramnghinglova, 2011
Litsea salicifolia Roxb. ex Nees.	Pain – leaves	Saikia et al., 2010
Luffa acutangula (L.) Roxb.	Cold and cough – fruits	Sunder et al., 2014
Lycopodium clavatum L.	Muscle contraction – plant	Bharati and Sharma, 2012
Mangifera indica L.	Constipation –fruit/dysentery, to expel placenta – fruit, seed and leaves.	Sharma and Sapcota, 2003; Sunder et al., 2014
Melia azedarach L.	Sprain/worms – leaves	Borthakur and Sarma, 1996; Salam et al., 2013
Mallotus philippinensis Muell.-Arg.	To kill intestinal worms and skin infection – seeds	Bharati and Sharma, 2012
Mentha spicata L	Removal placenta – paste/ Diarrhea and dysentery –whole plant/tonic – leaves	Borthakur and Sarma, 1996; Rajkumari et al., 2014; Salam et al., 2013
Mentha viridis L.	Fever –whole plants	Bharati and Sharma, 2012
Meyna laxiflora Robyns and *Acorus calamus* L.	Cough – seed/Diarrhea – fruit and rhizome	Sharma and Sapcota, 2003; Borthakur and Sarma, 1996
Mikania micrantha Kunth	Worms – leaves/cuts and wounds – leaves	Laskar et al., 2015; Lalramnghinglova, 2011
Millettia pachycarpa Benth.	Removal of insects from hair	Rajkumari et al., 2014
Millettia piscidia Wt.	Sores and worms – roots and fruits	Lalramnghinglova, 2011

TABLE 7.1   (Continued)

Scientific name	Disease and plant parts	References
Mimosa pudica L.	To improve weight and milk production – whole plants	Sunder et al., 2014
Momordica charantia L.	Diarrhea – fruits	Sunder et al., 2014
Moringa oleifera Lam.	Worms – root/wound, for good health and better lactation after delivery – leaves and stem bark	Laskar et al., 2015; Sunder et al., 2014
Musa spp	Snakebites and insect bites – juice	Lalramnghinglova, 2011
Musa balbisiana Colla	Placental discharge – leaves	Saikia et al., 2010
Musa paradisiaca L.	To cure diarrhea, snake bites, worms and blisters and hoof sore – whole plant/ constipation – petiole	Sunder et al., 2014; Salam et al., 2013
Mussaenda roxburghii Hk. f.	Snakebites – roots and stem bark	Lalramnghinglova, 2011
Nardostachys jatamansi DC.	Chronic fever and inflammation – leaves	Maiti et al., 2013
Nicotiana tabacum L.	Ectoparasite – leaves/broken horn, wound and tick infection – leaves	Saikia et al., 2010; Sunder et al., 2014
Ocimum gratissimum L.	Cold – leaves	Laskar et al., 2015
Oroxylum indicum (L.) Vent.	Fever and cough – root/ healing – bark	Laskar et al., 2015; Sharma and Sapcota, 2003
Oryza sativa L.	Retention of placenta and to let down milk – grains	Sunder et al., 2014
Paederia scandens L	Spleen – leaves/diarrhea and dysentery – leaves/dislocation of joints – leaves	Saikia and Borthakur, 2010; Rajkumari et al., 2014; Salam et al., 2013
Pasania spicata Qerst.	Blisters and sores – bark	Salam et al., 2013
Persicaria chinensis (L.) H. Gross	Maggot – leaves	Rajkumari et al., 2014
Phaseolus mungo L., & *Curcuma angustifolia* Roxb.	Skin – seeds	Saikia and Borthakur, 2010

TABLE 7.1   (Continued)

Scientific name	Disease and plant parts	References
Phyllanthus acidus Skeels	Skin – plant	Laskar et al., 2015
Phyllanthus niruri L.	To improve the body weight and milk	Sunder et al., 2014
Phytolacca acinosa Roxb.	Root – treating fever and joint pain.	Maiti et al., 2013
Picrasma javanica Blume	Increase cow milk, indigestion	Lalramnghinglova, 2011
Picrorhiza kurroa Royle ex Benth.	Cold, fever and appetizer. – root is mixed with stem bark of *Azadirachta indica*	Bharati and Sharma, 2012
Piper nigrum L.	Insect bites/snake bite – fruits	Saikia and Borthakur, 2010; Sunder et al., 2014
Plantago major L.	Healing – roots	Bharati and Sharma, 2012
Podocarpus neriifolius D. Don.	Centipede bites – bark	Lalramnghinglova, 2011
Polygonum strigosum R. Br.	Dysentery – bark	Saikia and Borthakur, 2010
Prunus armeniaca L.	Wounds – leaves	Salam et al., 2013
Prunus domestica L.	On maggot infested wounds – leaves	Saikia and Borthakur, 2010
Prunus persica (L.) Batsch.	Maggot kill/maggot and dysentery – leaves	Rajkumari et al., 2014; Salam et al., 2013
Psidium guajava L.	Diarrhea – leaves/dysentery – leaves	Laskar et al., 2015; Salam et al., 2013
Pterocephalus hookeri (C. B. Clarke) E. Pritzl.	Treatment of cough, chronic pain, gout and arthritis – whole plants	Maiti et al., 2013
Ranunculus sceleratus L.	Unconscious cattle – leaves	Salam et al., 2013
Rauvolfia serpentina (L.) Benth. ex Kurz.	Snake bite – bark	Bharati and Sharma, 2012
Rhododendron arboreum Sm.	Diarrhea and dysentery – flower	Bharati and Sharma, 2012
Rhus javanica L.	Diarrhea and dysentery – fruits	Salam et al., 2013
Ricinus communis L.	Foot ache – root/laxative – seeds/antipyretics/constipation – leaves	Laskar et al., 2015; Sharma and Sapcota, 2003; Borthakur and Sarma, 1996; Salam et al., 2013

TABLE 7.1   (Continued)

Scientific name	Disease and plant parts	References
Rubia cordifolia L.	Quick recovery in delivery – roots	Bharati and Sharma, 2012
Rubus ellipticus Sm.	Wound – young shoot/worm – shoots common cold and infectious fever	Bharati and Sharma, 2012; Salam et al., 2013; Maiti et al., 2013
Rubus idaeus L.	Fever, common cold, cough and lung diseases – stem	Maiti et al., 2013
Rumex maritimus L.	Dermatitis	Rajkumari et al., 2014
Saccharum officinarum L.	Remove placenta – Leaves	Laskar et al., 2015; Saikia and Borthakur, 2010; Rajkumari et al., 2014
Sapindus mukorossi Gaertn.	Leech bites, vermifuge/biocide – juice	Lalramnghinglova, 2011
Senecio scandens Buch.Ham. ex.D.Don.	Sores, ulcers, snakebites and worms – leaves	Lalramnghinglova, 2011
Schima wallichii Korth.	Sores, ulcers, snakebites and insect bites – bark	Lalramnghinglova, 2011
Scoparia dulcis L.	Snakebite, dog bite – roots	Laskar et al., 2015
Semecarpus anacardium L.f.	Antipyretic	Borthakur and Sarma, 1996
Swertia chirata (Roxb. ex Fleming) Karsten.	Deworming – fruits	Sunder et al., 2014
Sinopodophyllum hexandrum (Royle) T. S. Ying	Infection and indigestion – root and rhizome	Bharati and Sharma, 2012
Solanum kurzii L.	Mumps	Borthakur and Sarma, 1996
Spilanthes paniculata Wallich ex.DC.	Liver disorders – leaves	Laskar et al., 2015
Spondias pinnata (L.f.) Kurz.	Dysentery – bark	Laskar et al., 2015
Stephania hernandifolia Walp.	Water kept in bulbous root is sprinkled in the poultry farm to prevent from bird flu	Pradhan and Badola, 2008.
Sterculia villosa Roxb.	Dysentery – roots	Sharma and Sapcota, 2003
Sterculia urens Roxb.	Pleura – pneumonia – leaves	Lalramnghinglova, 2011

TABLE 7.1 (Continued)

Scientific name	Disease and plant parts	References
Streblus asper Lour.	Conjunctivitis –leaf and fruits	Sharma and Sapcota, 2003
Swertia chirata (Wall.) C. B. Clarke	Fever –fresh plant	Bharati and Sharma, 2012
Syzygium cumini (Duthie) N. P. Balakr.	Dysentery – bark/diarrhea – bark/Hematuria	Laskar et al., 2015; Borthakur and Sarma, 1996; Rajkumari et al., 2014
Tagetes patula L.	Cuts & wounds – leaves/ dyspepsia	Laskar et al., 2015; Borthakur and Sarma, 1996
Tamarindus indica L.	Applied to reduce wound swelling, Anorexia, flatulence, in muscle sprain, injury, mastitis and mouth ulcer – fruit leaves/ snakebites – seeds	Sunder et al., 2014; Lalramnghinglova, 2011
Terminalia arjuna (Roxb.) Wight &Arm.	Cold and fever – bark	Laskar et al., 2015
Terminalia bellirica (Gaertn.) Roxb.	Dysentery – fruits	Bharati and Sharma, 2012
Terminalia chebula (Roxb.) Retz.	Dysentery – fruit/diarrhea and dysentery – fruit or bark	Laskar et al., 2015; Bharati and Sharma, 2012
Terminalia citrina (Gaertn.) Roxb. ex Fleming	Anorexia	Rajkumari et al., 2014
Thalictrum foliolosum DC.	Used for treatment of inflammation and fever – roots	Maiti et al., 2013
Thunbergia coccinea Wall.	Wounds, sores, sickness and worms	Lalramnghinglova, 2011
Tinospora cordifolia (Willd.) Miers ex. Hk.f.	Snakebites and centipede bites/ dysentery – bark	Lalramnghinglova, 2011; Salam et al., 2013
Trigonella foenum-graecum L.	Hematuria – seed	Rajkumari et al., 2014
Urena lobata L., & *Spondias pinnata* (L. f.) Kurz	Fever – leaves	Laskar et al., 2015
Urtica dioica L.	Bone fractures – root, increase milk yield mixed with *Tamarindus indica* fruit/milk production – spines	Bharati and Sharma, 2012
Urginea indica L.	Skin – bulb	Laskar et al., 2015

TABLE 7.1 (Continued)

Scientific name	Disease and plant parts	References
Vigna mungo (L.) Hepper	Lactogogue	Rajkumari et al., 2014
Vitex negundo L	Wound – leaves/dermatitis/ eczema, scabies and skin infection – leaves	Borthakur and Sarma, 1996; Rajkumari et al., 2014; Salam et al., 2013
Vitex trifolia L.	Muscle sprain, injury and in mouth ulcer – tuber and leaves to wash the wart in poultry	Sunder et al., 2014
Wedelia biflora (L.) DC.	Broken horn, muscle sprain, injury and in snake bite – whole plants	Sunder et al., 2014
Xanthium strumarium L.	Wound –seed/diarrhea – leaves	Sharma and Sapcota, 2003; Salam et al., 2013
Xanthoxylum acanthopodium DC.	Skin infections – leaves	Salam et al., 2013
Xanthoxylum alatum Roxb.	Fowl lice and fish poison – leaves/twigs	Lalramnghinglova, 2011
Xanthoxylum armatum DC.	Anthelmintic	Borthakur and Sarma, 1996
Zea mays L.	Lactogogue	Rajkumari et al., 2014
Zingiber officinale Roscoe	Jiggery – rhizome mixed with fruits of *Piper longum* L., Cough – rhizome/constipation	Bharati and Sharma, 2012; Rajkumari et al., 2014
Ziziphus mauritiana Lam.	Burns on skin	Rajkumari et al., 2014

Prescriptions Used To Control Various Diseases

Disease	No of prescriptions (species)
Diuretic	1
Appetizer	10
Cough	13
Dysentery	35
Diarrhea	32
Dyspepsia	2
Indigestion	9

Prescriptions Used To Control Various Diseases

Disease	No of prescriptions (species)
Wound	27
Delivery/removal of placenta	13
Injury	5
Increase milk	18
Bone fracture	7
Animal bite	4
Insect bite	10
Foot/Foot mouth disease	5
Burn	3
Skin	12
Restorative	1
Mastitis/inflammation	8
Ulcer	4
Tonic/strength	5
Body ache/pain	6
Body weight	7
Worm/Endoparasite	28
Ringworm	1
Eye	5
Urinary infection/haematuria	7
Sore mouth	23
Fever	23
Ectoparasite/maggot	11
Scabies/itching	6
Unconscious cattle	1
Constipation	7
Stomachache	5
Pneumonia	1
Cut	7
Abscess	1
Broken horn	4
Control flies	1
Stop bleeding	3

Prescriptions Used To Control Various Diseases

Disease	No of prescriptions (species)
Blindness	1
Yoke gall	1
Hump	2
Sprain	5
Sickness	5
Carminative	1
Flatulence	2
Anthrax	2
Boils	2
Asthma	1
Snake bite	20
Bloat	1
Vitiated	1
Hardening	1
Jiggery/leech	5
Rabies	1
Tick	2
Cure diseases	3
Bronchitis	1
Cold	8
Muscle contraction/joint/ bone setting	3
Blisters	2
Spleen	2
Gout	1
Lung diseases	1
Infection	1
Mumps	1
Bird flu	1
Eczema	1
Biocide	1
Fish poison	3

KEYWORDS

- Andaman
- ethnoveterinary
- livestock health management
- northeast India

REFERENCES

1. Balaji, N. S., & Chakravarthi, P. V. (2010). Ethnoveterinary Practices in India: A Review, *Veterinary World, 3(12)*, 549–551.
2. Bharati, K. A., & Sharma, B. L. (2012). Plants used as ethnoveterinary medicines in Sikkim Himalayas, *Ethnobot Res Appl, 10*, 339–356.
3. Borthakur, S. K., Nath, K. K., & Sharma, T. R. (1998). Inquiry into old lead: Ethnoveterinary medicine for treatment of elephants in Assam. *Ethnobotany 10*, 70–74.
4. Borthakur, S. K., & Sharma, U. K. (1996). Ethnoveterinary medicine with special reference to cattle prevalent among the Nepalese of Assam. Jain, S. K. (Ed). Ethnobiology in Human Welfare, Deep Publication, New Delhi, pp. 197–199.
5. Cotton, C. M. (1996). Ethnobotany: Principles and Applications. John Wiley & Sons.
6. Jain, S. K., & Srivastava, S. (1999). Dictionary of Ethnoveterinary Plants of India. Deep Publications. New Delhi.
7. Jain, S. K., & Srivastava, S. (2001). Prospects of herbal drugs for ethnoveterninary practices (EVP) in North-East India. Nat. Sem. on Traditional Knowledge Base on Herbal Medicines and Plant Resources of North East India: Protection, Utilization and Conservation, Guwahati, Assam, India, p. 16.
8. Kanjilal, U. N., Kanjilal, P. C., & Das, A. (1938). Flora of Assam, vol. II. Bishen Singh and Mahendra Pal Singh, Dehradun.
9. Khatoon, R., Das, A. K., Singh, P. K., & Dutta, B. K. (2013). Etnthnoveterinary plants used by Kom tribe of Manipur, India, Bioresources and Trad. Knowledge of North East India, pp. 303–306.
10. Lalramnghinglova, H. (2011). Plants used in ethnoveterinary medicine including treatment of snake and insect bites in Mizoram. *Ethnobotany 23*, 57–63.
11. Laskar, S. A. K. A., Das, A. K., & Dutta, B. K. (2015). Plants used in ethno-veterinary medicine by Halam tribe settled in Hailakandi district of Southern Assam, India, *Intern. J. Curr. Res., 7*, 13136–13140.
12. Maiti, S., Chakravarty, P., Garai, S., Bandyopadhyay, S., & Chouhan, V. S. (2013). Ethno-veterinary practices for ephemeral fever of Yak: A participatory assessment by the Monpatribe of Arunachal Pradesh. *Indian J. Trad. Knowl. 12*, 36–39.

13. Mathias, E. (2001). Advantages and disadvantages in ethnoveterinary medicine (EVM): Introducing ethnoveterinary medicine. (http://www.ethnovetweb.com/whatisevm.pdf).

14. Mathias, E. (2010). Presentation at the conference on 'Ethnoveterinary medicine: Tradition, science, cultural richness,' Bologna.

15. Misra, K. K., & Kumar, K. A. (2004). Ethno-veterinary practices among the Konda Reddi of East Godavari district of Andhra Pradesh. *Stud. Tribes Tribals, 2(1)*, 37–44.

16. Namsa, N. D., Mandal, M., Tangjang, S., & Mandal, S. C. (2011). Ethnobotany of the Monpa ethnic group at Arunachal Pradesh, India. *J Ethnobiol Ethnomed* http://www.ethnobiomed.com/content/7/1/31.

17. Pradhan, B. K., & Badola, H. K. (2008). Ethnomedicinal plant use by Lepcha tribe of Dzongu valley bordering Khangchendzonga Biosphere Reserve, in North Sikkim, India, *Journal of Ethnobiology and Ethnomedicine, 4*, 22.

18. Prasad, D. V. (2014). Ethno-veterinary practices among the Nicobarese of Katchal Island. *J. Andaman Sci. Association, 19(1)*, 99–105.

19. Raikwar, A., & Prabhakar, M. (2015). Ethnoveterinary medicine: in present Perspective. *Int. J. Agric. Sci. & Vet. Med. 3(1)*, 44–49.

20. Rajkumari, R., Nirmala, R. K., Singh, P. K. Das A. K., Dutta, B. K., & Pinokiyo, A. (2014). Ethnoveterinary plants used by the Chiru tribes of Manipur, Northeast India, *Indian J. Trad. Knowl., 13*, 368–376.

21. Rastogi, S., Pandey, M. K., Prakash, J., Sharma, A., & Singh, G. N. (2015). Veterinary herbal medicines in India. *Methods in Pharmacol. 9*, 155–163.

22. Saikia, B., Sushanta, B., Saikia D., Gajurel, P. R., Rethy, P., & Das, A. K. (2010). Utilization of plants with reference to Ethno-veterinary herbal medicines of Sonitpur district, Assam, India. Presented in international conference at Mohanlal Sukhadia, University, Udaipur, 25–27 Nov.

23. Saikia, B., & Borthakur, S. K. (2010). Use of medicinal plants in animal healthcare-A case study from Gohpur, Assam, *Indian J. Trad. Knowl. 9(1)*, 49–51.

24. Salam, S., Jamir, N. S., & Singh, P. K. (2013). Ethnoveterinary plants of Ukhrul district, Manipur. *Ethnobotany 25*, 139–142.

25. Sapkota, D., & Sharma, U. K. (2000). Ethnoveterinary practices among the Nepalese dwellers of Assam- A survey, *Livestock International, 4(6)*, 9–12.

26. Schillhom Van Veen, T. W. (1996). Sense or Nonsense? Traditional methods of Animal disease prevention and control in Africa Savannah. In: Mc Corkle, C. M., Mathias, E., & Schillhorn Van Veen, T. W. (eds.) Ethnoveterinary Research and Development. Intermediate Technology Publications, Landon. p. 338.

27. Sharma, D. N. (2015). A report on animal health care in ancient India. Emeritus Scientist College of Veterinary and Animal Sciences, Palampur, HP.

28. Sharma, U. K. (2012). *Ethnoveterinary Plants of North east India* (book), Bishen Singh and Mahendrapal Singh, Dehradun, India.

29. Sharma, U. K., & Sapcota, D. (2003). Studies on some ethnoveterinary practices in Dhemaji district of Assam. *J. Natural Remedies, 3*, 73–77.

30. Somvanshi, R. (2006). Veterinary Medicine and Animal Keeping in Ancient India. *Asian Agri-History, 10*, 133–146.

31. Sunder, J., Kundu, A., & Kundu, M. S. (2014). Medicinal plant and ethno-veterinary practices used in South and North Andaman. *J. Andaman Sci. Ass. 19(1)*, 106–115.

32. Verma, S., & Singh, S. P. (2009). Current and future status of herbal medicines, *Veterinary World, 1(11)*, 347–350.
33. Warren, D. M. (1991). Using Indigenous Knowledge in Agricultural development Washington: World Bank Discussion Paper, No. 127, 46.
34. WHO. Int. World Health Organization. [Last accessed on 2014 Jul 15]. Available from: http://www.who.int/medicines/areas/traditional/definitions/en/.

CHAPTER 8

ETHNOBOTANY OF ANDAMAN AND NICOBAR ISLANDS

T. PULLAIAH,[1] BIR BAHADUR,[2] K. V. KRISHNAMURTHY,[3] S. JOHN ADAMS,[4] and ROBINDRA TERON[5]

[1]Department of Botany, Sri Krishnadevaraya University, Anantapur – 515003, A.P., India, E-mail: pullaiah.thammineni@gmail.com

[2]Department of Botany, Kakatiya University, Warangal, Telangana, India

[3]Consultant, R&D, Sami Labs Ltd. Peenya Industrial Area, Bangalore – 560058, Karnataka, India

[4]Department of Pharmacogonosy, R&D, The Himalaya Drug Company, Makali, Bangalore, India

[5]Department of Life Science and Bioinformatics, Assam University, Diphu Campus, Karbi Anglong, Diphu, Assam – 782462

CONTENTS

Abstract 208
8.1   The Andamans: People and Their Culture 208
8.2   Tribal Diversity in Andamans (7.5%) 211
8.3   Ethnomedical Plants of Andamans 215
8.4   Other Uses of Plants.. 234

8.5   Ethnic Food Plants and Ethnic Foods of the
      Andaman and Nicobar Islands 238
Keywords 245
References 246

ABSTRACT

The Andaman archipelago comprises of about 570 islands and encompasses an area of about 6,340 square miles. This chapter detail the ethnic tribes of Andaman and Nicobar Islands which include Great Andamanese, Onges, Jarawas, Sentinelese, Nicobarese and Shompen. The usage of plants for food, medicine and other uses by these ethnic people is given. In the Andamans studies on ethnic foods revealed minimal processing and no great efforts are devoted for preparing the foods. Plants foods of the Jarawas and Sentineleses are trivial and only few plants are consumed by them, the preparation methods are not known/not documented which suggest most foods are eaten raw. More ethnobotanical exploration is needed to analyze and document the ethnic foods consumed by tribal communities of the Andamans.

8.1   THE ANDAMANS: PEOPLE AND THEIR CULTURE

The Andaman archipelago comprises of about 570 islands and encompasses an area of about 6,340 square miles (Krishnakumar, 2009), situated in a north-south direction between 6° and 14° North and 92° and 94° East at the mouth of the Bay of Bengal (Awasthi, 1991). The Andamans are divided into two main groups of islands, Great Andaman and Little Andaman, separated by the Duncan passage (Figure 8.1). The Great Andaman is further subdivided into three separate groups: North Andaman, Middle Andaman, and South Andaman (Sekhsaria and Pandya, 2010). The entire land surface of the Andamans is hilly, enclosing narrow valleys; the tendency of slope is from east to west. The islands have typical tropical maritime climatic situation with average annual rainfall of 3100 mm, temperature ranges from 20 to 32°C and high relative humidity (70–92%). These islands are rich in floral

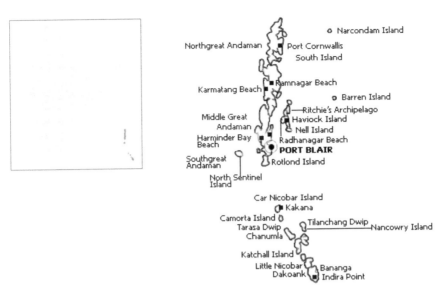

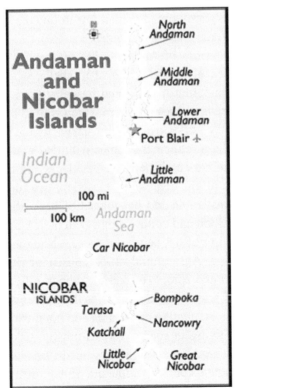

FIGURE 8.1 Map of the Andamans.

biodiversity which represents elements of both North-East India and Indonesia-Myanmar regions (Balakrishnan and Ellis, 1996).

The Andaman Islands is home to indigenous tribes who are divided by two categories: the indigenous tribal people and the outsiders. Latter who are settled in the territory due to the fact of colonial rule, include Bengali, Tamil, Malayali, Telugu, Oriya, North Indian and others (Majumdar, 1975). The blend of these two classes of people constitutes a colorful ethnicity to the people's profile of Andamans. The indigenous tribes are generally dark in color, short in stature with peppercorn hairs belonging to Negrito stock and represented by the Great Andamanese, the Onges, the Jarawas and the Sentinelese (Sharief, 2007). The aboriginal population of the Andaman Islands, along with the Semangs of Malaysia, the Aetas of the Philippines, and the few population groups of Papua New Guinea who morphologically resemble the African pygmies, are the remnants of the 'Negrito' populations of Southeast Asia (Kashyap et al., 2003). Formerly, the Onge tribe was semi-nomadic, roaming around the shores of the island in response to different seasons (Bhargava, 1983).

The aboriginal tribes of Andaman are known for their skills in arts and crafts. They excel in crafts related to shells, wood, cane and bamboo. Apart from this, mat making and basketry form an integral part of their culture. There is no specific attire which is used by the people of the Andamans and they still move around naked living in the inaccessible coastal areas. A slight refinement comes with the Jarawas where they use only adornments of bark and shell, like necklaces, armbands, waist bands, etc. But, however, all the ceremonial occasions are adorned by necklaces made of shell, waistbands and headbands of bark fiber. Thus, they still preserve their tradition and culture along with their language and religion. The main occupation of the people of these islands includes agriculture, forestry and fishing. Agricultural crops consist of rice, coconuts, betel (areca nuts), fruits and spices (turmeric), rubber, oil palms and cashews. During the khariff season, paddy becomes the prime field crop. Fishery is also another major occupation of the area and not meant for domestic use. Aboriginal tribes living in coastal forests mostly make best use of their surrounding forest produce for their daily needs, for example, fuel, fodder, edibles and others items but also come out of the forest towards sea coasts and utilize its resources too, to meet their basic requirements. Among other tangible culture of the Andaman, food system of the aboriginal tribes adds to the ethnic and cultural heritage of the region. Over the years, the interactions of native food systems and that of the migrants favored amalgamation and evolution of diverse food cultures which helped in identification of more new local food resources in this small archipelago (Singh et al., 2013). Dagar and Dagar (1999) gave a detailed account of plants and animals used by the Negrito and Mongoloid tribals of Andaman and Nicobar Islands in their routine life for food, shelter, dugout canoe making, taboos, rituals and medicines (Figure 8.1).

8.2 TRIBAL DIVERSITY IN ANDAMANS (7.5%)

8.2.1 GREAT ANDAMANESE

A small group of about 100 persons inhabiting little Andaman Islands. The Great Andamanese are traditionally non-vegetarian. Their staple food consists of fish, pig, crab, dugong, shellfish, turtle egg, and tubers, etc. The people are finely skilled in arts and crafts and therefore, are able to utilize several plant materials for their hunting tools. The Great Andamanese produce their string (bole) from the bark fiber of the climber *Anodendron paniculatum*. The fiber is also used to make string for harpoon lines, bowstrings, and turtle nets. Stem pieces of 1/2 or 1 m are taken by the Great Andamanese during fishing traps which is claimed that the obnoxious odor of the wood wards off attacks of large fishes and crocodiles. The eggs of birds are also collected for consumption. Besides that, various plants and plant products are gathered and consumed either in raw form or cooked as vegetable. Twenty-four plants have been reported to be used by the Andamanese as source of food. They are fond of seeds of *Entada scandens, E. pursaetha*, pith of *Caryotas obolifera*, two species of *Dioscorea* (yam) (Patnaik, 2006). Certain edible fruits of *Terminalia catappa, Carica papaya, Annona squamosa, Acacia pennata, Artocarpus omeziana, Artocarpus integrifolia, Ficus nervosa, Moringa pterygosperma, Psidium guajava, Bruguiera gymnorrhiza, Calamus viminalis, Cocos nucifera, Pandanus andamanensium, Musa sapientum* var. *simiarum, Nypa fruticans, Manilkara littoralis, Citrus medica, Atalantia monophylla, Mangifera comptospermum, Mangifera indica*, etc. are often consumed by the Great Andamanese (Awasthi, 1991). The people are expert in honey hunting and they employ various plant materials during the hunt. Paste, juice, and vapors of *Polyalthia jenkinsii*, obtained by chewing the leaves and sprayed by mouth on honeybees, are used to disperse these insects during honey collection. When the Great Andamanese raid a hive, they strip off the leaves and chew the stem; the liquid thus extracted is smear over their body. The same juice is used also to disperse the attacking bees. Bees are at once repelled by the obnoxious odor of the juice emitted in a fine spray from the mouth. Sometimes they use the chewed stalks to drive off the last defenders of the hive.

8.2.2 ONGES

Onges are pure hunter-gatherers and as they were formerly semi-nomadic, they never took any interest in cultivation. Of course, they do not destroy edible plants; on the contrary, they try to protect useful plants. They take only the required number of edible plants while the remaining is left for regeneration. This shows their natural interest in the conservation of the flora. The Onges eat mostly natural food in which the island abounds. They are very fond of jackfruit, yams, *Pandanus* species. The leaves of *Pandanus* sometime provide roofing for Onge shelters. They particularly like pilchards. They catch mollusks, Crustacea, lobsters, crayfish and crabs, even some kind of hermit crab. They eat cicada too. They collect the pupae which are supposed to be a great threat. It is noteworthy to mention that in the indigenous diet items of the Onge menu birds, crocodiles, lizards, jungle cats, bats, rats and snakes are not included because as per Onge beliefs they harbor spirit of dead or malevolent spirits. Onge tribals can consume even slightly toxic fruits or seeds, viz., *Abrus precatorius*, *Barringtonia asiatica*, *Cycas rumphii* and *Dioscorea glabra* after mild processing through boiling or roasting. Probably by heating the plant parts, the toxic properties are destroyed (Tanaka, 1976) which makes them less harmful to be consumed. The three food plants of the Onge tribe, viz, *Cycas rumphii*, *Dioscorea glabra*, and *Pandanus* are also used by the natives of southeastern Asian countries (Bhargava, 1983). Moreover, the procedures employed in cooking and consuming are similar to those of other Asian tribes (Anonymous, 1948–1972; Burkill, 1951; Smitinand, 1972; Tanaka,

1976; Bhargava, 1983). At present, the tribals are rapidly developing a taste for the well-cooked food of the civilized world. Wheat flour, rice, and fruits of *Cocos nucifera* have recently been added to their diet.

8.2.3 JARAWAS

Jarawas, also known as *Ang*, are considered to be the original inhabitants of the Andaman with the other Negrito tribes (Sarkar, 2008). They entirely depend on forest and marine sources for survival. Diet of the Jarawa includes varieties of fruits, tubers, honey, mollusk, fish, and animals like pig, wild boars, monitor lizard and turtle. Besides, honey was an important item of food for the Jarawas. Normally, men hunt crabs by hitting arrows when these were encountered in water or mudflats. The women use net for trapping the crabs and often dug out the crabs from burrows. The women and children usually caught fishes from shallow waters, in streams and near shoreline, by hand-nets. Jarawa women collected turtles' eggs from the sandy beach in a bay area. The turtle nesting grounds were detected near the edge of tidal flat (high water mark), where grass grew. The women and children used to collect marine mollusks like trochus, turbo, giant clams, cowries, etc., from the inter-tidal areas of coral beds on open seashore or mouth of bay area. All kinds of fruits are eaten fresh, and a great portion is consumed on the gathering spot itself, except *Pometia pinnata*, *Baucaria sapida*, and *Cycas*, which are gathered in large quantities and carried to the camp. Men, especially the young ones, climb high up the trees to collect jackfruit, which becomes abundant during the peak dry season of the year. During this period jackfruit comprised a considerably high portion of their food, more at camps in interior parts of forest and less in coastal areas. Traditionally, food was cooked in pit ovens called *aalaav*; those were made inside or outside their huts for roasting food. Such ovens are mostly used to cook pig meat and jackfruit. After three to four hours the cooked food is taken out for consumption. In recent times, it has been observed that most of the time they boil pig meat and other items of food. Boiling is done in *buchu* or aluminum vessels either supplied by the AAJVS (Andaman Aadmi Janjati Vikas Samiti) or procured from the villages. The males process pig meat; cooking the meat in pit ovens is also done by them, while boiling meat in a *buchu* is not a gender specific job.

It has generally been observed that the males consume larger part of pig meat. If it is monitor lizard, only the males consume it without giving any share to the females.

The Jarawas are more dependent on animal foods for protein and fat. This is supplemented by a wide variety of plant foods that provide reasonable quantity of carbohydrates and vitamins. The Jarawas more often consume fruits and honey found in the forests rather than digging for tubers and roots (see Table 8.2). The Jarawas use fruits, nuts, seeds, leaves, tubers and roots of different plants as secondary source of diet. They eat many kinds of seeds and tubers, some are eaten raw and some are processed before eating. Most of these seeds and tubers are gathered and transported to the camp by women, while men and children occasionally help them when the seeds are abundant. Members of Botanical Survey of India collected information about 58 plants which provide food to the Jarawas. Frequently used ones are *Artabotrys speciosus*, *A. chaplasha*, *A. lakoocha*, *Baccaurea ramiflora*, *Alamus andamanicus*, *Cycas rumphii*, *Dioscorea bulbifera*, *D. vexans*, *D. glabra*, *Diospyros andamanica*, *Ficus racemosa*, *Garcinia cowa*, *Mangifera andamanica*, *Pinanga manii*, *Donax canaeformis*, *Pometia pinnata* and *Terminalia catappa*.

8.2.4   SENTINELESE

Sentinelese is a small tribal group of about 100 people of Negrito race inhabiting North Sentinel. The Sentinelese culture is based on observations during contact attempts in the late 20th century. They are noted for resisting attempts at contact by outsiders and their hostile attitude towards the strangers. Unlike the Andamanese, Onge and Jarawa, the Sentinelese have refused to have contact with outsiders, and seemingly as a result remain culturally intact and healthy. Repeated attempts by the administration to make friendly overtures to them have resulted only in arrows fired from trees or beaches on the island's periphery. Their language remains unclassified. The Sentinelese maintain an essentially hunter-gatherer society, obtaining their subsistence through hunting, fishing, and collecting wild plants; there is no evidence of any agricultural practices or producing fire (Raghunathan, 1976). Food consists primarily of plant stuffs gathered in the forest, coconuts, which are frequently found on the beaches as flotsam, pigs, and, presumably, other wildlife (which apart from sea turtles is limited to some smaller birds and invertebrates). Fruits of *Pandanus* and *Sapodilla* remain their staple food. Wild honey is also seen to be widely collected by the Sentinelese.

8.2.5 NICOBARESE

Nicobarese is a tribe group of about 22,000 people. It is a Mangoloid race inhabiting Nicobarese group of islands in Bay of Bengal. Linguistically of non-Khmer branch of Austro-Asiatic family.

8.2.6 SHOMPEN

Shompen is a small tribal group of 223 persons of Mongoloid race inhabiting the Great Nicobar Island in Bay of Bengal. *Shompens* are the aboriginal inhabitants of Great Nicobar Island. They probably migrated into this area, several hundred years ago from Malaysian regions and got admixtured with *Nicobarese* tribes at later stages. They are one of the Mongoloid aborigines. They are semi-nomadic, food gatherers and hunters with stone age civilization; live in small groups in dense interior forests of the island and exclusively depend on forest resources and sea products for most of their sustenance. The Shompens build temporary huts propped on stilts 2–6 m above ground. Inside the huts, crude mats made from pandanus and cane strips are used and leaves of *Leea grandiflora* Kurz. serves bed sheets, while a piece of bamboo is often used as pillow. The Shompens prepare indigenous dugouts or canoes called 'horis,' which are of two types. Small canoes having carrying capacity of two or three persons are used for crossing creeks and rivers. Big canoes having carrying capacity of 2–7 persons are used for transportation and fishing in the sea. These canoes which vary in size from 6 to 10 ft., are generally fixed with outrigger for balance and moved using paddles.

8.3 ETHNOMEDICAL PLANTS OF ANDAMANS

Ethnic tribes of Andaman and Nicobar Islands use various plants or plant parts as a source of food, shelter, clothing, medicine, timber and for other miscellaneous purposes (Table 8.1 and 8.2). Ethnic tribes inhabiting the interior forest of the Islands are mainly forest people and their relationship

TABLE 8.1 Ethnomedicinal Plants Used by Ethnic Tribes of Andamans

S. No.	Name of the plant species	Parts Used	Purpose	Reference(s)
1	*Abrus precatorius* L.	Root, leaves, seeds	Antidiarrheic, emetic, alexeteric, antidysenteric, asthma, snake bite, contraceptive	Ghosh, 2004a,b, c
2.	*Abrus pulchellus* Wall. ex Thw.	Roots	Colic infections	Ghosh, 2004a
3	*Acacia andamanica* Nielsen	–	Premature ejaculation, astringent	Ghosh, 2004a, c
4	*Acalypha indica* L.	Leaves	Purgative	Verma et al., 2010
5	*Acorus calamus* L.	Rhizome	Headache, cold	Sharief et al., 2005
6	*Actopanes canniformis* (Forst.) K.Schum.	Stem, root	Fever	Elanchezhian et al., 2007; Sharief and Rao, 2007
7	*Adenia cardiophylla* (Masters) Engler	Whole plant	Bodyache, ringworm, conjunctivitis	Ghosh, 2004a
8	*Adenia nicobarica* King		Body pains	Bhargava, 1981
9	*Adenia trilobata* (Roxb.) Engler	–	Headache, snake-bite, stomach trouble	Ghosh, 2004a
10	*Adenostemma lavenia* (L.) Kuntze	Leaves	Dental problems	Verma et al., 2010
11	*Aegle marmelos* (L.) Correa		Stomach pains and disorders	Bhargava, 1981
12	*Aerva lanata* Juss.	Leaves	Fever	Verma et al., 2010
13	*Aganosma marginata* (Roxb.) G.Don	–	Emmenogogue, fever, tonic, urogenital	Ghosh, 2004a, c
14	*Ageratum conyzoides* L.	Leaves	Fever, throat pain, conjunctivitis	Sharief, 2007; Verma et al., 2010
15	*Allamanda cathartica* L.	–	Febrifuge	Ghosh, 2004a
16	*Alstonia kurzii* Hook. f.	Bark, root, leaf	Fever	Elanchezhian et al., 2007; Sharief and Rao, 2007

TABLE 8.1 (Continued)

S. No.	Name of the plant species	Parts Used	Purpose	Reference(s)
17	*Alstonia macrophylla* Wall.	Bark, root, leaves, root bark	Fever, gastric disorder, swelling, bone fracture, stomachache, urinary infections, skin diseases	Chakraborty and Rao, 1988; Dagar and Dagar, 1991; Das et al., 2006; Elanchezhian et al., 2007; Sharief and Rao, 2007; Verma et al., 2010
18	*Alyxia reinwardtii* var. *meiantha* (Stapf) Markgraf	Leaf	Headache	Ghosh, 2004a
19	*Amomum aculeatum* Roxb.	Leaves, stem	Cough, fever, scar	Sharief, 2007
20	*Amomum fenzlii* Kurz.	Roots, flowers	Malarial fever, stomach disorders	Das et al., 2006
21	*Ampelocissus barbata* (Wall.) Planch.	—	Swellings, boils, sprains, cuts, cholera, rheumatism	Ghosh, 2004a
22	*Anamirta cocculus* (L.) Wight & Arn	Root	Fever, dyspepsia, menstrual troubles	Ghosh, 2004a, c
23	*Ancistrocladus attenuatus* Dyer	—	Dysentery, malaria	Ghosh, 2004a
24	*Ancistrocladus tectorius* (Lour.) Merr.	Leaves, stem bark	Antimalarial, fracture	Ghosh, 2004a; Sharief et al., 2005
25	*Angiopteris lygodiifolia* Roscust	Young leaves	Cough, cold	Sharief, 2007
26	*Annona reticulata* L.	Leaves	Bone fracture	Verma et al., 2010
	Annona squamosa L.	Juice	Snake bite	Verma et al., 2010
27	*Anodendron manubrium* Merr.	Leaves	For abortion	Sharief, 2007
28	*Anodendron paniculatum* A.DC.	Leaves	For abortion	Awasthi, 1991

TABLE 8.1 (Continued)

S. No.	Name of the plant species	Parts Used	Purpose	Reference(s)
29	*Anthocephalus indicus* A. Rich.	Branches	Shafts of arrows	Awasthi, 1991
30	*Ardisia solanacea* Roxb.	Root, leaves	Blood clot, hemorrhage, chest pain, wash uterus after child birth, antiabortion	Elanchezhian et al., 2007; Sharief, 2007; Sharief and Rao, 2007; Verma et al., 2010
31	*Areca catechu* L.	Fruit	Constipation, stimulant, stomach disorder	Awasthi, 1991; Sharief, 2007
32	*Areca triandra* Roxb.	Fruits, stem	Menstrual problems	Sharief, 2007
33	*Argemone mexicana* L.	Latex	Conjunctivitis	Verma et al., 2010
34	*Argyreia hookeri* Cl.	Leaves	Swelling, hydrocele	Awasthi, 1991; Sharief, 2007
35	*Aristolochia tagala* Chamisso	Whole plant	Snake bite, stimulate menstrual flow	Ghosh, 2004a,b,c
36	*Asparagus racemosus* Willd.	Roots	Menstrual flow, burning sensation in urine, jaundice	Ghosh, 2004a,c; Sharief et al., 2005
37	*Atalantia monophylla* DC.	—	Respiratory problems, rheumatism	Ghosh, 2004a
38	*Azadirachta indica* A.Juss.	Leaves, bark	Cuts, wounds	Awasthi, 1991; Sharief, 2007
39	*Barringtonia asiatica* (L.) Kurz	Leaves	Bone fracture, wounds	Gupta et al., 2004; Verma et al., 2010
40	*Bauhinia stipularis* Korth.	—	Dysentery, febrifuge	Ghosh, 2004a
41	*Bougainvillea spectabilis* Willd.	—	Cold remedies	Ghosh, 2004a
42	*Breyeneia retusa* (Dennst.) Alston	Leaves	Body pain, fever	Verma et al., 2010
43	*Bridelia cinnamomea* Hook.f.	—	Astringent	Ghosh, 2004a
44	*Bruguiera gymnorrhiza* Lam.	Twig tips	Fatigue	Verma et al., 2010
45	*Byttneria andamanensis* Kurz	Bark	Hair wash	Ghosh, 2004a

TABLE 8.1 (Continued)

S. No.	Name of the plant species	Parts Used	Purpose	Reference(s)
46	*Byttneria grandiflora* DC.	Leaves	Used at the time of delivery	Ghosh, 2004a,c
47	*Caesalpinia andamanica* (Prain) Hattink	—	Tonic, antiperiodic, colic, red eye	Ghosh, 2004a
48	*Caesalpinia bonduc* (L.) Roxb.	—	Antidote, cirrhosis, cough, diarrhea, emmenagogue, hematochezia, jaundice, swelling	Ghosh, 2004a,b
49	*Caesalpinia cristata* L.	—	Toothache, antiperiodic, snakebite, colic, fever, pimple, malaria, tonic, swelling	Ghosh, 2004a
50	*Caesalpinia hymenocarpa* (Prain) Hattink	—	Tonic	Ghosh, 2004a
51	*Callicarpha longifolia* Lam.	Leaves	Cuts, wounds	Verma et al., 2010
52	*Calophyllum inophyllum* L.	Leaves	Bone fracture, pain in eye, stye	Verma et al., 2010; Bharati et al., 2015
53	*Calycopteris floribunda* (Roxb.) Lam.	—	Astringent, laxative	Ghosh, 2004a
54	*Camellia sinensis* (L.) Kuntze	Leaves	Centipede bite, scorpion sting	Sharief et al., 2005
55	*Canarium commune* L.	Leaves	Headache	Sharief, 2007
56	*Canarium euphyllum* Kurz	Resin	Repel insects	Bhargava 1981; Sharief, 2007
57	*Canavalia ensiformis* (L.) DC.	Seeds	Skin disease	Sharief et al., 2005
58	*Capparis sepiaria* L.	—	Alterative, fever, tonic	Ghosh, 2004a
59	*Capparis zeylanica* L.	—	Anodyne, antihydrotic, boil, cholera, colic, sedative, sore, stomachic, swelling	Ghosh, 2004a
60	*Cardiospermum halicacabum* L..	—	Diuretic, emetic, purgative, buboes, sore eyes, aperients, rheumatism, nervous disorders	Ghosh, 2004a

TABLE 8.1 (Continued)

S. No.	Name of the plant species	Parts Used	Purpose	Reference(s)
61	*Carica papaya* L.	Fruit	Prophylactic	Sharief, 2007
62	*Caryota mitis* Lour.	Young shoots	Vomiting, stomachache	Sharief, 2007
63	*Casearia grewiaefolia* Vent.	Leaves	Diarrhea, dysentery	Verma et al., 2010
64	*Cassia alata* L.	Leaves	Ringworm	Bharati et al., 2015
65	*Cassia sophera* L.	Leaves	Hypertension, giddiness	Bharati et al., 2015
66	*Casuarina equisetifolia* L.	—	Insect repellant	Bhargava, 1981
67	*Cayratia pedata* (Lam.) Juss. ex Gagnep.	—	Headaches	Ghosh, 2004a
68	*Cayratia trifolia* (L.) Domin.	—	Fever, itch, rhinosis, sore	Ghosh, 2004a
69	*Celastrus paniculatus* Willd.	Leaves	Opium antidote, stimulant, rheumatic pain, leprosy, abortion, leucoderma, bitter, paralysis, beriberi	Ghosh, 2004a,c
70	*Centella asiatica* (L.) Urban.	Whole plant	Cuts, wounds, fracture	Sharief et al., 2005
71	*Chromolaena odorata* L.	Leaves	Cuts, wounds, leech bite	Sharief et al., 2005; Sharief, 2007; Verma et al., 2010
72	*Cissampelos pariera* L.	—	Eye diseases, snake-bite, febrifuge, diarrhea, colic, tonic, diuretic	Ghosh, 2004a,b
73	*Cissus discolor* Bl.	—	Sore eyes, snake bite	Ghosh, 2004a
74	*Cissus elongata* Roxb.	—	Sores, cuts, wounds, insect bites, swelling, scabies, fever, antipriodic	Ghosh, 2004a
75	*Cissus pentagona* Roxb.	—	Headache, boils, stomachache	Ghosh, 2004a

TABLE 8.1 (Continued)

S. No.	Name of the plant species	Parts Used	Purpose	Reference(s)
76	*Citrus medica* L.	Fruit	Constipation, antibiotic, stomach disorder	Awasthi, 1991; Elanchezhian et al., 2007; Sharief, 2007
77	*Claoxylon indicum* Reinw. ex Bl.	Leaves	Cuts, wounds, eye injury, cough	Verma et al., 2010; Bharati et al., 2015
78	*Clematis smilacifolia* Wall. subsp. *andamanica* Kapoor	—	Cordage	Ghosh, 2004a
79	*Clerodendron inerme* (L.) Gaertn.	Leaves	Bone fracture	Verma et al., 2010
80	*Clitoria ternatea* L.	Root, seeds	Epilepsy, snake bite, leucorrhoea	Ghosh, 2004a,b,c
81	*Coccinia grandis* (L.) J.Voigt	Fruits	Scabies, small pox, febrifuge	Ghosh, 2004a
82	*Cocculus hirsutus* (L.) Diels	—	Snake & insect bite, skin allergies	Ghosh, 2004a,b
83	*Cocculus pendulus* (J. R., & G. Forst.) Diels	Leaves, fruits	Febrifuge, promotes menstruation	Ghosh, 2004a,c
84	*Cocos nucifera* L.	Fruit	Dental problems	Verma et al., 2010
85	*Colubrina asiatica* (L.) Brongn.	Leaves	Abortifacient, headache, fever, bone fracture, pneumonia, gynecological disorders	Ghosh, 2004a; Verma et al., 2010
86	*Combretum latifolium* Bl.	—	Tonic	Ghosh, 2004a
87	*Connarus semidecandrus* Jack.	Root	Colic	Ghosh, 2004a
88	*Corchorus aestuans* L.	Leaves	Body pain	Verma et al., 2010
89	*Cordia grandis* Roxb.	Leaves	Stomachache	Verma et al., 2010
90	*Costus speciosus* (Koeing) Sm.	Leaves, rhizome	Stomach disorder; diarrhea, headache, purgative, tonic, anthelmintic, diarrhea, eye trouble, sudorific, snake bite	Das et al., 2006; Elanchezhian et al., 2007; Sharief and Rao, 2007

TABLE 8.1 (Continued)

S. No.	Name of the plant species	Parts Used	Purpose	Reference(s)
91	*Crotalaria pallida* Ail.	Leaves	Snake bite	Sharief et al., 2005
92	*Croton argyratus* Blume	Seeds	Laxative, stomach disorders	Elanchezhian et al., 2007; Sharief and Rao, 2007
93	*Cryptolepis buchanani* Schultes	Roots, fruits, seeds	Chills and edema, snake bite	Ghosh, 2004a,b
94	*Cryptolepis sinensis* (Lour.) Merr.	Stems, leaves	Snakebites, traumatic injury, scabies	Ghosh, 2004a,b
95	*Cucumis callosus* (Rottl.) Cogn	Fruit	Constipation	Verma et al., 2010
96	*Cupania jackiana* Hiern	Leaves	Conjunctivitis	Verma et al., 2010
97	*Curcuma longa* L.	Rhizome	Fracture, eye pain	Sharief et al., 2005
98	*Curcuma zedoaria* (Christm.) Roscoe	Rhizome, leaves	Cold, cough	Sharief, 2007
99	*Cuscuta reflexa* Roxb.	–	Purgative	Ghosh, 2004a
100	*Cyanthillium cinereum* (L.) H.Robs.	Leaves	Pain in eye	Bharati et al., 2015
101	*Cyathosperma viridiflorum* Griff.	–	Tonic, aphrodisiac	Ghosh, 2004a
102	*Cymbidium aloefolium* (L.) Sw.	Plant	Ear pain	Sharief et al., 2005
103	*Daemonorops kurziana* Becc.	Stem., leaves	Sedative, tonic	Ghosh, 2004a
104	*Datura metel* L.	Leaves	Swas, bodyache during fever, snake bite	Bharati et al., 2015; Verma et al., 2010
105	*Dendrobium crumenatum* Sw.	Leaves	Fever	Verma et al., 2010

TABLE 8.1 (Continued)

S. No.	Name of the plant species	Parts Used	Purpose	Reference(s)
106	*Desmodium umbellatum* (L.) DC.	Leaves	Fever	Bhargava, 1981, 1983; Sharief, 2007
107	*Desmos cochinchinensis* Lour.	Fruits	Lactation	Ghosh, 2004a,c
108	*Dioscorea alata* L.	Tuber	Digestive problems, kidney and spleen disorders	Ghosh, 2004a
109	*Dioscorea bulbifera* L.	Tuber	Contraceptive	Ghosh, 2004a,c
110	*Dioscorea esculenta* (Lour.) Burkill	Tuber	Kidney trouble	Ghosh, 2004a
111	*Dioscorea hispida* Dennst.	Tuber	Syphilitic sores, arthritis, rheumatic pain	Ghosh, 2004a
112	*Dioscorea vexans* Prain & Burk	Tuber	Antifertility, arthritis, asthma, eczema, chronic cough, diarrhea and diabetes and regulate metabolism.	Das et al., 2006
113	*Dischidia bengalensis* Colebr.	Leaves, twigs	Mumps, sores, bone fracture	Elanchezhian et al., 2007; Sharief and Rao, 2007
114	*Dischidia nummularia* R.Br.	–	Eczema, herpes, boils, goiter, diuretic	Ghosh, 2004a
115	*Donax canaeformis* (G.Forst.) K.Schum.	Root, stem, leaves	Body pain, stomach pains and disorders, fever, gynecological disorders, abdominal and spinal pain	Bhargava, 1981; Sharief, 2007; Sharief and Rao, 2007
116	*Dracaena angustifolia* Roxb.	Leaves	Stomach pain	Sharief, 2007
117	*Drynaria quercifolia* L.	Plant	Body pain	Verma et al., 2010
118	*Drypetes assamica* (Hook.f.) Pax & Hoffm.	Leaves	Chest pain, snake bite	Sharief, 2007
119	*Entada rheedei* Spr.	Root	Astringent, snake bites	Ghosh, 2004a,b

TABLE 8.1 (Continued)

S. No.	Name of the plant species	Parts Used	Purpose	Reference(s)
120	*Erycibe expansa* Wall. ex G.Don	Leaves	Skin rash, labor delivery	Ghosh, 2004a,c
121	*Erythrina orientalis* (L.) Merr.	Bark	Fever	Awasthi, 1991; Sharief, 2007
122	*Eupatorium odoratum* L.	Leaves	Wounds	Awasthi, 1991
123	*Euphorbia atoto* Forst.f.	Leaves	Cuts, wounds, rheumatism, ulcers, sores	Verma et al., 2010
124	*Euphorbia hirta* L.	Leaves	Cuts, wounds	Gupta et al., 2004; Verma et l., 2010
125	*Euphorbia longan* Steud.	Leaves	Rheumatism	Verma et al., 2010
126	*Ficus ampelas* Burm.	Leaves	Bone fracture	Verma et al., 2010
127	*Ficus hispida* L.f.	Leaves	Flatulence	Verma et al., 2010
128	*Ficus microcarpa* L.f.	Stem, leaf	Fracture, joint pain	Bharati et al., 2015
129	*Ficus tinctoria* G. Forst.	Stem, leaves	Fracture, joint pain	Bharti eet al., 2015
130	*Flagellaria indica* L.	Plant	Diuretic	Ghosh, 2004a
131	*Ganophyllum falcatum* Blume	Leaves	Abdominal pain	Bharati et al., 2015
132	*Garcinia nervosa* Miq.	Leaves, roots	Body pain, washing uterus after child birth	Elanchezhian et al., 2007
133	*Globba marantina* L.	Leaves	Conjunctivitis	Verma et al., 2010
134	*Glochidion calocarpum* Kuna	Seed, bark leaf	Skin diseases, fever	Elanchezhian et al., 2007; Sharief and Rao, 2007
135	*Gloriosa superba* L.	Tuber, root	As an aid to child birth and for abortion, snake bite	Ghosh, 2004a,b,c
136	*Glycosmis arborea* DC.	Leaves	Chronic headache	Sharief, 2007
137	*Gossypium herbaceum* L.	Leaves	Burning micturition	Bharati et al., 2015

TABLE 8.1 (Continued)

S. No.	Name of the plant species	Parts Used	Purpose	Reference(s)
138	*Gouania tilifolia* Lamk.	Stems	Internal injuries, fractures	Gupta et al., 2004
139	*Grewia acuminata* Juss.	Leaves	Parturition	Verma et al., 2010
140	*Guettardia speciosa* L.	Leaves	Stomachache	Verma et al., 2010
141	*Gymnema latifolium* Wall. ex Wight	Leaves	Emetic, snake bite	Ghosh, 2004a,b
142	*Harrisonia brownie* A. H. L.Juss.	–	Diarrhea	Ghosh, 2004a
143	*Heritiera littoralis* Dryand	Leaves	Stimulant	Sharief, 2007
144	*Hernandia ovigera* L.	Leaves, bark, seeds	Headache, tumor, epilepsy, fits, anti-inflammatory, purgative, cuts, wounds	Das et al., 2006
145	*Hernandia peltata* Sesse & Moc.		Headache	Bhargava, 1981
146	*Hibiscus tiliaceus* L.	Leaves	Stomach disorder, stimulant, urinary troubles	Awasthi, 1991; Sharief, 2007; Verma et al., 2010
147	*Hippocratea grahamii* Wight	Root	Tonic, emmenagogue, post partum	Ghosh, 2004a
148	*Hornstedtia fenzlii* (Kurz.) K.Schum.	Root, flower	Wash the uterus after child birth	Sharief and Rao, 2007
149	*Horsfieldia glabra* (Bl.) Warb.	Fruits	Abdominal pain	Sharief, 2007
150	*Hoya globosa* Hook.f.	–	Poisonous fish stings, gonorrhea, wounds, varicose ulcers	Ghosh, 2004a
151	*Ichnocarpus frutescens* (L.) W.TAiton	Seeds, stem leaves	Rheumatism, urticarial	Ghosh, 2004a
152	*Ipomoea aquatica* Forssk.	Plants	Weakness, nervousness	Ghosh, 2004a
153	*Ipomoea nil* (L.) Roth	–	Anthelmintic	Ghosh, 2004a

TABLE 8.1 (Continued)

S. No.	Name of the plant species	Parts Used	Purpose	Reference(s)
154	*Ipomoea pes-caprae* (L.) Sweet	Leaves	Headache, edema, rheumatism, sores, ulcers, boils	Bhargava, 1981; Ghosh, 2004a; Verma et al., 2010
155	*Ipomoea pes-tigridis* L.	Leaves	Blood dysentery, burns, scalds, snake bite	Ghosh, 2004a,b
156	*Jacquemontia paniculata* (Burm.)H.Hallier	–	Swellings	Ghosh, 2004a
157	*Jasminum cordifolium* Wall.	Leaves	Toothache	Ghosh, 2004a
158	*Jasminum sambac* (L.) Aiton	Flowers	Ear, nose, throat diseases	Ghosh, 2004a
159	*Kaempferia rotunda* L.	Rhizome	Gastric problems, giddiness	Sharief et al., 2005
160	*Kaempferia siphonantha* King ex. Baker	Tuber	Fever, stomach pain	Das et al., 2006
161	*Knema andamanica* (Warb.) de Wilde	Leaves, bark	Throat pain, cough	Sharief, 2007
162	*Lasianthus andamanicus* Hook.f.	Fruit	Antidote	Sharief, 2007
163	*Leea grandifolia* Kurz	Leaves	Fever	Elanchezhian et al., 2007; Sharief and Rao, 2007
164	*Leea indica* Merr.	Leaves	Cuts, wounds	Verma et al., 2010
165	*Lepidopetalum montanum* (Bl.) Radlk.	Leaves	Stomachache	Gupta et al., 2004
166	*Luffa cylindrica* (L.) M.Roemer	Fruits, leaves	Purgative, emetic, febrifuge, snake bite	Ghosh, 2004a,b
167	*Macaranga indica* Wight	Leaves	Antiemetic, stomachache	Verma et al., 2010
168	*Macaranga nicobarica* N. P Balakr. & P. Chakr.	Leaves	Stomach disorder	Elanchezhian et al., 2007; Sharief and Rao, 2007

TABLE 8.1 (Continued)

S. No.	Name of the plant species	Parts Used	Purpose	Reference(s)
169	*Macaranga peltata* (Roxb.) Mull.Arg.		Stomach pains and disorders	Bhargava, 1981
170	*Macaranga tanarius* (L.) Mull. Arg.	Leaves	Indigestion, abdominal pain	Bharati et al., 2015
171	*Mallotus peltatus* (Geisel.) Mull. Arg.	Leaves	Menstrual pain, stomach disorders	Sharief, 2007; Sharief and Rao, 2007
172	*Mallotus phillipensis* (Lam.) Mull.-Arg.	Fruits, bark, leaves, roots, seed	Anthelmintic, abdominal pain, skin diseases, cuts, wounds	Das et al., 2006
173	*Melastoma malabathricum* L.	Leaves, stem, roots	Wounds	Elanchezhian et al., 2007; Sharief and Rao, 2007
174	*Merremia umbellata* subsp. *orientalis* (H.Hallier) van Oostrum	Leaves	Purgative, snake bite, thrush, diuretic, anthelmintic	Ghosh, 2004a
175	*Microsorium punctatum* L.	Leaves	Snake bite	Verma et al., 2010
176	*Millingtonia hortensis* L.	Leaves	Headache, bodyache, fever	Sharief et al., 2005
177	*Momordica charantia* L.	Leaves	Sprue, asthma, skin affections	Ghosh, 2004a
178	*Momordica cochinchinensis* Spreng.	—	Abscesses, mumps, edema, rheumatism	Ghosh, 2004a
179	*Morinda citrifolia* L.	Leaves, roots, fruit	Cuts and wounds, stomach pains and disorders, bone fracture, bodyache	Bhargava, 1981; Gupta et al., 2004; Verma et al., 2010; Bharati et al., 2015
180	*Mucuna gigantea* (Willd.) DC.	Shoots, seeds	Sprain, aphrodisiac, purgative	Sharief, 2007

TABLE 8.1 (Continued)

S. No.	Name of the plant species	Parts Used	Purpose	Reference(s)
181	*Myristica andamanica* Hook.f.	Leaves, twigs	Sickness, bleeding	Sharief, 2007
182	*Myristica elliptica* Wall.	Seed, bark	Skin diseases	Elanchezhian et al., 2007
183	*Myristica peltata* Wall. ex Hook.f.	Seeds, bark	Skin diseases	Sharief and Rao, 2007
184	*Nypa fruticans* Wurmb.	Leaves, roots	Roofing, hunting crocodiles	Awasthi, 1991
185	*Ochrosia oppositifolia* K.Schum.	Leaves	Gynecological disorders	Verma et al., 2010
186	*Ocimum sanctum* L.	Leaves	Cough, cold, fatigue	Awasthi, 1991; Gupta et al., 2004; Sharief, 2007; Verma et al., 2010
187	*Ophiorrhiza nicobarica* N. P. Balakr.	Leaves	Wounds	Elanchezhian et al., 2007; Sharief and Rao, 2007
188	*Oplismenus compositus* (L.) Beauv.	Plants	Snake bite	Verma et al., 2010
189	*Orophea katschallica* Kurz	-	Insect repellent	Bhargava, 1981; Sharief, 2007
190	*Oroxylum indicum* Vent.	Leaves	Injury	Bharati et al., 2015
191	*Oxalis corniculata* L.	Whole plant	Fracture	Sharief et al., 2005
192	*Paedaria foetida* L.	Leaves	Prodtitis, gout, dysentery, flatulence, eye infections, toothache, ringworm, malaria, fracture	Ghosh, 2004a; Bharraati et al., 2015
193	*Paedaria scandens* (Lour.) Merr.	–	Digestive, antirheumatic, stomachic, tonic	Ghosh, 2004a
194	*Pandanus andamanensis* Hort. ex Balf.f.	Leaves	Body pain	Sharief, 2007
195	*Pandanus lerum* Jones	Leaves	Fatigue	Verma et al., 2010

TABLE 8.1 (Continued)

S. No.	Name of the plant species	Parts Used	Purpose	Reference(s)
196	*Parabaena sagittata* Miers	Leaves	Snake bite	Verma et al., 2010
197	*Paramignya andamanica* (King) Tan	Leaves, fruits	Cough, bronchitis	Ghosh, 2004a
198	*Parsonsia alboflavescens* (Dennstedt) Mabberley	Leaves	Leg swellings, disinfectant, tuberculosis, vulnerary, febrifuge, rheumatism	Ghosh, 2004a
199	*Passiflora foetida* L.	Leaves	Conjunctivitis	Verma et al., 2010
200	*Peperomia pellucida* (L.) H. B. K.	Whole plant	Cuts, wounds, headache, fever	Sharief et al., 2005
201	*Passiflora foetida* L.	–	Snake bite, hypertension, anti-inflammatory, diabetes, bone fracture, itching, wounds	Ghosh, 2004a
202	*Peperomia pellucida* H. B. K.	Juice	Diarrhea, dysentery, urinary troubles	Verma et al., 2010
203	*Phyllanthus amarus* Schumm. & Thonn.	Leaves, plant, root	Bites of centipedes and snakes, antidote, stomachache, fever, jaundice, allergy, body pain, boils and sores, diarrhea, dysentery, gonorrhea	Awasthi, 1991; Gupta et al., 2004; Elanchezhian et al., 2007; Sharief, 2007; Verma et al., 2010
204	*Phyllanthus andamanicus* Balakr. & Nair	Leaves	Diuretic	Das et al., 2006
205	*Phyllanthus emblica* L.	Fruits, leaves	Weakness after abortion, anti-emetic	Sharief et al., 2005; Verma et al., 2010
206	*Phyllanthus fraternus* Webster	Leaves, root	Allergy; boils and sores, diarrhea, dysentery, gonorrhea, stomachache	Verma et al., 2010
207	*Phyllanthus niruri* L.	Plant	Jaundice	Sharief et al., 2005
208	*Physalis minima* L.	Leaves	High fever, constipation	Gupta et al., 2004; Verma et al., 2010

TABLE 8.1 (Continued)

S. No.	Name of the plant species	Parts Used	Purpose	Reference(s)
209	*Piper betle* L.	Stem, leaves, petioles	Headache, cold, cough, body pain, constipation, wounds, boils, lumbago, stimulant, male contraceptive, bone fracture	Ghosh, 2004a,c; Sharief et al., 2005; Sharief, 2007; Verma et al., 2010
210	*Piper longum* L.	Fruits	Throat lozenges, uterine hemorrhage	Ghosh, 2004a,c
211	*Pipturus argenteus* (Forst.f.) Wedd.	Leaves	Muscular swellings	Verma et al., 2010
212	*Plumeria rubra* L.	Bark, leaves, latex	Dysentery, intestinal worms, bone fractures, blisters, sores, tongue cleaning	Gupta et al., 2004; Sharief et al., 2005; Verma et al., 2010
213	*Pongamia pinnata* (L.) Pierre	Leaves, stem bark, twigs	Malaria, fever, back pain, chronic headache, toothache, teeth cleaning	Bhargava, 1983; Awasthi, 1991; Sharief et al., 2005; Sharief, 2007
214	*Pothos scandens* L.	Stem, leaves	Asthma, small pox, post partum, worms, convulsions, asthma	Ghosh, 2004a
215	*Premna serratifolia* L.	Leaves, fruit	Body pain, cough	Bhargava, 1981, 1983; Awasthi, 1991; Sharief, 2007
216	*Pseudavaria prainii* (King) Merr	Leaves	Headache, abdominal pain	Sharief, 2007
217	*Punica granatum* L.	Leaves	Cholera, chest pain	Verma et al., 2010; Bharati et al., 2015
218	*Pycnarrhena longifolia* (Decne ex Miq.) Bece.	Roots	Tonic, cicatrizant, snake bite	Ghosh, 2004a,b
219	*Pyrossia lanceolata* (L.) Ferw.	Stem, leaf	Fracture, joint pain	Bharati et al., 2015
220	*Rauvolfia sumatrana* Jack	Leaves	Injury	Bharati et al., 2015
221	*Rhizophora apiculata* Bl.	Respiratory roots, leaves	Fish bootee, antidote	Awasthi, 1991; Sharief, 2007

TABLE 8.1 (Continued)

S. No.	Name of the plant species	Parts Used	Purpose	Reference(s)
222	*Ricinus communis* L.	Leaves	Ear pain, burning micturition	Verma et al., 2010; Bharati et al., 2015
223	*Rinorea bengalensis* (Wall.) O.Kuntze	Bark	Chest pain, cold, cough, dysentery	Awasthi, 1991
224	*Rinorea macrophylla* (Decne) O.Kuntze	Leaves, bark	Lactation	Awasthi, 1991; Sharief, 2007
225	*Samanea saman* Merr.	Leaves	Conjunctivitis	Verma et al., 2010
226	*Sarcostemma acidum* (Roxb.) Voigt	–	Lactation	Ghosh, 2004a
227	*Sargassum wightii* Grev.	Plant	Malaria	Awasthi, 1991
228	*Scaevola koenigii* Vahl		Cough	Bhargava, 1981
229	*Scaevola sericea* Vahl	Fruits, leaves	Headache, cough; rheumatic pain, fever, bodyache	Bhargava, 1981, 1983; Sharief, 2007
230	*Schefflera elliptica* (Bl.) Harms	Leaves	Fracture	Sharief et al., 2005
231	*Semecarpus kurzii* Engler	Leaf, fruit, resin	Anthelmintic, malarial fever, injuries, allergy of skin	Das et al., 2006; Elanchezhian et al., 2007; Sharief and Rao, 2007
232	*Senna occidentalis* (L.) Link (Syn.: *Cassia occidentalis* L.)	Seeds, leaves	Centipede bite, bodyache during fever, fever	Sharief et al., 2005; Verma et al., 2010
233	*Sida acuta* Burm.f	Leaves	Hairfall	Gupta et al., 2004
234	*Smilax bracteata* C.Presl.	Leaves	Uterine tract problem	Ghosh, 2004c
235	*Smilax glabra* Roxb.	Leaves, fruits	Urogenital diseases	Ghosh, 2004c.

TABLE 8.1 (Continued)

S. No.	Name of the plant species	Parts Used	Purpose	Reference(s)
236	*Smilax ovalifolia* Roxb.	Roots	Uterine diseases	Ghosh, 2004a,c
237	*Smilax zeylanica* L.	Roots	White discharge	Ghosh, 2004a,c
238	*Solanum nigrum* L.	Leaves	Bodyache during fever	Verma et al., 2010
239	*Spilanthes paniculata* Wall. ex DC.	Plant	Toothache	Sharief et al., 2005
240	*Stephania andamanica* Diels	–	Anthelmintic, sedative	Ghosh, 2004a
241	*Stephania japonica* (Thunb.) Miers	Leaves	Leucorrhoea, birth control	Ghosh, 2004a,c
242	*Sterculia rubiginosa* Vent.	Leaves	Cough, fever	Verma et al., 2010; Bharati et al., 2015
243	*Sterculia prviflora* Roxb.	Leaves	Injury	Bharati et al., 2015
244	*Strychnos andamanensis* Hill.	Roots	Snake bite	Ghosh, 2004b
245	*Strychnos minor* Dennst.	Roots	Prolapse of uterus	Ghosh, 2004a
246	*Strychnos wallichiana* Stendel	Roots	Rheumatism, ulcer, fever, epilepsy	Ghosh, 2004a
247	*Syzygium samarangense* (Bl.) Merr. & Perry	Leaves	Fever, headache	Sharief, 2007
248	*Tabernaemontana crispa* Roxb.	Leaves, fruit	Dizziness, injury, dysentery, stomachache, ulcers, sores	Gupta et al., 2004; Verma et al., 2010; Bharati et al., 2015
249	*Tamarindus indica*	Leaves	Diarrhea, dysentery	Verma et al., 2010
250	*Tetrastigma lanceolarium* (Roxb.) Planch.	–	Headache, fever, boils, dropsy	Ghosh, 2004a
251	*Thespesia populnea* (L.) Sol. ex Corr.	Leaves	Constipation	Bhargava, 1983; Sharief, 2007

TABLE 8.1 (Continued)

S. No.	Name of the plant species	Parts Used	Purpose	Reference(s)
252	*Thottea tomentosa* (Bl.) Ding Hou	Whole plant	Chest pain, headache, cough, cold	Sharief, 2007
253	*Tinospora cordifolia* (Willd.) Hook.f. & Thoms.	Roots, whole plant	Asthma, rheumatism, febrifuge, snake bite, sexual impotency	Ghosh, 2004a,b,c
254	*Tinospora glabra* (Burm.f.) Merr.	–	Febrifuge, tetanus, jaundice	Ghosh, 2004a
255	*Tournefortia ovata* Wall. ex G.Don	Roots, whole plant	Purgative, snake bite, influenza, insect stings, female problems	Ghosh, 2004a,b,c
256	*Trichosanthes bracteata* (Lamk.) Voigt	Whole plant	Throat infection, diarrhea, dysentery	Sharief, 2007; Verma et al., 2010
257	*Triumfetta repens* (Bl.) Merr. & Rolfe			
258	*Triumfetta rhomboidea* Jacq.	Leaves	Cough	Verma et al., 2010
259	*Tylophora indica* (Burm.f.) Merr.	Leaves, roots	Snake bite, body pain	Ghosh, 2004a; Verma et al., 2010
260	*Uncaria sessilifructus* Roxb.	Leaves	Diarrhea, dysentery, urinary tract problems	Ghosh, 2004a,c
261	*Urena lobata* L.	Leaves	Conjunctivitis	Sharief et al., 2005
262	*Vitex trifolia* L.	–	Insect repellant	Bhargava, 1981
263	*Vigna unguiculata* (L.) Walp. ssp. *cylindrica* (L.) van Esltine	Seeds	Fistula, jaundice, tumor, small pox	Ghosh, 2004a
264	*Wedelia biflora* DC.	Leaves	Cuts and wounds, headache	Bhargava, 1981, 1983; Sharief, 2007
265	*Zingiber officinale* Rosc.	Leaves	Cough	Verma et al., 2010
266	*Zingiber zerumbet* (L.) J. E.Sm	Rhizome	Cold, cough, headache, giddiness	Sharief et al., 2005

with forest is in a balanced state. They live in cohesion with the nature with least or negligible disturbance to the fragile ecosystem. The tribes depend completely on the forest and marine resources for their livelihood. The semi-nomadic nature of these tribes within the forest area, allow them to use the resources judiciously without over exploiting them.

Dagar (1989) documented uses of 73 plant species as folk medicine used by Nicobarese tribals of Car Nicobar Island. Dagar and Dagar (1991) reported the use of 65 plant species as folk medicine among the Nicobarese of Katchal Island. Dagar and Dagar (1999) gave a detailed account of plants and animals used by Negrito and Mongoloid tribals of Andaman and Nicobar Islands in their routine life for food, shelter, dugour canoe making, taboos, rituals and medicines. Kumar et al. (2006) gave the ethnobotanical profile of 197 species used by the Nicobarese tribe. Prasad et al. (2008) reported that rural folk of North Andamans are using 72 plant species for curing 42 ailments. Ethnomedicinal uses of 289 plant species used by the aborigines in Andaman & Nicobar Islands have been documented by Pandey et al. (2009). Rasingam et al. (2012) gave the details of 11 plant species used as herbal tooth sticks used by the Chota Nagpuri and Tamil inhabitants of Andaman and Nicobar Islands. Chander et al. (2014) reported use of 150 medicinal plant species to treat 47 different medicinal uses, divided into nine categories of use. Chander et al. (2015a) recorded the use of 132 medicinal plant species for treating 43 ailments among Nicobrese of Nancowry group of Islands. Chander et al. (2015b) reported uses of 34 medicinal plant species to treat a total of 16 ailments by the Nicobarese inhabiting Little Nicobar Island of Andaman & Nicobar Archipelago. Chander et al. (2015c) documented the use of 78 medicinal plant species to treat 38 different ailments among Karens of Andaman & Nicobar Islands. Other publications on ethnomedicinal plants of Nicobarese include Dagar (1989) and Dagar and Dagar (1996, 2003).

8.4   OTHER USES OF PLANTS

Ethnic tribes of Andaman and Nicobar Islands use plants for various other purposes which are given in Table 8.2.

TABLE 8.2 Miscellaneous Ethnobotanical Uses by Ethnic Tribes of Great Nicobar Islands

S. No.	Name of the plant species	Parts Used	Purpose	Reference(s)
1	*Actephila excelsa* Mull. Arg.	Stem	Poles, beams & thatching sticks	Elanchezhian et al., 2007
2	*Anaxagorea javanica* Bl.	Stems	Rudders	Awasthi, 1991
3	*Ancistrocladus extensus* Wall. ex Planch.		Arrows	Bhargava, 1981
4	*Anodendron paniculatum* A.DC.	Bark	String	Bhargava, 1981; Awasthi, 1991
5	*Antidesma coriaceum* Tul.	Leaves	Honey bee dispersal	Awasthi, 1991
6	*Artocarpus gomezianus* Wall. ex Trec.	Trunk	Dugout canoes	Awasthi, 1991
7	*Barringtonia asiatica* (L.) Kurz	Fruit, trunk	Fish poison, canoe	Elanchezhian et al., 2007
8	*Bombax insigne* Wall.	Silky fibers	Stuffing pillows	Awasthi, 1991
9	*Calamus andamanicus* Kurz.	Leaves, cut stem	Mats, quench thirst	Awasthi, 1991
10	*Calamus longisetus* Griff.	Leaves	Roofing	Awasthi, 1991
11	*Calamus palustris* Griff.		Huts construction	Bhargava, 1981
12	*Canarium denticulatum* Bl.	Trunk	Dugout canoes	Awasthi, 1991
13	*Canarium euphyllum* Kurz.	Resin, trunk	Mosquito repellent, dugout canoes, covering binding of arrows	Bhargava, 1981, 1983
14	*Ceiba pentandra* (L.) Gaertn.	Trunk	Dugout canoes	Awasthi, 1991
15	*Ceriops tagal* (Perr.) C. B.Rob.	Trunk, bark	Pillars, dye	Awasthi, 1991
16	*Cocos nucifera* L.	Rachis of leaves	Broom sticks	Awasthi, 1991
17	*Crinum asiaticum* L.	Leaves, stem bark	Roofing, pillow covers	Awasthi, 1991
18	*Daemonorops manii* Becc.	Shoot apex	To cover female genitals	Bhargava

TABLE 8.2 (Continued)

S. No.	Name of the plant species	Parts Used	Purpose	Reference(s)
19	*Desmos dasymaschalus* (Bl.) Safford	Branches; tree trunk	For making arrows for fish hunting; pillar in construction	Bhargava 1981, 1983
20	*Dinochloa scandens* O. Kuntze	Stem, twig pieces	Making floor of hut, as fishing harpoons, as ear ornament	Elanchezhian et al., 2007
21	*Donax cannaeformis* (G.Forst.) K.Schum.	Stems peelings, leaves	Basket making, mats, purify drinking water	Bhargava 1983; Awasthi, 1991
22	*Drypetes longifolia* (Bl.) Pax & Hoffm.	Trunk	Poles, pillars	Awasthi, 1991
23	*Ficus fulva* Reinw. ex Blume	Bark fiber	Cordage	Elanchezhian et al., 2007
24	*Ficus retusa* L. var. *nitida* Thunb.	Bark fiber	Cordage	Awasthi, 1991
25	*Garcinia andamanica* King	Trunk	Poles and pillars	Bhargava, 1983
26	*Garcinia nervosa* Miq.	Branches	Paddle of canoe	Elanchezhian et al., 2007
27	*Genianthus laurifolius* Hook.f.	Bark	Nets, bowstrings, fastening of adzes	Awasthi, 1991
28	*Haematocarpus validus* (Miers) Bakf.	Flexible stems	Tie poles, traps for hunting deer and boar	Awasthi, 1991
29	*Hernandi peltata* Meissn.	Trunk	Dugout canoes	Awasthi, 1991
30	*Ixora brunnescens* Kurz.	Trunk	Rudders	Awasthi, 1991
31	*Korthalsia rogersii* Becc.	Flexible stems	Tie poles	Awasthi, 1991
32	*Liciuala peltata* Roxb.	Leaves	For making umbrellas	Bhargava, 1983; Awasthi, 1991
33	*Mallotus resinosus* Merr.	Stem	Poles, beams & thatching sticks	Elanchezhian et al., 2007
34	*Mangifera camptospermum* Pierra	Wood	To make dugout canoe	Awasthi, 1991

TABLE 8.2 (Continued)

S. No.	Name of the plant species	Parts Used	Purpose	Reference(s)
35	*Manilkara littoralis* (Kurz.) Dub.	Wood	For making bow	Bhargava, 1981, 1983
36	*Meladorum macranthum* Kurz.	Branches, bark	Shafts of arrows, hog spears, as apron by men	Awasthi, 1991
37	*Nypa fruticans* Wurmp	Leaves	Thatching	Elanchezhian et al., 2007
38	*Orophea hexandra* Bl.	Logs	Fuel	Awasthi, 1991
39	*Orophea katschallica* Kurz.	Leaves	Honey bee dispersal	Bhargava, 1983
40	*Pandanus leram* Jones	Leaves	Thatching	Elanchezhian et al., 2007
41	*Pandanus tectorius* Sol. ex Warb.	Leaves	Thatching	Bhargava, 1983
42	*Phaeanthus andamanicus* King	Wood	Bows, rudders	Awasthi, 1991
43	*Polyalthia jenkinsii* Hook.f. & Thoms.	Leaves	Honey bee repellant	Awasthi, 1991
44	*Pseuduvaria prainii* (King.) Merr.	Branches	Rudders	Awasthi, 1991
45	*Pterocarpus dalbergioides* Roxb.	Trunk	Sounding boards	Awasthi, 1991
46	*Pterygota alata* R.Br	Wood	Firewood	Elanchezhian et al., 2007
47	*Sagaraea elliptica* (A.DC.) Hook.f. & Thoms.		Bows	Bhargava, 1981
48	*Semecarpus kurzii* Engler	Stems	Poles, beams and thatching sticks	Elanchezhian et al., 2007
49	*Sterculia macrophylla* Vent.	Trunks	Dugout canoes	Awasthi, 1991
50	*Xylocarpus granatum* Koen.	Trunks, fruits	Pillars, toys	Awasthi, 1991
51	*Zingiber squarrosum* Roxb.	Petioles	Chewed to alleviate thirst	Bhargava, 1983

8.5   ETHNIC FOOD PLANTS AND ETHNIC FOODS OF THE ANDAMAN AND NICOBAR ISLANDS

8.5.1   DIVERSITY OF FOOD PLANTS

There are limited reports on ethnic food plants of indigenous tribes of the region. Works on the culture and tradition as well as ethnobotany of the aboriginal tribes of the Andamans has been carried out by a few anthropologists who have made some references to plants used by the tribal folks (Klos, 1902; Chak, 1967; Singh, 1975; Cipriani, 1996; Balakrishnan, 1996; Kashyap et al., 2003; Patnaik, 2006; Singh et al., 2007; Krishnakumar, 2009; Seksharia and Pandya, 2010). Some authors reported dietary utilization of plant resources by indigenous people of Andaman and Nicobar Islands (Thothathri, 1966; Awasthi, 1991; Sangal, 1971; Chengappa, 1958; Joshi, 1975; Sahni, 1953; Anonymous, 1948–1972; Bhargava, 1981, 1983; Raghunathan, 1976; Watt, 1990; Zama, 1976; Shareif, 2007; Singh and Singh, 2012). The chief reason for scarce ethnobotanical information could be because only the Great Andamanese and Onge regions are accessible for outsiders while the Jarawa and Sentinelese peoples are still hostile (Awasthi, 1991). The indigenous tribes of the Great Andamans have great affinity towards wild foods, particularly they are acquainted to consumption of wild fruits. Perhaps, with long association with forest and meticulous observation of plants and animals, they have gained knowledge on the poisonous and non-poisonous forest products. Some of the foods are eaten raw while some are eaten either in cooked form or eaten roasted. The people are also aware of quenching their thirst through chewing stems of certain plants like *Flagellaria indica* or sometimes chew petioles of *Zingiber squarossum* to alleviate their thirst. Available data on food plants of the indigenous tribes of the Great Andamans is presented in Table 8.3. A total of 61 edible plants belonging to 37 botanical families have been compiled. A glance of the enumeration reflects the foods are minimally processed and no great efforts are devoted for preparing the foods. Plants foods of the Jarawas and Sentineleses are almost negligible; of the few plants consumed by them, the preparation methods are not known which suggest most foods are eaten raw.

TABLE 8.3 Diversity of Food Plants and Preparation by Ethnic Tribes of Andamans

Sl. no.	Plants	Family	Parts used	Food preparation and consumption			
				Great Andamanese	Onges	Jarawa	Sentinelese
1.	Abrus precatorius L.	Fabaceae	Ripe pods	–	Roasted and eaten	–	–
2.	Acacia pennata Willd.	Mimosaceae	Fruits	Eaten raw	–	–	–
3.	Calamus andamanicus Kurz.	Arecaceae		–	–	NK	–
4.	Annona squamosa L.	Annonaceae	Fruits	Daily diet	–	–	–
5.	Artabotrys speciosus Kurz. ex Hook.f. & Thoms.	Annonaceae	Fruits	–	–	NK	–
6.	Artocarpus chaplasha Roxb.	Moraceae		–	–	NK	–
7.	Artocarpus gomeziana Wall. ex Trec.	Moraceae	Fruits	Eaten raw when ripe; young fruits eaten boiled as vegetable	–	NK	–
8.	Artocarpus integrifolia L.	Moraceae	Fruits	Eaten as vegetable	–	–	–
9.	Artocarpus lakoocha Roxb.	Moraceae	Fruits	–	–	–	–
10.	Atalantia monophylla	Rutaceae	Fruits	Eaten raw	–	–	–
11.	Baccaurea ramiflora Lour.	Euphorbiaceae		–	–	NK	–
12.	Barringtonia asiatica (L.) Kurtz.	Lecythidaceae	Seed		Eaten roasted	–	–
13.	Bombax insigne Wall.	Bombacaceae	Nut kernel		Eaten raw	–	–
14.	Bruguiera gymnorhiza (L.) Lamk.	Rhizophoraceae	Fruits	Eaten raw	–	–	–

TABLE 8.3 (Continued)

Sl. no.	Plants	Family	Parts used	Food preparation and consumption			
				Great Andamanese	Onges	Jarawa	Sentinelese
15.	Calamus viminalis Willd.	Arecaceae	Fruits	Eaten raw	–	–	–
16.	Carica papaya L.	Caricaceae	Fruits	Daily food	–	–	–
17.	Caryota mitis Lour.	Arecaceae	Stem	Eaten raw	–	–	–
18.	Cocos nucifera L.	Arecaceae	Kernel	Eaten raw	–	–	–
19.	Cycas rumphii Miq.	Cycadaceae	Fruits and tender leaves, seeds	Daily food	Cooked as vegetable	NK	–
20.	Desmodium umbellatum (L.) DC.	Fabaceae	Fruits	–	Roasted and eaten	–	–
21.	Dioscorea bulbifera L.	Dioscoreaceae	Tuber	–	–	NK	–
22.	Dioscorea glabra Roxb.	Dioscoreaceae	Tuber	–	Eaten raw or boiled	NK	–
23.	Dioscorea vexans Prain & Burkill	Dioscoreaceae	Tuber	–	–	NK	–
24.	Diospyros andamanica (Kurz) Bakh	Ebenaceae		–	–	NK	–
25.	Donax canniformis (G.Forst.) K.Schum.	Marantaceae		–	–	–	–
26.	Dracaena augustifolia Roxb.	Dracaenaceae	Fruits	–	Eaten roasted	–	–
27.	Ficus hispida L.f.	Moraceae	Fruits	–	Eaten roasted	–	–
28.	Ficus nervosa Heyne ex Roth	Moraceae	Fruits	Eaten raw	–	–	–

TABLE 8.3 (Continued)

Sl. no.	Plants	Family	Parts used	Food preparation and consumption				
				Great Andamanese	Onges	Jarawa	Sentinelese
29.	*Ficus racemosa* L.	Moraceae		–	–	NK	–
30.	*Flagellaria indica* L.	Flagellariaceae	Stem	–	Chewed and eaten raw	–	–
31.	*Garcinia andamanica* King.	Clusiaceae	Fruits	Eaten raw	–	–	–
32.	*Garcinia cowa* Roxb. ex DC.	Clusiaceae		–	–	NK	–
33.	*Heritiera littoralis* Aiton	Sterculiaceae	Seed, leaves	–	Seeds eaten roasted, leaves used in preparation of Ogne tea	–	–
34.	*Hibiscus tiliaceus* L.	Malvaceae	Leaves	–	Beverage, taken as tea	–	–
35.	*Ipomoea sepiaria* Roxb.	Convolvulaceae	Tuber	Eaten roasted	–	–	–
36.	*Magnolia andamanica* (King) Raju & Nayar	Magnoliaeeae	Leaves	Meat is baked in leaves	–	–	–
37.	*Mallotus peltatus* (Geisel.) Muell.-Arg.	Euphorbiaceae	Leaves	–	Eaten raw; treats abdominal pain	–	–
38.	*Mangifera andamanica* King	Anacardiaceae		–	–	NK	–
39.	*Mangifera comptospermum* Pierre	Anacardiaceae	Fruits	Eaten raw	–	–	–

TABLE 8.3   (Continued)

Sl. no.	Plants	Family	Parts used	Food preparation and consumption			
				Great Andamanese	Onges	Jarawa	Sentinelese
40.	Mangifera indica L.	Anacardiaceae	Fruits	Eaten raw	–	–	–
41.	Manihot esculenta Crantz	Euphorbiaceae	Tubers	Eaten roasted or cooked for vegetable	–	–	–
42.	Manilkara littoralis (Kurz) Dubard	Sapotaceae	Fruits	Eaten raw	Eaten	–	–
43.	Moringa pterygosperma Gaertn.	Moringaceae	Fruits and leaves	Cooked for vegetables	–	–	–
44.	Musa sapientum L.	Musaceae	Fruits and inflorescent	Ripe fruit eaten raw, inflorescence and immature fruits cooked as vegetables	–	–	–
45.	Nypa fruticans Wurmb.	Arecaceae	Fruit kernels	Eaten raw	–	–	–
46.	Oroxylum indicum (L.) Kurz	Bignoniaceae	Fruits	–	Eaten raw	–	–
47.	Pandanus andamanensium Kurz.	Pandanaceae	Fruits	Staple food	–	–	–
48.	Pandanus tectorius Sol. ex Warb.	Pandanaceae	Fruits	–	Staple food.	–	Staple foods
49.	Phoenix paludosa Roxb.	Arecaceae	Stem pith and inflorescence	Cooked as vegetables	–	–	–
50.	Pinanga manii Becc.	Arecaceae		–	–	NK	–

TABLE 8.3 (Continued)

Sl. no.	Plants	Family	Parts used	Food preparation and consumption			
				Great Andamanese	Onges	Jarawa	Sentinelese
51.	*Pometia pinnata* J. R. Forst. & G. Forst.	Sapindaceae	Fruits	—	—	Eaten raw	—
52.	*Pongamia pinnata* (L.) Pierre.	Fabaceae	Seeds	—	Eaten raw	—	—
53.	*Premna serratifolia* L.	Verbenaceae	Fruits	—	Eaten after mixing with rice	—	—
54.	*Psidium guajava* L.	Myrtaceae	Fruits	Eaten raw	—	—	—
55.	*Pterospermum diversifolium* Blume	Sterculiaceae	Leaves	Meat is baked in leaves of this species	—	—	—
56.	*Rhaphidophora pertusa* Schott	Araceae	Leaves	Leaves cooked with immature fruits of *Artocarpus gomeziana*, reduce sourness	—	—	—
57.	*Rhizophora apiculata* Blume	Rhizophoraceae	Fruits	—	Eaten boiled	—	—
58.	*Sarcostigma wallichii* Baill.	Icacinaceae	Fruits	Eaten raw	—	—	—
59.	*Tamarindus indica* L.	Caesalpiniaceae	Tender pods	Usually cooked with fish.	—	—	—
60.	*Terminalia catappa* L.	Combretaceae	Fruits, Nut kernel	Eaten raw	Eaten raw	NK	—
61.	*Trichosanthes tricuspidata* Lour.	Cucurbitaceae	Fruits	—	Eaten roasted	—	—

8.5.2 DIETARY SYSTEMS AND CULINARY METHODS

Seafoods form the dominant component of the food system of the Andamanese. They also consume both red and white meat. Being hunters by origin, the people of the islands hunt birds and wild animals and feast on them. Before the use of fire was known to them, foods are said to be consumed in raw form. The region is rich in biodiversity and the inhabitants mainly survive through means of forest and forest products. Forest food includes mango (*Mangifera* sp.), banana (*Musa* sp.), orange (*Citrus* sp.), pineapple (*Ananas comosus*), guava (*Psidium guajava*). Fruits of *Pandanas leram, P. odaratissimus* and *P. tectorius* are common to all the indigenous tribes which also form the staple food of the Andamans. Some forest produce like roots and inner stems of certain wild palm (*Pinanga manii*) known as *komba* are also collected for food. All parts of plants (leaves, tender stem, roots, flowers, unripe fruits, spikes and immature seeds) are consumed. Traditional vegetables are consumed after minimal processing *viz.* cleaning, washing, boiling, frying, grinding, mixing and drying. The cuisines include *chutney*, fried items, pickles, boiled vegetables, roasted tender stem and mix vegetables. *Eryngium foetidum, Moringa oleifera, Hibiscus sabdariffa* and *Piper serpentum* are used to enhance taste and flavor of dietary preparations. The vegetables are also used in making of household snacks like *pakora*, soup, *muruku, vada* and *maththi*. Immature fruits of perennial trees are also used for culinary preparations but their less popularity was primarily due to cumbersome processes of product preparation and lack of availability (Singh and Singh, 2012). There exist differences among local communities for preference of traditional vegetables which might be due to differences in dietary habits and associated food traditions (Majumdar, 1975; Singh et al., 2013).

Ethnic tribes of the Andamans also exploit animal resource as source of food. Small animals and snakes are occasionally hunted for food. Along with this, folks supplement their diet with a variety of marine products, ranging from octopus (known as *koe*) to multiple varieties of fish. Sea turtles (*Eretmochelys* sp.) and their eggs are also relished. The tribes are fond of hunting and hunt almost all the small animals such as small rodents, snakes, birds, etc. For hunting larger animals such as wild boars, monkeys and crocodiles, they usually form well-organized groups. Crocodile hunting is very rarely undertaken as it involves grouping of almost all the men and grown-up boys of a band and is a rather dangerous task. Sometimes, the total effort put in at times may result in just injuring the crocodile and in such case the hunt becomes unproductive. Both men and women gather all sorts of edible leaves and root matter; insects and larvae are often included in their collection. Fishing technology is well developed as they have variety of fishing spears which they use in the shallow coral bedded sea fronts where the waters are clear and fish are visible; use of fish net is a common practice. They use outrigger canoes which are large and capable for venturing into deep sea, but generally they use it for short trips along the coast to visit other settlements or nearby islands.

8.5.3 FOOD SYSTEMS AND CULTURE

The Onges prefer to catch sea cow *Dugong dugon* (a mammal belonging to order Sirenia) for delicious meat and they place the lower jaw of the animal in front of their house to ward off evil spirits. The Great Andamanese are very much aware of the poison of the climber *Anodendron paniculatum*. The leaves of this plant when eaten by pregnant women is said to cause abortion as the watery-milky juice of the plant is said to be septic. Aromatic resin of *Canarium euphyllum* is used by the Great Andamanese for burning during certain ceremonies. The people are very much fond of consuming the fruits of *Carica papaya* while the dried, crushed leaves are used as a substitute for tobacco. The Great Andamanese prepare tea from the mature leaves of *Hibiscus tiliaceus*, which are boiled in water to get an extract. The tea which blends into a colored and flavored drink is also used for stomach disorders.

KEYWORDS

- Andamans
- ethnobotany
- ethnofood plants
- ethnomedicinal plants
- Nicobar Islands
- traditional knowledge

REFERENCES

1. Anonymous (1948–1972). The Wealth of India-Raw Materials, Vols. 1–9; Council of Scientific & Industrial Research; New Delhi.
2. Awasthi, A. K. (1991). Ethnobotanical Studies of the Negrito Islanders of Andaman Islands, India: The Great Andamanese. *Economic Bot. 45 (2)*, 274–280.
3. Balakrishnan, N. P., & Ellis, J. L. (1996). Andaman and Nicobar Islands. In: Hajra et al. (eds.). Flora of India, Part 1. Botanical Survey of India, Calcutta, India.
4. Bharati, P. L., Prakash, O., & Jadhav, A. D. (2015). Plants used as traditional medicine by the Nicobari tribes of Andaman & Nicobar Islands. *Int. J. Bioassays 4(12)*, 4650–4652.
5. Bhargava, N. (1981). Plants in folk life and folklore in Andaman and Nicobar Islands. In: S. K.Jain (ed.) Glimpses of Indian Ethnobotany. Oxford & IBH Publishing, New Delhi, pp. 329–345.
6. Bhargava, N. (1983). Ethnobotanical studies of the tribals of Andaman & Nicobar Islands, India I: Onge. *Econ. Bot. 37(1)*, 110–119.
7. Chak, B. L. (1967). Green islands in the sea. Publication Division, Ministry of Information and Broadcasting, Government of India, Delhi.
8. Chakraborty, T., & Balakrishnan, N. P. (2003). Ethnobotany of Andaman and Nicobar Islands, India – A review. *J. Econ. Taxon. Bot. 27(4)*, 869–893.
9. Chakraborty, T., & Rao, M. K. V. (1988). Ethnobotanical studies of Shompens of Great Nicobar Island. *J. Econ. Taxon. Bot. 12*, 39–54.
10. Chander, M. P., Kartick, C., Gangadhar, J., & Vijayachari, P. (2014). Ethnomedicine and healthcare practices among Nicobarese of Car Nicobar – an indigenous tribe of Andaman and Nicobar Islands. *J. Ethnopharmacol., 158 part A*, 18–24.
11. Chander, M. P., Kartick, C., & Vijayachari, P. (2015a). Herbal medicine & healthcare practice amng Nicobarese of Nancowry group of Isalands – an indigenous tribe of Andaman & Nicobar Islands. *Indian J. Med. Res. 141(5)*, 720–740.
12. Chander, M. P., Kartick, C., & Vijayachari, P. (2015b). Medicinal plants used by the Nicobarese inhabiting Little Nicobar Island of the Andaman and Nicobar Archipelago, India. *J. Altrn. Complement. Med. 21(7)*, 373–379.
13. Chander, M. P., Kartick, C., & Vijayachari, P. (2015c). Ethnomedicinal knowledge among Karens of Andaman & Nicobar Islands, India. *J. Ethnopharmacol. 162*, 127–133
14. Chengappa, B. S. (1958). Working Plan for the Forests of the Andaman Islands, 1942–57, Port Blair: Andaman and Nicobar Administration.
15. Cipriani, L. (1996). The Andaman Islanders. Weiden-feld and Nicolson, London.
16. Dagar, H. S. (1989). Plant folk medicines among Nicobarese tribals of Car Nicobar Islands, India. *Econ. Bot. 43*, 215–224.
17. Dagar HS. (1989). Plants in folk medicine of the Nicobarese of Bampoka Island. *J Andaman Sci Assoc 5*, 69–71.
18. Dagar, H. S., & Dagar, J. C. (1991). Plant folk medicines among the Nicobarese of Katchal Islands, India. *Econ. Bot. 45*, 114–119.
19. Dagar, H. S., & Dagar, J. C. (1996). Ethnobotanical studies of the Nicobarese of Chowra Islands of Nicobar group of Islands. *J. Econ. Taxon. Bot. Additional Series, 12*, 381–388.

20. Dagar, J. C., & Dagar, H. S. (1999). Ethnobotany of aborigines of Andaman-Nicobar Islands. Surya International, Dehra Dun.
21. Dagar, H. S., & Dagar, J. C. (2003). Plants used in ethnomedicine by the Nicobarese of islands in Bay of Bengal, India. *J. Econ. Taxon. Bot. 27*, 73–84.
22. Das, S., Sheeja, T. E., & Mandal, A. (2006). Ethnomedicinal uses of certain plants from Bay Islands, *Indian J. Trad. Knowl. 5*, 207–211.
23. Elanchezhian, R., Senthilkumar, R., Beena, S. J., & Suryanarayana, M. A. (2007). Ethnobotany of Shompen – a primitive tribe of Great Nicobar Island. *Indian J. Trad. Knowl. 6(2)*, 342–345.
24. Ghosh, A. (2014a). Survey of ethno-medicinal climbing plants in Andaman and Nicobar Islands, India. *Int. J. Pharm. Life Sci. 5(7)*, 3671–3677.
25. Ghosh, A. (2014b). Traditional phytotherapy treatment for snakebite by tribal people of Andaman and Nicobar Islands, India. *Indian J. Fundamental Appl. Life Sci. 4(2)*, 130–132.
26. Ghosh, A. (2014c). Climbing plants used to cure some gynecological disorders by tribal people of Andaman and Nicobar Islands, India. *International J. Pharmacy and Life Sci. 5(5)*, 3531–3533.
27. Gupta, S., Porwal, M. C., & Roy, P. S. (2004). Indigenous knowledge on some medicinal plamts among the Nicobari tribe of Car Nicobar Island. *Indian J. Trad. Knowl. 3(3)*, 287–293.
28. Joshi, M. C. (1975). Census of India 1971, Choura-A socio-economic survey. Government of India, New Delhi.
29. Kashyap, V. K., Sitalaximi, T., Sarkar, B. N., & Trivedi, R. (2003). Molecular Relatedness of the Aboriginal Groups of Andaman and Nicobar Islands with Similar Ethnic Populations. *Int. J. Hum. Genet, 3(1)*, 5–11.
30. Kloss, C. B. (1902). Andamans and Nicobars. Vivek Publishing House, New Delhi.
31. Krishnakumar, M. V. (2009). Andaman Islands: Development or Despoliation? *The Intern. J. Res. into Island Cultures*, 3, 104–117.
32. Kumar, B. K., Kumar, T. Selvun, B. Sajibala, R. S. C. Jairaj, S. Mehrotra and P. Pushpangadan. (2006). Ethnobotanical heritage of Nicobarese tribe. *J. Econ. Taxon. Bot. 30 (2)*, 331–348.
33. Majumdar, R. C. (1975). Penal settlements in Andamans. New Delhi: Ministry of Education and Social Welfare, Govt. of India Press, McGraw-Hill. pp. 251–258.
34. Pandey, R. P., Rasingam, L., & Lakra, G. S. (2009). Ethnomedicinal plants of the Aborigines in Andaman & Nicobar Islands, India. *Nelumbo 51.*
35. Patnaik, R. (2006). The Last Foragers: Ecology of Forest Shompen. In: P Dash Sharma (Ed.): Anthropology of Primitive Tribes. New Delhi: Serial Publications, pp. 116–129.
36. Prasad, P. R. C., Reddy, C. S., Raza, S. H., Dutt, C. B. S. (2008). Folklore medicinal plants of North Andaman Islands, India. *Fitoterapia 79*, 458–464.
37. Raghunathan, K. (1976). Andaman and Nicobar Islands. Recordings of the Medico Botanical Survey Team (CCRIMH-New Delhi), Publ. 19. (Cyclo-styled).
38. Rao, P. S. N., Vinod Maina & Tiggaa, M.. (2001). The plants of sustenance among the Jarawa aboriginies in the Andaman Islands. *J. Forestry 24(3)*, 395- 402.
39. Rasingam, L., Jeeva, S., & Kannan, D. (2012). Dental care of Andaman and Nicobar folks: medicinal plants used as toothstick. *Asian Pacific J. Trop. Biomed.* S1013–S1016.

40. Sahni, K. C. (1953). Botanical exploration in the Great Nicobar. *Indian Forester,* *79*, 3–16.
41. Sampathkumar, V., & Rao, P. S. N. (2003). Dye yielding plants of Andaman & Nicobar Islands. *J. Econ. Taxon. Bot.* 27(4), 827–838.
42. Sangal, P. M. (1971). Forest food of the tribal population of Andaman and Nicobar Islands. *Indian Forester.* *97*, 646–650.
43. Sekhsaria, P., & Pandya, V. (2010). The Jarawa tribal Reserve Dossier: Cultural and biological diversities in the Andaman Islands. UNESCO, Paris.
44. Sharief, M. U. (2007). Plants folk medicine of *Negrito* tribes of Bay Islands. *Indian J. Trad. Knowl., 6 (3),* 468–476.
45. Sharief, M. U., Kumar, S., Diwakar, P. G., & Sharma, T. V. R. S. (2005). Traditional phytotherapy among Karens of Middle Andaman. *Indian J. Trad. Knowl. 4 (4),* 429–436.
46. Sharief, M. U., & Rao, R. R. (2007). Ethnobotanical studies of Shompens – A critically endangered and degenerating ethnic community in Great Nicobar Island. *Curr. Sci. 93(11),* 1623–1628.
47. Singh, R. (1975). Arrows speak louder than words: The last Andaman Islanders. *Natl. Geogr. 148,* 66–91.
48. Singh, S., & Singh, D. R. (2012). Species diversity of vegetables crops in Andaman and Nicobar Islands: efforts and challenges for utilization. In: Singh D. R. et al. (eds.): Souvenir on Innovative technologies for conservation and sustainable utilization of island biodiversity. CARI, Port Blair. pp. 120–129.
49. Singh, S., Singh, D. R., Singh, L. B., Chand, S., & Roy, S. D. (2013). Indigenous Vegetables for Food and Nutritional Security in Andaman and Nicobar Islands, India. *Intern. J. Agriculture and Food Sci. Technol., 4(5),* 503–512.
50. Thothathri. K. (1966). The tonyoge plant of Little Andaman. *Indian Forester, 92,* 530–532.
51. Verma, C., Bhatia, S., & Srivastava, S. (2010). Traditional medicine of the Nicobarese. *Indian J. Trad. Knowl. 9,* 779–785.
52. Watt, G. (1990). A dictionary of the economic products of India. 6 vol. Periodical Experts, New Delhi. (Reprinted in 1972).
53. Zama, L. (1976). Forestry in the Andamans. *Yojana 20,* 56–61.

CHAPTER 9

DOCUMENTATION AND EXCHANGE OF ETHNOBOTANICAL KNOWLEDGE

C. L. RINGMICHON[1] and BINDU GOPALAKRISHNAN[2]

[1]K.V. Pendharkar College, Dept. of Botany, Dombivli (E), Thane Dist., Mumbai, Maharashtra, E-mail: ringmi2005@rediffmail.com

[2]Department of Botany, Mithibai College, Vile Parle (W), Mumbai-56, E-mail: bindu_phd@rediffmail.com

CONTENTS

Abstract 249
9.1   Introduction 250
9.2   Ethnobotanical Studies of Different Tribes of North-East India....252
9.3   Documentation and Exchange of Ethnobotanical
       Knowledge in North-East India 253
Keywords 262
References 262

ABSTRACT

Documentation of ethnobotanical knowledge is gaining significant importance. It is an important instrument for research dealing with medicines, cultivation, vegetations etc. North East India is rich in biodiversity. It constitutes the states of Arunachal Pradesh, Assam, Manipur, Meghalaya,

Mizoram, Nagaland, Sikkim and Tripura. The people of these regions still depend on nature for their livelihood. They possess vast Knowledge of their surrounding flora and fauna. This knowledge is documented by many research scholars with the help of the ethnic tribes. The documentation shows the potentials of the ethnobotanical studies with particular reference to biodiversity conservation of the important folk medicinal plants, edible plants which are used for treating various ailments and diseases in their daily life. Thus, the ethnobotanical knowledge will remain alive for generation after generation.

9.1   INTRODUCTION

Documentation of ethnobotanical knowledge is gaining significant importance. This is mainly to preserve protect and commercialize traditional knowledge, example culture, medicine, religion etc. The WIPO Traditional Knowledge Documentation Toolkit provides useful practical guidance on how to undertake a Traditional Knowledge documentation exercise (http://www.wipo.int/export/sites/www/tk/en/resources/pdf/tk_toolkit_draft.pdf).

Documenting ethnobotanical knowledge may help preserve knowledge. Today, the cultural survival of many indigenous communities is threatened, and some traditional systems of disseminating knowledge may already be lost. Modern lifestyles and the disruption of traditional ways of life may cause younger generations to lose interest in learning about traditional medicine. Traditional languages used to pass down information may no longer be as widely understood. Documenting such information may help preserve this knowledge for future generations. Documentation can be a vital step in facilitating research on Traditional Medicinal safety and efficacy. In addition, documentation may assist with clinical practice and teaching. Given the important role traditional medicine plays in providing health care, documenting ethnomedicinal plants may help improve public health. For example, in South Africa, the Research Group for Traditional Medicines has established a database to improve research on Traditional Medicine (WIPO FFM, supra note 119).

Documenting ethnobotanical knowledge may also be useful for defensive protection of traditional medicine. Defensive protection prevents third parties from improperly obtaining IP rights over ethnomedicinal plants.

For example, the Indian government provided information to the European Patent Office to invalidate a patent granted on the anti-fungal properties of Neem, a traditional Indian medicine. The Indian government presented documentation of the traditional use of Neem, and the patent was revoked in 2008. However, defensive protection does not prevent third parties from using this knowledge. In fact, providing information that traditional knowledge medicine constitutes prior can prevent from any hypocrisy. The most prominent example of defensive protection has been the Traditional Knowledge Digital Library (TKDL) established by the Indian government [European Patent Office (EPO), India's Traditional Knowledge Digital Library (TKDL): A powerful tool for patent examiners].

North east India is mega biodiversity area. However, this region is still unexplored and informations available are rudimentary and scanty. The present chapter focuses on the various documentations carried out in North east India (Figure 9.1).

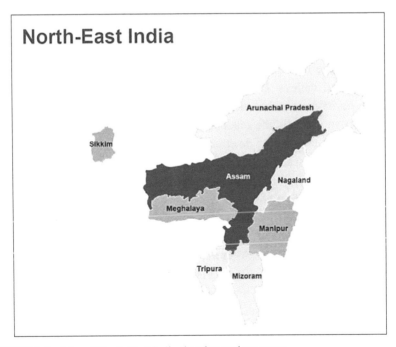

FIGURE 9.1   Map of North-East India showing various states.

The North East states comprises of Arunachal Pradesh, Assam, Manipur, Meghalaya, Mizoram, Nagaland, Sikkim and Tripura. It lies between 21°34 'N to 29°50 'N latitude and 87°32 'E to 97°52 'E longitudes. It covers an area of ca 262060 sq. km. The states are characterized by diverse physiographic, ranging from plains, plateaus and mountains with associated valleys, categorized into the Eastern Himalayas, Northeast hills (Patkai-Naga Hills and Lushai Hills) and Brahmaputra and the plains of Barak valley. Besides ethnic and cultural diversity, it is one of the mega biodiversity regions in the world which falls under the Himalaya and the Indo-Burma biodiversity hotspots. They are the major biomes recognized in the world. It is one of the richest reservoirs of plant diversity and supporting about 50% of India's biodiversity. It receives moderately high rainfall and the average minimum and maximum are 1650 mm and 6320 mm, respectively. There are approximately 225 tribes hailing from the Northeast region, out of the total 450 tribes that are found in the country (Chatterjee et al., 2006; Mao et al., 2009).

9.2   ETHNOBOTANICAL STUDIES OF DIFFERENT TRIBES OF NORTH-EAST

Majority of the tribal communities resides in the hills and some parts of the plains and valleys. Being rich in biodiversity and also known for its valuable heritage of herbal medicinal remedies, they attract the attention of the tourists and equally the academicians or researchers for various reasons. There is a huge potential to do ethnobotanical research in the region, primarily, because, half of the total Indian tribal communities lives and practices their cultures in its own unique way (Dutta and Dutta 2005; Lokho, 2012). Notable reports and several works has been done on Ethnomedicinal plants used by the different tribal communities from Northeast India, include the Apatani, Arunachal Pradesh (Kala, 2005), North Cachar hills (Sanjem et al., 2008), Tai-Khamyangs of Assam (Sonowal and Barua, 2011), Santhals (Bodding, 1925–1927, 1940), Miris (Hajra and Baishya, 1997), Karbis (Jain and Borthakur 1980; Teron and Borthakur, 2008), Tinsukia, Assam (Buragohain, 2011), Mishing (Singh et al., 1996), Khasi and Jaintia (Joseph and Kharkongor, 1997), Garo (Vasudeva and Shanpru, 1997), Assamese, Manipuri, Naga (Islam 1996; Rao, 1997; Jamir, 1999), Meitei in Manipur

(Singh and Singh 1996), Zou tribe in Manipur (Gangte et al., 2013), Imphal-East District, Manipur (Leishangthem and Sharma, 2014), Naga tribes in Manipur (Ringmichon et al., 2011), Mao Naga tribe in Manipur (Lokho, 2012), Khasi and Garos, Meghalaya (Neogi et al., 1989), Mizoram (Rai and Lalramnhinglova, 2010a, b), Angami-a, Nagaland (Megoneitso and Rao, 1983), Lotha, Nagaland (Jamir et al., 2008), Reang, Tripura (Shil and Choudhury, 2009), Sikkim (Singh et al., 2002), etc.

9.3   DOCUMENTATION AND EXCHANGE OF ETHNOBOTANICAL KNOWLEDGE IN NORTH-EAST INDIA

Lokho (2012) describes that the Naga tribals have a great heritage of oral traditions which involves beliefs and practices associated with nature, plants and animals which have a very rich culture and traditional practices which is unique from one tribe to the other. The diversity of the ethnic tribes among the Nagas presents a vast scope of ethnobotanical researches. There are 31 different Naga tribes: Angami, Chakeshang, Ao, Sema, Rengma, Lotha, Chang, Konyak, Sangtam, Phom, Zeliang, Mao, Maram, Tangkhul, Maring, Anal, Mayan-Monsang, Lamkang, Nockte, Haimi, Htangun, Ranpan, Kolyo, Kenyu, Kacha, Yachimi, Kabui, Uchongpok, Makaoro, Jeru and Somra (Horam, 1975). But, only a few accounts on ethnobotany mainly emphasized on medicinal and wild edible plants used by the Angami-a (Megoneitso and Rao, 1983), Nagaland (Rao and Jamir, 1982a, 1982b), Zeliang (Jamir and Rao, 1990), Zeme (Rout et al., 2010), Lotha (Jamir et al., 2008), Mao (Mao and Hyneiwta, 2009; Mao, 1993, 1998), Nagaland (Chankija, 1999), etc., has been reported by few research-ers. The Naga tribes live and spread out in the state of Nagaland, Naga hills in Manipur, North Cachar and Mikir hills, Lakhimppur, Sibsagar and Nowgong in Assam, north-east of Arunachal Pradesh, Somrat tract and across the border into Burma. Borborah et al. (2014), also reported that use of the members of the genus *Allium* L. in Northeast India is quite sig-nificant from the perspective of ethnopharmacology. The pharmacological aspect of the genus *Allium* L. have been clinically evaluated since long due to its typical flavor and ethnomedicinal importance. Several species of *Allium* L. have been reported from northeast India having ethnobotanical uses and are very popular among the ethnic groups either as spice/veg-etables or in folk medicine.

Ethnobotanical appraisal of Hill-Tiwas of Assam is reported for the first time (Teron and Barthakur, 2014). Rout et al. (2012) surveyed and collected information on traditional uses of plants by the Dimasa tribe of Assam for curing and treating different diseases like urinary disorder, diarrhea, malaria etc. Among the plant types, like herbs were the most frequently used, ferns and Cycads also find usage in their traditional heal-ing. In another study, Rout et al. (2010), had revealed that the Zeme Naga from Assam are using 8 species of medicinal plants for the treatment of diarrhea. An exhausted survey for anti-malarial plants in seven districts of Assam with the personal discussions and group interviews with the tradi-tional practitioners revealed that the 22 plant species could be a potential source of new antimalarial therapies (Gohain et al., 2015).

A survey was carried out by first hand questioning among traditional health practitioners and educated people for the treatment of different reproductive health related disorders and diseases by the rural people of Rangia Sub-division of Kamrup District, Assam. The survey also focuses 22 plant species used for the treatment of 11 different reproductive disor-ders, leucorrhea, excess uterine bleeding, infertility in female, night fall or wet dream, vomiting at the time of pregnancy, gonorrhea, easy delivery of baby, increase of breast milk, irregular menstruation, and infertility in male and female contraception (Choudhary et al., 2011). Gam and Nath (2012) focused on conservation of plant diversity through traditional beliefs and religious practices of rural Mishing tribes in Majuli river Island, Assam. It has been reported that there is definite traditional customs and rituals which play a vital role in conservation of natural resources through strin-gent customary laws, e.g., the wild leafy vegetables like, *Sarchoclamys pulcherrima* Goud., *Ficus glomeroata* L., *Ficus hispida* L., *Meliosma sim-plifolia* Roxb. etc. are necessary to cook with pork in their ritual activities. These species also may be related to cut fats of pork. Deori et al. (2007) has reported that *Sujen*, a popular local rice beer has a very important role in the socio-cultural life of Deori tribe of Assam and it is also used in all their festive occasions and celebrations. The plant species used in the preparation of *Mod pitha* (natural starter) for brewing *Sujen*. Methodology of rice beer preparation and various plant materials used in starter culture preparation by some tribal communities of North-east India: A survey has been also reported by Das et al. (2012).

Kala (2005), investigated the wealth of medicinal plants used by the Apatani tribe of Arunachal Pradesh, who traditionally settled seven villages in the Ziro valley of lower Subansiri district. He documented 158 medicinal plant species which were distributed across 73 families and 124 genera, Asteraceae was the most dominant family (19 species, 11 genera), followed by Zingiberaceae, Solanaceae, Lamiaceae and Araceae for curing various ailments and further it discussed in the changing socio-economic contexts. Khongsai et al. (2011), revealed about the vast diversity of herbal medicinal plants used by the various tribes of Arunachal Pradesh. The common medicinal plants used by *Apatani, Mongpa, Sinpho* and *Tangsa* tribes were studied and around 28 species were listed mostly herb used for medicine. The *Padam, Ngishi* and *I-Idu* tribes were also commonly used about 56 plants species as medicine from 29 families. They believed that dreadful diseases like cancer and diabetes can be treated with local herbal plants. Thus, the author focuses on potentials of ethnobotanical research for conservation and documentation of traditional medicinal knowledge for further availability and utilization to the benefit of mankind. Shanker et al. (2012) surveyed folk medicinal plants used by folk healers of Mishing tribe in few places of Lakhimpur and Dhemaji district of Assam and East Siang district of Arunachal Pradesh for the malaria, jaundice and female menstruation problems which are the prominent diseases in the community. The rural populations among the Monpa ethnic group in Arunachal Pradesh have a rich knowledge of forest- based natural resources and consumption of wild edible plants as an integral part of selecting socio-cultural life. The documentation study also revealed that it can be used as an ethnopharmacological basis for selecting plants for future phytochemical and pharmaceutical studies reported by Namsa et al. (2011). The folk medicinal food plants used among the indigenous people of East Siang district of Arunachal Pradesh was studied for the nutraceutical point of view and 36 plants species has been identified (Payum et al., 2014). More than 500 dye-yielding plant species like *Daphne papyracea* is also documented by Mahanta and Tiwari (2005). This plant being traditionally used by the Monpa tribe of West Kameng and Tawang districts for preparing dye as well as for making hand-made paper for painting and writing scripts in monasteries. The Apatanis, Khamptis, Tangsas, Wanchos and Monpas have been using species like *Rubia cordifolia, Rubia sikki-mensis, Woodfordia fruticosa, Colquhounia coccinea*, etc., for dyeing. It is also informed that some of these mentioned species possess ethno-medic-inal and fiber-yielding properties in addition to natural dyeing and was being used in traditional health care practices, rope-making, fish poison-ing, etc. The study was done in order to explore the availability of natural dye-yielding plants in Arunachal Pradesh as well as to document the indig-enous knowledge, and procedures related to preparation of natural dyes by the tribal societies in the state (Mahanta and Tiwari, 2005).

The ethno-medicinal plants used by the native practitioners of Chandel district, Manipur were reported by Deb et al. (2011). Ringmichon et al. (2011) reported that Naga tribes of Manipur prefer to dwell at hilltops and inhospitable terrians isolated from the main civilization and for all their needs they completely depend on nature. During illness they believe in using herbal remedies rather than the allopathic medicines as they have a vast knowledge of their surrounding flora and fauna. Lokho (2012) reported about the Mao Nagas who are settled as agriculturalist and heav-ily depended upon the nature. They live at the hill forest where they prac-ticed organic farming since time immemorial and consumed the products which are free from hazardous elements that keep them healthy. The Mao folk medicinal plants, which, can be used to discover new compounds for developing modern medicine were studied. The studies show that there is an urgent need for conservation and management of these pre-cious medicinal plants for sustainable use and scientific study so as to harvest its constituents to cater the needs of vibrant healthcare products in future. Ningombam et al. (2014) observed that traditional healers of Manipur were found to play great role in the primary healthcare systems and curing some diseases with greater success and greater preference from the people than that of modern medications. They also stressed that there is a common cultural understanding regarding spirituality and healing that harbors trusts between the patients and the *Maiba* and *Maibi*. The findings revealed herbal remedies have many advantages like easily availability, easier to prepare and in addition to that it can be used home prepared remedies and moreover it was also linked to family influence and tradi-tional, spiritual, dual heath care and socioeconomic status. Leishangthem and Sharma, (2014) revealed that a total of 50 medicinal plants, belonging to 26 families were recorded for the treatment of different diseases viz. asthma, arthritis, cough, fever, diabetes, dysentery, gastric and indigestion, jaundice, toothache, skin diseases, etc. It was suggested that the high diversity of bio-resources needs to be conserved for livelihood sustenance of the future generation. Yumnam et al. (2012), emphasized that Manipur is a rich source of medicinal plants and a large number of medicinal plant species were used in the ethnomedicinal treatment for different diseases. A study was carried out by Singh et al. (2014) at Andro Village in Imphal East district (Manipur), inhabited by a scheduled caste community known as 'Lois'. The Andro Village have a very good knowledge about the treatment of various diseases and ailments with plants. A total of 29 medicinal plant species belonging to 27 genera and distributed over 19 families were found to be used by the schedule caste community of Andro in the treatment of rectum disease-piles. Ningombam and Singh, (2014), witnessed that *Phlogacanthus thyrsiformis* (Roxb. ex Hadrw.) Mabb., locally known as *Nongmangkha* is a quite popular as an ethno-botanical important plant for the *meetei* community. It was gathered from 68 informants using semi structure questionnaires on the utilization, taboos, folk medicine and conservation of the species. The plant forms an integral part of rites and rituals, myths, food items, taboos, medicinal, customs and traditions with the *meetei* community. Folk medicinal uses are cold, cough, influenza, easy delivery of child birth, abortion, irregular menstruation, diarrhea, dysentery, cholera, high blood pressure control, boils, small pox, skin problems, sprains, body ache, constipation and burns. The plant also found to be grown in every house who owns a kitchen garden. It is also reported that superstitious belief, which is still practiced by local people till today is not to pluck any part of the plant on Sunday. In another study, survey was done by Singh and Huidrom (2013) in Central Valley of Manipur. It was found that Meitei community in the study area extensively used *Justicia adhatoda* L. as ethno-medicine as well as food plant. Gurumayum and Soram (2014), claimed that Manipur state as a whole lies in the Indo-Burma Biodiversity hot spot owing to which harbors diverged plants supporting about 50% of India's biodiversity. Mao Naga tribe inhabits the Mao area, located at a unique geographic, climatic and topographical area in Senapati district of Manipur. An ethno-medicinal survey has been conducted with the help of local volunteers and accordingly this paper has a record of 45 plant species being used in traditional medicine belonging 41 genera and 28 families for treating diarrhea and dysentery.

Kayang et al. (2005), evaluated that the traditional knowledge is the best starting point for effective in situ conservation, which requires accurate and up to date information of the status of medicinal plant populations, the extent and nature of plant use by local communities and the capacity of the resource base to support different economic activities. Sajem and Gosai (2006) documented the traditional knowledge of medicinal plants that are in use by the indigenous Jaintia tribes residing in few isolated pockets of northeast India. During the study done through structured questionnaires in consultations with the tribal practitioners revealed that 39 medicinal plant species belonging to 27 families and 35 genera are used. Hyniewta and Kumar (2008), worked on Herbal remedies among the Khasi traditional healers and villager folks in Meghalaya. Laloo and Hemlatha (2011) reported that in the state Meghalaya 58 plant species are used to treat diarrhea and dysentery. Singh et al. (2014), documented pharmaceutically important plant resources used in primary health care of ethnic Garo tribes from Eastern Himalayas (Nokrek Biosphere Reserve [NBR], India) in order to document information on medicinal plants and to maximize the collection of indigenous knowledge of Garo tribes. A total of 157 plant species representing 134 genera and 81 families were found to be commonly used in the treatment of 67 health-problems. Mir et al. (2014) studied diversity of endemic and threatened ethnomedicinal plant species in Meghalaya and suggested that plants play a vital role in the healthcare of the local tribal people in Meghalaya. Traditional remedies were also part of the cultural and spiritual life of these people. The result shows, total of 131 species, including 36 endemic and 113 species under different threat categories were found. It was also found that the indigenous community holds substantial knowledge on ethnomedicinal plants that plays an important role in assisting the primary healthcare needs of the people. These plants would be of much benefit, if evaluated and introduced in the modern scientific health care system. However, the decline in population due to overharvesting and habitat destruction of these plants calls for necessary measures for their effective conservation. Study conducted by Sharma et al. (2014) to highlight the indigenous uses of medicinal plants by Garo tribe in North Garo Hills, Meghalaya, showed a total of 66 medicinal plants belonging to 61 genera and 40 families were used ethnomedicinally.

In Mizoram Bhardwaj and Gakhar (2005), indicated that 17 species, belonging to 14 families are used by the native people for the cure of cuts and wounds. It is also revealed that the plant not only contain antiseptic value but also have regenerative and healing properties, sticking property of paste of bark was also observed in Laki tree. Lafakzuala et al. (2007) enumerated and discussed the ethnobotanical aspect of the plants used by the tribal of Mizoram.

A survey of ethnomedicinal plants occurring in the tribal area of Mizoram was conducted by Rai and Lalramnghinglova (2010) and reported 159 ethnomedicianl plant species belonging to 134 genera and 56 families. Rai and Lalramnghinglova (2010a, b) also stated that this the first-hand information of certain ethnomedicinal plants from an Indo-Burma hotspot region (Mizoram).

Shanker et al. (2012) stated that Mizoram is inhabited by Mizo tribe and they use various herbal preparations for treating various ailments. Records of 25 folk medicinal claims used by Mizo tribe which are popularly used in various formulations and their uses have been described. Hazarika et al. (2012) reported the wild edible fruits of Mizoram, used as an ethno-medicine. Report by Shanker and Rawat (2013) deals with the traditional healing herbs used by Mizo tribe in the treatment of several ailments viz. fever, ringworm, itching, worm infestation, dysentery, diarrhea, high blood pressure, jaundice, ulcer, scabies, kidney stone, piles, fistula, dandruff etc. in the Aizawl and Mamit districts of Mizoram. Lalmuanpuii et al. (2013) documented the traditional practice and knowledge of medicines/naturopathy among the Mizo ethnic group of Lunglei district. A total of 82 medicinal plant species belonging to 42 families and 76 genera were documented along with their parts used, methods of preparation and types of ailments treated. It was revealed that there is a positive relationship between age and traditional knowledge and practice; while a negative relationship between educational level and traditional knowledge and practice was observed.

Changkija (1999) documented an account of 109 plant species that have medicinal uses among the tribes of Nagaland. Jamir et al. (2012) recorded

52 species of medicinal herbs being used by various Naga tribes. Zhasa et al. (2015) explored the indigenous knowledge on utilization of available plant biodiversity which have been utilized for treatment and cure of human ailment by eight Naga tribes, i.e., Angami, Zeliang, Ao, Lotha, Sangtam, Konyak, Chakhesang, Rengma, and Khiamniungam in 20 villages of 9 districts of Nagaland. About 241 plant species belonging to 142 families were recorded for traditional medicine used by eight Naga tribes.

Singh et al. (2015), reported the ethnomedicinal plants and traditional healing practices used for the treatment of jaundice by the four Naga tribes namely *Angami, Lotha, Sumi* and *Zeliang* inhabiting in *Kohima, Wokha, Zunheboto* and *Peren* districts of Nagaland state. Bhuyan et al. (2015) reported that an extensive study on Traditional practice of medicinal plants by 4 major tribes of Nagaland was conducted in different localities from districts of the state. The tribes undertaken for study were Ao, Angami, Lotha, Sema, residing in Nagaland. The study comprises 257 species of ethnomedicinal plants belonging to 85 families.

In Sikkim Pradhan and Badola (2008) described the ethnomedicinal plants used by Lepcha tribe of Dzongu valley, bordering Khangchenzonga Biosphere reserve. It not only depicted the value of medicinal plants and rich ethnomedicinal knowledge, but also on agroclimatic zone for the cultivation of herbal plant species. Bantawa and Rai (2009), discussed the traditional practices among Jhankri, Bijuwa and Phedangma on locally available plants material to cure various ailments and disorders. Das et al. (2012) reported a large number of plants, plant extracts, and decoctions used by ethnic and rural people in treatment of various ailments. Panda (2012), found that the traditional healers act as health care actors for treating arthritis, fracture, jaundice, diarrhea and respiratory diseases of children with other persistence, long lasting chronic health conditions with the used of medicinal plants. Sharma (2013) carried out an ethnobotanical study in Darjeeling Himalayas to document plants used against skin diseases. During the field survey, ethnomedicinal information of 91 species of medicinal plants belonging to 53 families was compiled from different habitats of the study area. Application of plants against skin diseases included various forms of preparation.

Majumdar et al. (2006) studied the medicinal plants prescribed by different tribal and non-tribal medicine men of Tripura. Sen et al. (2011)

highlighted the traditional knowledge of medicinal plants being used by the tribe in West and South district of Tripura. It also mentioned about the uses of plants in primary health care system. Nineteen different tribes in Tripura, depend on natural resources at a great extent. This paper documented 113 medicinal plant species from 56 families along with their botanical name, local name, family name, habit, medicinal parts used, and traditional usage of application. Tribes of Tripura have rich traditional knowledge on plant based medicine. Different parts of the plants in crude form/plant extracts/decoctions/infusion or pastes are employed in diverse veterinary and human diseases by the tribes of Tripura in daily life. Dipankar et al. (2012), reported the indigenous ethno-medicinal knowledge of Darlong community in Tripura. It revealed their traditional usage of diverse plant species as both deterrent and therapeutic agent for different ailments. The study comprises customary usage of 39 plant species belonging to 38 genera and 24 families, along with their local name and various parts used.

The field study conducted by Debnath et al. (2014) over the Mog and Reang communities of Sabroom and Santirbazar Subdivision of Tripura to find out ethno-medicinal knowledge and plant parts utilizing in their various ailments. In the investigation total 51 species were identified belonging to 34 families. The data revealed that both the communities extensively use herbal medicine for the treatment of 30 different ailments. They frequently used these species to retrieve from different common ailments like rheumatism, jaundice, diarrhea, tumor, cough, blood sugar, fever and others. Das et al. (2014) documented a total of 55 ethnomedicinal plants belonging to 42 families and 49 genera having antifertility property. Pandey and Mavinkurve (2014) prepared an inventory of ethnomedicinal plants used by the Chakma tribe of Tripura state, India. Chakma people are mostly residing in deep forest and depend on their own traditional health care system. The survey was conducted during 2012 in Agartala, Tripura by interviewing the local health practioners of the different villages of the state, a total of 19 angiosperms and one pteridophyte have been documented for folklore medicinal plants used by *Chakma tribes* of Tripura.

Roy Choudhury et al. (2015) indicated that a total of 75 species of plants under 68 genera belonging to 43 families were collected during the study for the treatment of 15 disease categories.

Thus in nutshell the documentation and exchange of ethnobotanical knowledge in North east India is vast due to rich biodiversity. Still it is unexplored as many parts of the northeast India need to be studied and documented. Thus the exchange of knowledge may reach manifold. It will also keep this ethnobotanical knowledge alive for generation after generations. The purpose of research on traditional herbal medicine is not only for drug development but also for quality control and mechanism study of herbs.

KEYWORDS

- biodiversity
- edible plants
- ethnic people
- ethnobotany
- medicinal plants
- North East India
- traditional healer
- tribes

REFERENCES

1. Bantawa, P., & Rai, R. (2009). Studies on ethnomedicinal plants used by traditional practitioners, *Jhankri, Bijuwa and Phedangma* in Darjeeling Himalaya. *Nat. Prod. Radiance 8(5)*, 537–541.
2. Bhardwaj, S., & Gakhar, S. K. (2005). Ethnomedicinal plants used by the tribals of Mizoram to cure cuts & wounds. *Indian J. Trad. Knowl. 4(1)*, 75–80.
3. Bhuyan, S. I., Mewiwapangla & Laskar, I. (2014). Indigenous Knowledge and traditional use of medicinal plants by four major tribes of Nagaland, North East India. *Intertl. J Innovative Sci, Engin Technol 1(6)*, 481–484.
4. Bodding, P. O. (1925–1927). Studies in Santal medicine and connected folklore, II Santal Medicine. *Mem. Asiat. Soc. Bengal 10(2)*, 133–426.
5. Boddding, P. O. (1940). Studies in Santal medicine and connected folklore. *Memiors Asiat. Soc. Bengal 10*, 427–502.
6. Borborah, E., Dutta, B., & Borthakur, S. K. (2014). Taditional uses of *Allium* L. species from North East India with special reference to their Pharmacological activities. *American J. Phytomed. Clinical Therapeut. 2(8)*, 1037–1051.

7. Buragohain, J. (2011). Ethnomedicinal Plants used by the ethnic communities of Tinsukia district of Assam, India. *J. Rec. Res. Sci. and Technol, 3(9)*, 31–42.

8. Chankija, S. (1999). Folk medicinal Plants of the Nagas in India. *Asian Folk Studies, 58*, 205–230.

9. Chatterjee, S., Saikia, A., Dutta, P., Ghosh, D., Pangging, G., & Goswami, A. K. (2006). Biodiversity Significance of North East India. WWF-India, New Delhi.

10. Choudhary, N., Mahanta, B., & Kalita, J. C. (2011). An ethnobotanical survey on medicinal plants used in reproductive health related disorders in Rangeia subdivision, Kamprup district, Assam. *Intern. J. Sci. Advanced Technol. 1 (7)*, 154–159.

11. Das, A. J., Deka, S. C., & Miyaji, T. (2012). Methodology of rice beer preparation and various plant materials used in starter culture preparation by some tribal communities of North-east India: A survey. *Intern. Food Res. J. 19(1)*, 101–107.

12. Das, B., Talukdar, A. D., & Choudhury, M. D. (2014). A few traditional medicinal plants used as antifertility agents by ethnic people of Tripura, India. *Intern. J. Pharm. Pharmaceut. Sci. 6(3)*, 47–53.

13. Das, T., Mishra, S. B., Saha, D., & Agarwal, (2012). Ethnobotanical survey of medicinal plants used by Ethnic and rural people in Eastern Sikkim Himalaya region. *Intern. J. Ayurved Herbal Med. 2(2)*, 253–259.

14. Deb, L., Singh, K. R., Singh, K. R., Singh, K. B., & Thongam, B. (2011). Some ethno-medicinal plants used by the Native practitioners of Chandel district, Manipur, India. *Inter. Res. J. Pharm. 2(12)*, 199–200.

15. Debnath, B., Debnath, A., Shilsharma, S., & Paul, C. (2014). Ethnomedicinal knowledge of Mog and Reang communities of South district of Tripura, India. *Indian J. Advances plant Res. 1(5)*, 49–54.

16. Deori, C., Begum, S. S., & Mao, A. A. (2007). Ethnobotany of *Sujen*- A local rice beer of Deori tribe of Assam. *Indian J. Tradit. Knowl. 6(1)*, 121–125.

17. Dipankar, D., Lalsimawii, D., Abhijit, S., Mandakranta, R., & Datta, B. K. (2012). Traditional Ethno-medicinal plants use by the Darlong tribes in Tripura, Northeast India. *Intern J Ayurved Herbal Med. 2(6)*, 954–966.

18. Dutta, B. K., & Dutta, P. K. (2005). Potential of ethnobotanical studies in North East India: An overview. *Indian J. Trad. Knowl. 4(1)*, 7–14.

19. European Patent Office [EPO], India's Traditional Knowledge Digital Library (TKDL): A powerful tool for patent examiners.

20. Gam, N. K., & Nath, P. C. (2012). Conservation of plant diversity through traditional beliefs and religious practices of rural Mishing tribes in Majuli river Island, Assam, India. *Indian J. Fund. Applied Life Sc. 2(2)*, 62–68.

21. Gangte, H. E., Thoudam, N. S., & Zomi, G. T. (2013). Wild edible plants used by the Zou tribe in Manipur, India. *Int.Scientific Res. 3(5)*, 1–8.

22. Gohain, N., Prakash, A., Gogoi, K., Bhattacharya, D. R., Sarmah, N., Dahutia, C., & Kalita, M. C. (2015). An ethnobotanical survey of anti-malarial plants in some highly malaria affected districts of Assam. *Intern. J. Pharm. Pharmaceut. Sc. 7 (9)*, 147–152.

23. Gurumayum and Soram (2014). Some Anti-diarrhoeic and anti-dysenteric ethno-medicinal plants of Mao Naga tribe community of Mao, Senapati district, Manipur. *Intern J Pure Applied Biosc. 29*, 147–155.

24. Hajra, P. K., & Baishya, A. K. (1997). Ethnobotanical notes on the Miris (Mishings) of Assam plains. In: Jain SK (Ed.) Contribution to Indian Ethonobotany, Scientific Publishers, Jodhpur. pp. 161–168.

25. Hazarika, T. K., Lalramchuana & Nautiyal, B.P (2012). Studies on wild edible fruits of Mizoram, India used as ethnomedicine. *Genet. Resour. Crop. Evol.* DOI 10.1007/s 10722–012–9799–5

26. Horam, M. (1975). Naga Polity, B. R. Publ. Corp. Delhi.

27. http://www.wipo.int/export/sites/www/tk/en/resources/pdf/tk_toolkit_draft.pdf

28. Hynniewta, S. R., & Kumar, Y. (2008). Herbal remedies among the Khasi traditional healers and the villager folks in Meghalaya. *Indian J Tradl Knowl. 7(4)*, 581–586.

29. Islam, M. (1996). Ethnobotany of certain underground parts of plants of North Eastern Region, India. *J. Econ. Taxon. Bot. Adl. Ser. 12*, 338–343.

30. Jain, S. K., & Borthakur, S. K. (1980). Ethnobotany of the Mikirs of India. *Econ. Bot. 34(3)*, 264–272.

31. Jamir, N. S. (1999). Ethnobotanical studies among Naga tribes in Nagaland. In: B. Kharbuli, D. Syiem & H. Kayang (eds.). Biodiversity North East India Perspective, North Eastern Biodiversity Research Cell, North Eastern Hill University, Shillong. 128–140.

32. Jamir, N. S., & Rao, R. R. (1990). Fifty new or interesting medicinal plants used by the Zeliang of Nagaland (India), *Ethnobotany 2*, 11–18.

33. Jamir, N. S., Lanusunep & Pongener, N. (2012). Medico-herbal medicine practiced by the Naga tribes in the state of Nagaland (India). *Indian J. Fundamen Applied Life Science. 2(2)*, 328–333.

34. Jamir, N. S., Takatemjen & Limasemba. (2008). Traditional knowledge of Lotha-Naga tribes in Wokha district, Nagaland, *Indian J. Tradit. Knowl. 9(1)*, 45–48.

35. Joseph, J. A., & Kharkongor, P. A. (1997). A preliminary ethnobotanical survey in Khasi and Jaintia Hills, Meghalaya. In: *Contribution to Indian Ethonobotany*, ed. S. K. Jain, Scientific Publishers, Jodhpur. pp. 187–194.

36. Kala C. P. (2005). Ethnomedicinal botany of the Apatani in the Eastern Himalayan region of India. http://www.ethnobiomed.com/content/1/1/11.

37. Kayang, H. Kharbuli, B., Myrboli, B., & Syiem, D. (2005). Medicinal plants of Khasi Hill of Meghalaya, India. *Bioprospecting & Ethnopharmacol. 1*, 75–80.

38. Khongsai, M., Saikia, S. P., & Kayang, H. (2011). Ethnomedicinal plants used by different tribes of Arunachal Pradesh. *Indian J. Trad. Knowl. 10(3)*, 541–546.

39. Lafakzuala, R., Lalramnghinglova, H., & Kayang, H. (2007). Ethnobotanical usage of plants in Western Mizoram. *Indian J. Trad. Knowl. 6(3)*, 486–493.

40. Lalmuanpuii, J., Rosangkima, G., & Lamin, H. (2013). Ethno-medicinal practices among the Mizo ethnic group in Lunglei district, Mizoram. *Science Vision 13(1)*, 24–34.

41. Laloo, D., & Hemalatha, S. (2011). Ethnomedicinal plants used for diarrhea by tribals of Mehalaya, Northeast India. *Pharmacognosy Reviews 5(10)*, 147–154.

42. Leishangthem, S., & Sharma, L. D. (2014). Study of some important medicinal plants found in Imphal-East district, Manipur, India. *Intern J. Scienti. Res. 4 (9)*, 1–5.

43. Lokho, A. (2012). The folk medicinal plants of the Mao Naga in Manipur, North East India. *Intertl J. Scientific and Research Publication, 2(6)*, 1–8.

44. Mahanta, D., & Tiwari, S. C. (2005). Natural dye-yielding plants and indigenous knowledge on dye preparation in Arunachal Pradesh, northeast India. *Curr. Sci. 88(9),* 1474–1480.

45. Majumdar, K., Saha, R. Datta, B. K., & Bhakta, T. (2006). Medicinal plants prescribed by different tribal and non-tribal medicine men of Tripura. *Indian J. Trad. Knowl. 5(4),* 559–562.

46. Mao A. A. (1993). A preliminary report on the folklore Botany of Mao Naga of Manipur (India), *Ethnobotany 5,* 143–147.

47. Mao A. A. (1998). Ethnobotanical observation of Rice Beer 'Zhuchu' preparation by the Mao Naga tribe from Manipur (India), *Bull. Bot. Surv. India. 40,* 53–57.

48. Mao, A. A., & Hynniewta, T. M. (2009). Plants used as Agricultural seasons indicator by Mao Naga tribe, Manipur, India, *Ind. J Tradit Knowl. 10(3),* 578–580.

49. Mao, A. A, Hyniewta, T. M., & Sanjappa, M. (2009). Plant Wealth of Northeast India with reference to ethnobotany, *Ind. J. Tradit. Knowl. 8(1),* 96–103.

50. Megoneitso & Rao R. R. (1983). Ethnobotanical studies in Nagaland, sixty two medicinal plants used by the Angami-a Naga, *J. Econ. Taxon. Bot. 4(1),* 167–172.

51. Mir, A. H., Krishna Upadhaya, K., & Hiranjit Choudhury, H. (2014). Diversity of Endemic and Threatened Ethnomedicinal Plant Species in Meghalaya, North-East India. *Intern. Res. J. Environment Sci. 3(12),* 64–78.

52. Namsa, N. D., Mandal, M., Tangjang, S., & Mandal, S. C. (2011). Ethnobotany of the Monpa ethnic group at Arunachal Pradesh, India. *J. Ethnobiol. Ethnomed.* http://www.ethnobiomed.com/content/7/1/31.

53. Neogi, B., Prasad M. N. V., & Rao R. R. (1989). Ethnobotany of some weeds of Khasi and Garo Hills, Meghalaya, Northeastern India, *J. Economic Botany. 43(4),* 471–479.

54. Ningombam, D. S., Devi, S. P., Singh, P. K., Pinokiyo, A., & Thongam, B. (2014). Documentation and assessment on knowledge of Ethno-medicinal ptactioners; A case study on Local Meetei healers of Manipur. *J. Pharm. Biolog. Sci. 9(1),* 53–70.

55. Ningombam, D. S & Singh, P. K. (2014). Ethnobotanical Study of *Phologacanthus thyrsiformis* Nees: A conserved Medicinal Plant of Manipur, Northeast India. *Intern. J. Herbal Medicine 1 (5),* 10–14.

56. Panda, A. K. (2012). Medicinal plants used and primary health care in Sikkim. *Intern. J. Ayurved Herbal Med. 2(2),* 253–259.

57. Pandey, A., & Mavinkurve, R. G., 2014. Ethno-botanical usage of plants by the Chakma community of Tripura, Northeast India. *Bulletin Environ. Pharmacol. Life Sci. 3(6),* 11–14.

58. Payum, T., Das, A. K., & Shanker, R. (2014). Nutraceutical folk food used among indigenous people of east siang district of Arunachal Pradesh, India. *Am J. Pharm Tech Res. 4(4),* 696–701.

59. Pradhan, B. K., & Badola, H. K. (2008). Ethnomedicinal plant used by Lepcha tribe of Dzongu valley, bordering Khangchenzonga Biosphere reserve, in North Sikkim, India. *J. Ethnobiol. Ethnomed. 4(22),* 1–18.

60. Rai, P. K., & Lalramnhinglova, H. (2010a). Lesser Known Ethnomedicinal plants of Mizoram, North East India: An Indo-Burma hotspot region, *J. Medicinal Plants Res. 4(13),* 1301–1307.

61. Rai, P. K., & Lalramnghinglova, H. (2010b). Ethnomedicinal plant resources of Mizoram, India: Implication of traditional knowledge in Health care system. *Ethnobotanical Leaflets 14*, 274–305.

62. Rai, P. K., & Lalramnghinglova, H. (2011). Ethnomedicinal plants of India with special reference to an Indo-Burma hotspot region: An overview. *Ethnobotany Research & Apllications 9*, 379–420.

63. Rao, R. R. (1997). Ethnobotanical studies on some Adivasi tribes of North East India with special reference to the Naga people. In: Contribution to Indian Ethnobotany, ed.S. K. Jain, Scientific Publishers, Jodhpur. pp. 209–223.

64. Rao, R. R., & Jamir, N. S. (1982a). Ethnobotanical studies in Nagaland 1. Medicinal plants, *Econ. Bot. 36*, 176–181.

65. Rao, R. R., & Jamir, N. S. (1982b). Ethnobotanical studies in Nagaland 2. Fiftyfour Medicinal plants used by Nagas, *J. Econ. Taxon. Bot. 3 (1)*, 11–17.

66. Ringmichon, C. L., Shimpi, N. S., & Gopalkrishnan, B. (2011). Some noteworthy antipyretic herbal remedies used by Naga tribes in Manipur. *Ethnobotany 23*, 82–85.

67. Rout, J., Sanjem, A. L., & Nath, M. (2010). Traditional Medicinal Knowledge of the Zeme (Naga) tribe of North Cachar Hills District, Assam on the treatment of Diarrhoea. *Assm. Univ. J. Sci. and Tech. Biol. and Environ. Sci. 5(1)*, 63–69.

68. Rout, J., Sajem, A. L., & Nath, M. (2012). Medicinal plants of North Cachar hills district of Assam used by Dimasa tribe. *Indian J. Trad. Knowl. 11 (3)*, 520–527.

69. Sajen, A. L., & Gosai, K. (2006). Traditional use of medicinal plants by the Jaintia tribes in North Cacha hills district of Asssam. *J. Ethnobiol. Ethnomed.* Doi: 10.1186/1746–4269-2-33

70. Sanjem, A. L., Rout, J., & Nath, Minaram, (2008). Traditional Tribal knowledge and Status of some Rare and Endemic medicinal Plants of north Cachar Hills District of Assam, Northeast India, *J. Ethnobotanical Leaflets 12*, 261–275.

71. Sen, S., Chakraborty, R., De, B., & Devanna, N. (2011). An ethnobotanical survey of medicinal plants used by ethnic people in west and South of Tripura, India. *J Forestry Res. 22(3)*, 417–426.

72. Shanker, R., Lavekar, G. S. Deb, S., & Sharma, B. K. (2012). Traditional healing practice and folk medicines used by Mishing community of North east India. *J. Ayurved Integr. Med. 3(3)*, 124–129.

73. Shanker, R., & Rawat, M. S. (2013). Medicinal Plants Used in Traditional Medicine in Aizawl and Mamit Districts of Mizoram. *J. Biol. Life Sci. 4(2)*, 95–102.

74. Shankar, R., Rawat, M. S., Majumdar, R., Baruah, D., & Bharali, B. K. (2012). Medicinal plants used in traditional medicine in Mizoram. *World J. Sci. Technol. 2(12)*, 42–45.

75. Sharma, B. C. (2013). Ethnomedicinal plants used against skin diseases by indigenous population of Darjeeling Himalayas, India. *Indian J. Fundamen. Applied Life Sci. 3(3)*, 299–303.

76. Sharma, M., Sharma, C. L., & Marak, P. N. (2014). Indigenous uses of medicinal plants in north Garo hills, Meghalaya, NE India. *Res. J. Recent Sci. 3*, 137–146.

77. Shil, S., & Choudhury, M. D. (2009). Ethnomedicinal Importance of Pteridophytes used by Reang tribe of Tripura, North East India. *J. Ethnobotanical Leaflets 13*, 634–643.

78. Singh, B., Borthakur, S. K., & Phukan, S. J. (2014). A survey of ethnomedicinal plants utilized by the Indigenous people of Garo hills with special reference to the Nokrek Biosphere Reserve (Meghalaya), India. *J. Herbs, Spices & Medicinal Plants 20(1)*, 1–30.

79. Singh, J., Bhuyan, T. C., & Ahmed, A. (1996). Ethnobotanical studies on the Mishing tribes of Assam with special reference to food and medicinal plant. *J. Econ. Tax. Bot. Addl. Ser. 12*, 350–356.

80. Singh, K. P., & Singh, H. B. K. (1996). Superstition in botanical folklore with reference to Meitei culture. *Econ. Tax. Bot. Addl. Ser. 12*, 367–372.

81. Singh, H. B., Prasad, P., & Rai L. K. (2002). Folk Medicinal Plants in the Sikkim Himalayas of India. *Asian Folklore studies 61*, 295–310.

82. Singh, K. J., & Huidrom, D. (2013). Ethnobotanical uses of medicinal plant, *Justicia adhatoda* L. by Meitei community of Manipur, India. *J. Coastal Life Med. 1(4)*, 322–325.

83. Singh, N. P., Gajurel, P. R., Panmei, R., & Rethy, P. (2015). Indigenous healing practices and ethnomedicinal plants used against jaundice by some Naga tribes in Nagaland, India. *Pleione 9(1)*, 40–48.

84. Singh, T. T., Sharma, H. M., Devi, A. R., & Sharma, H. R. (2014). Plants used in the treatment of piles by the Scheduled caste community of Andro village in Imphal East District, Manipur (India). *J Plant Sci 2(3)*, 113–119.

86. Sonowal, R., & Barua, I. (2011). Ethnomedical Practices among the Tai-Khamyangs of Asssam, India. *J. Ethno. Med. 5(1)*, 41–50.

87. Teron, R., & Borthakur, S. K. (2008). Traditional Knowledge relating to use of flora and fauna as indicators in predicting annual seasons among *Karbi* tribe of Assam. *Indian J. Trad. Knowl., 8(4)*, 518–524.

88. Vasudeva, M. K., & Shanpru, R. (1997). Some plants in the life of Garos of Meghalaya. *In* Jain SK (Ed.) Contribution to Indian Ethonobotany, Scientific Publishers, Jodhpur: pp. 179–186.

89. WIPO FFM, supra note 119.

90. Yumnam, R. S., Devi, C. O., Abujam, S. K., & Chetia, D. (2012). Study on the Ethnomedicinal System of Manipur. *Intern J Pharmaceut and Biol Archives. 3(3)*, 587–591.

91. Zhasa, N. N., Hazarika, P., & Tripathi, Y. C. (2015). Indigenous Knowledge on utilization of plant biodiversity for treatment and cure of diseases of Human beings in Nagaland, India: A case study. *Intern. Res. J. Biol. Sci. 4(4)*, 89–106.

CHAPTER 10

QUANTITATIVE ETHNOBOTANY: ITS IMPORTANCE IN BIOPROSPECTING AND CONSERVATION OF PHYTORESOURCES

CHOWDHURY HABIBUR RAHAMAN

Department of Botany, Visva-Bharati University, Santiniketan – 731235, West Bengal, India, E-mail: habibur_cr@rediffmail.com, habibur_cr@yahoo.co.in

CONTENTS

Abstract 270
10.1 Introduction 271
10.2 Methods and Techniques Used in Collection
     of Ethnobotanical Data and Its Quantitative Analysis 274
10.3 Phytoresources and Quantitative Ethnobotany 278
10.4 Progress in Quantitative Ethnobotanical Research
     and Its Future Prospects 283
10.5 Conclusion 285
Keywords 286
References 286

ABSTRACT

Quantitative Ethnobotany or quantification in Ethnobotany encompasses the statistical analysis of folk knowledge about utilization of local phytoresources. Appropriate quantitative tools are used in ethnobotany to analyze the collected data for more objectivity in ethnobotanical research. There is a growing interest among the ethnobotanists worldwide in improving the traditional type of compilation of their ethnobotanical works by employing suitable quantitative indices in data collection, analysis and interpretation of results. Over the last few decades, ethnobotanists have been using more than one hundred quantitative indices for determination of consensus among the informants, use value, cultural significance, conservation priorities of the plant resources, etc. This approach in ethnobotany has also been tested as effective tool in selection of ethnobotanical claims as good candidate for bioprospecting and new drug discovery. For this reason, scientists rely mostly upon the ethnobotanical information or lead for development of various natural products like pharmaceuticals, nutraceuticals, cosmetics, etc. Taking the leads from ethnobotany as well as traditional herbal medicine, many novel natural products including drugs have been designed worldwide by the coordinated efforts of ethnobotanists, phytochemists, pharmacologists and clinical persons.

Suitable ethnobotanical tools are also being employed successfully for management and conservation of plant resources at local as well as regional level. In the field of Ethnoecology, scientists have devised the unique quantitative technique like Local Conservation Priority Index (LCPI) or Conservation Priority Index (CPI) by using some quantitative indices from ethnobotany and ecology for assessing the conservation priorities of plant species used in local folk communities. It has now been considered as an effective tool in the field of ethnoecology for successful management and conservation of local phytoresources. In this article, the application and importance of six quantitative indices commonly used in ethnobotanical research worldwide for bioprospecting and conservation of phytoresources, have been discussed with special emphasis on Indian ethnobotany. Finally, the progress and future prospects of this branch of Ethnobotany has been briefed here in this review.

10.1   INTRODUCTION

Man lives in close vicinity of the nature and human beings are constantly being nurtured by its different types of components including plants. Since the dawn of civilization, plants have been playing pivotal role for the growth and development of the human society by providing the food, shelter and health care. In ancient time, people developed the practices of various usages of plant wealth for their subsistence, existence and survival, and also for reducing the hardship of their struggling life. Those traditional practices of plant usages had been established into specific systems of knowledge through trial and error method over a period of time. Traditional knowledge regarding various kinds of plant usages are the basis of Ethnobotany. Ethnobotany is now understood by the scientists as a scientific discipline which explores the relationship between people in a culture and plants in an environment. The term 'Ethnobotany' was first coined by Harshberger in 1895 (Harshberger, 1896). It can be defined as the total natural and traditional relationship and interactions between men, domesticated animals and their surrounding plant wealth (Jain, 1987). Ethnobotany has now been established as a multi-disciplinary subject and it deals with the studies among traditional people for recording their unique traditional knowledge about plant wealth and for search of new resources of herbal drugs, edible plants and other aspects of plants (Mudgal and Jain, 1983). During last few decades, scientific studies in the field of ethnobotany have been ensued on various lines covering ethnobotany of specific tribes, of certain regions, of particular plant groups or diseases and on many other miscellaneous sub- or interdisciplinary approaches throughout the World including India (Schultes, 1979; Etkin, 1988; Heinrich et al., 1992; Moerman, 1996; Jain and Patole, 2001; Jain, 2004, Ignacimuthu et al., 2006; Albuquerque et al., 2007; Savithramma et al., 2007; Tabuti, 2008; Kim and Song, 2013; Saqib et al., 2014).

Ethnobotany is a multidisciplinary subject and research activity today in this academic field requires a variety of skills in different interrelated subjects, especially in Botany, Anthropology and Linguistic. Botanical training is essential for the identification and preservation of plant specimens; anthropological training helps to understand the cultural concepts around the perception of plants; linguistic training equally helps to transcribe the local terms and to understand the syntax, and semantics. Since the beginning of ethnobotanical research, it was noticed that the ethnobotanical works mostly embodied the documentation of the plant knowledge without or rarely with a little bit statistical analysis. Such documentation works in ethnobotany were largely subjective type and data compilations there in all the works were very traditional one without employing the suitable statistical indices for more objectivity in research. But from the beginning of the 20th century, the field of ethnobotany saw the transformation from the raw compilation of data to a greater methodological and conceptual reorientation. This is in fact the beginning of academic ethnobotany. In the recent past, to add more objectivity in the field of ethnobotanical research, scientists have been employing different statistical indices during data analysis. And thus, the 'Quantitative Ethnobotany' was identified globally as a distinct approach in the field of ethnobotanical research. The term Quantitative Ethnobotany was first introduced by Balee in 1986 and it was then popularized among the ethnobotanists by Prance and his associates (1987) throughout the world. Use of the quantitative techniques for analysis of the collected data has become increasingly popular among the ethnobiologists day-by-day. 'Quantitative Ethnobotany' involves in measuring the importance of plants and vegetation to the people in a culture or community, in a comparative manner. Richness and reliability of traditional plant knowledge can successfully be assessed by appropriate quantitative ethnobotanical tools. Quantitative Ethnobotany can be defined as an approach where different quantitative techniques are employed to analyze and interpret the recorded data for getting more precise objectivity in ethnobotanical research. It has been defined as "application of quantitative techniques to the direct analysis of contemporary plant use data" (Phillips and Gentry, 1993). Other workers perceived it as quantification in ethnobotany which includes aspects related to the analysis of people's knowledge about the uses of plant species. It embodies the use of quantitative indices or techniques and/or the application of statistical analysis (Medeiros et al., 2011).

Quantitative approaches aim to describe the variables quantitatively and analyze the data statistically. It provides more objectivity to the ethnobotanical research that helps in comparative analysis of ethnobotanical data for identification of more important plant species used by the people in a particular culture or community. It also add new dimension to the conservation strategies of phytoresources by providing differential pattern of utilization of plant species, forest resources or vegetation in a region. Ethnobotany highlights the exact pattern of utilization of resources which gives clear indication towards management planning of local phytore-sources and thus plays a very important role in conservation prioritization of plant species in a region which are identified as rare and most accept-able species in a culture. Ethnobotanical research and its quantitative approaches are now considered as the most efficient tool for management, sustainable utilization and conservation of phytoresources in a particular area (Figure 10.1).

Scientists all over the world are engaged in exploring new life-saving drugs and biomolecules, taking the lead from traditional herbal knowl-edge. Quantitative techniques perfectly determine the most important as well as most reliable medicinal species used in a community, and they rightly guide scientists to select the good candidates among the list of statistically analyzed plant species for bioprospecting. In the present chapter, an attempt has been made to discuss the role of quantitative ethnobotany in bioprospecting and conservation of plant resources.

Quantitative ethnobotanical research

Selection of appropriate quantitative tools

↓

Identification of important species

Bioprospecting of natural products

Conservation of plant resources

➤ Development of new drug
➤ Enhanced production of desired phytochemicals through biotechnological approaches

➤ Management planning of local phyto-resources through ethno-conservation approaches
➤ Conservation prioritization of rare and most acceptable plant species in a culture

FIGURE 10.1 Diagrammatic outline for selection of important species for both bioprospection and conservation through quantitative analysis.

10.2   METHODS AND TECHNIQUES USED IN COLLECTION OF ETHNOBOTANICAL DATA AND ITS QUANTITATIVE ANALYSIS

The methods and techniques commonly employed in ethnobotanical research have been discussed in briefly in this chapter. Informants are the instrumental here for collection of data as the basic information about traditional knowledge are collected from them. Many techniques are available to conduct the interviews, ranging from individual approaches to research conducted with groups of people. Interviews are one of the most basic procedures used to collect the data in ethnobiological studies. According to the objectivity of the study, suitable statistical tools are selected and accordingly the procedures of interview are employed to obtain the purposeful data from a specific study. The "interviews" generally employed in ethnobotanical research for data collections are structured, unstructured, semi-structured, and informal.

In structured interviews, previously planned questions are asked to each informant independently which help in codification or categorization of the answers and thus allows rapid production of materials for analysis in an advantageous way. In unstructured interviews, the informant is requested to speak about some topic of researcher's interest without any preplanned questions. In case of semi-structured interviews, although the questions are partially framed by the investigator before conducting actual field research, they are largely flexible and allow more attention to be paid to issues that might arise during the interview. If it is not possible to interview the same informant twice, semi-structured interviews are the best tool to use. The "open" side of this technique allows the interviewees to answer the questions according to their own conceptions. This type of interview is similar to an unstructured interview but differs in that it is totally beyond the investigator's control. Various participatory methods like participatory rural appraisal (PRA) and rapid rural appraisal (RRA) are also employed for data collection by the researchers in ethnobiological and ethnoecological research (Lulekal et al., 2008; Woodward et al., 2012). Some of the ecological methods have successfully been applied in ethnobotanical research for measurements of species diversity and richness (Begossi, 1996; Hanazaki et al., 2000; Begossi et al., 2002; Peroni and Hanazaki, 2002).

Since the 1990s, a number of quantitative techniques have been proposed for ethnobotanical data analysis, and till date many authors have adopted them in their research program. Phillips (1996) has reviewed the techniques used in ethnobotanical research considering the degree of subjectivity of the study and discussed the quantitative techniques under three major types: (i) informant consensus, (ii) subjective allocation, and (iii) aggregation of uses. In the recent past, Hoffman and Gallaher (2007) have analyzed the important indices of ethnobotanical research and used the term Relative Cultural Importance which includes different techniques like use value, fidelity level, importance value, cultural significance, total use value, etc. Recently Medeiros et al. (2011) have reviewed 87 quantitative techniques and explained them under three major groups as cited by Phillips (1996).

In a recent study, Mathur and Sundaramoorthy (2013) have mentioned 120 different indices and categorized them into several groups like consensus methods, use value methods, ethno-medicine methods, relative importance methods, equitability methods, methods related to food, and ecological methods for analyzing the ethnobotanical data. One has to fully understand the assumptions that are made when adopting a specific quantitative technique to analyze the data. A researcher will adopt suitable indices according to his/her goal of the study and data interpretation.

Some important quantitative indices have been described below which are widely used in ethnobotanical research, especially in bioprospecting of ethnomedicinal plants and conservation of local phytoresources.

10.2.1   FACTOR OF INFORMANT CONSENSUS (FIC)

Over the last ten years the most widely used tool in quantitative analysis of ethnobotanical data, is the factor of informant consensus (Fic). The current formula of this index has been proposed by Heinrich et al. (1998) based on a definition first introduced by Trotter and Logan in 1986. To use Fic, first it is necessary to classify different health disorders and illnesses into broad disease categories. The main objective of this tool is to identify the important species used in particular disease categories (grouping of similar health disorders and illnesses into a broad group) where there is consensus on the use of plant species among the informants. The level of homogeneity between information provided by different informants is calculated using this index. It is calculated as $Fic = Nur - Nt/(Nur - 1)$, where, Nur is the number of use reports from informants for a particular plant-usage category and Nt is the number of taxa or species used for that usage category for all informants. Here value ranges between 0 and 1, where '1' indicates the highest level of informant consent. For instance, if few taxa are used by the informants, then a high degree of consensus among the informants is reached.

Interpretation of the Fic results may provide clue for drug development by selecting plant species with high Fic value. It also highlights the use-pressure for particular species used in the locality and thus also helps to assess its threat status.

10.2.2 FIDELITY LEVEL (FL)

It can be defined as the ratio between the number of informants who inde-pendently reported the use of a species for a major purpose and total num-ber of informants who mentioned the plant for any use. It is the percentage of informants claiming the use of a species for a main purpose. The for-mula of Fidelity level is $Fl = Np/N \times 100$, where, Np is the number of informants that reported a particular use of a plant species, and N is the number of informants that reported the plant for any use (Friedman et al., 1986). This index is also employed to identify the main use among differ-ent uses of a species.

10.2.3 USE VALUE

To compare the relative importance of each species, the use value is calcu-lated (adapted from the proposal of Rossato et al., 1999) using the follow-ing formula: $UV = \Sigma U/n$, where, UV is the use-value of a species; U is the number of citations of that species; and n is the total number of informants cited that species. The use-value of a species is based only on the impor-tance attributed by each informant.

10.2.4 CULTURAL IMPORTANT INDEX

Importance of a species in the culture of a particular geographic area can be calculated with the help of different indices like Relative Frequency of Citation (RFC) (Shah et al., 2015), Relative Importance Index (RI) (Albuquerque et al., 2007a, b), Cultural Agreement Index (CAI) (Bruschi et al., 2011), Cultural Importance Index (CI) (Pardo-de-Santayana et al., 2007), etc.

10.2.5 IMPORTANCE VALUE INDEX (IVI)

In order to establish conservation priorities of a species based on indicators from pharmaceutical products, a complex and effective tool like Importance Value Index (IVI) is used by the researchers (Dhar et al., 2000; Melo et al., 2009). It is expressed by the formula: $IVI = RI + SI$, where RI = relative importance of a species; SI = sensitivity index. Now, $SI = [(SR \times NR)/(SR \times NR)] \times 100$, where SR = sensitivity rank, considers attributes related to the manner in which a species is harvested and the degree of anthropogenic pressure to which it is subjected; NR = naturalness rank, concerns the origin of the species from where it is procured for use as raw materials in industry). Here, value of this index varies from 1 to 3.

10.2.6 CONSERVATION PRIORITY INDEX (CPI) OR LOCAL CONSERVATION PRIORITY INDEX (LCPI)

CPI is a unique tool specially devised by the ethnobotanists and ecologists taking selective indices from ethnobotany as well as ecology for assessment of conservation priorities of the plant species (Martinez et al., 2006; Lucena et al., 2013). The LCPI is a bit simplified and modified index used in ethnobotanical research (Oliveira et al., 2007) to identify the occurrence status of the local flora. The LCPI is determined by the formula: $LCPI = CR + DA + RD$, where, CR is Citation Richness (numbers of use-categories for each species); DA refers to the Degree of Attention (frequency of occurrence of the species in the locality) and RD is meant for Relative Density of the species. Scoring used to calculate the LCPI is given in Table 10.1.

TABLE 10.1 Scores to Calculate LCPI

Parameter	Scores
Citation Richness (CR)	**1–10**
2 points are summed for each use-category reported	
Degree of attention (DA)	**1–10**
High (frequency of occurrence ≥60%)	1
Moderate (frequency of occurrence ≥20% and <60%)	4
Low (frequency of occurrence <20%)	7
Weak (not encountered)	10
Relative density (RD)	**1–10**
Very low	10
Low	7
Medium	4
High	1

10.3 PHYTORESOURCES AND QUANTITATIVE ETHNOBOTANY

10.3.1 BIOPROSPECTING OF PHYTORESOURCES AND QUANTITATIVE ETHNOBOTANY

The identification and evaluation of biological material found in nature to obtain new products is known as bioprospecting (Artuso, 2002). There is a worldwide resurgence of interest in ethnobotanical as well as ethnomedicinal studies now to meet the growing needs of agro-industries, herbal drug industries, conservation and development of plant genetic resources. Scientists in the world have now been concentrated upon ethnomedicinal plants for its scientific validation through various scientific studies including bioprospecting. Bioprospecting is the process for searching of new gens or compounds from unknown sources. It can be classified into three major areas of studies like chemoprospecting, gene prospecting and bionic prospecting which include discovery and development of new drugs, production of pharmaceuticals, agro-chemicals, cosmetics, food additives, improved crop varieties, proteins, enzymes, GMOs, GM foods, etc. Bioprospecting is done through (a) taxonomy guided lead, (b) phytochemistry guided lead, and (c) ethno guided lead. The ethno guided lead gives more positive result than other two in the field of drug development. For this reason, ethnomedicines are getting more importance in the scientific world for development of various pharmaceuticals. A schematic presentation of the steps involved in developing phytomedicines, starting from the ethnoguided lead is given below (Figure 10.2). It is estimated that approximately 25% of the world's pharmaceutical products find a significant degree of origin in indigenous communities. Ethnobotanical approach to bioprospecting has led to the development of at least 88 modern pharmaceuticals, among them tubocurarine, a muscle relaxant, and quinine, an antimalarial compound, are very familiar (Baker et al., 1995; Cox, 1994; Farnsworth, 1994). The ethnobotanical approach can be considered as the practice of using traditional healers' knowledge to select important organisms for testing against a broad range of diseases (Cox, 1994; Slish et al., 1999). Taking the leads from traditional medicine as well as ethnomedicine many new drugs have been designed worldwide by the coordinated efforts of ethnobotanists, phytochemists, pharmacologists and clinical persons.

Once indigenous people share information or genetic material with the modern world, they effectively lose control over those resources, regardless of whether or not they are compensated. The Convention on Biological

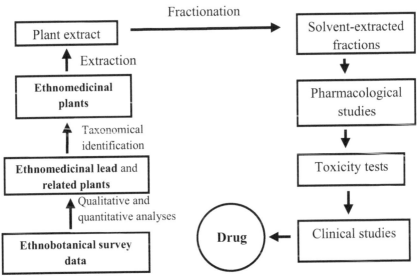

FIGURE 10.2 Steps involved in drug development from ethnomedicinal lead.

Diversity (CBD) offers a multilateral facade for addressing conservation and sustainable use of biodiversity. It also says that states have sovereign rights over their natural resources, and that terms and conditions for access to these materials are within the domain of national legislation. The Convention also recognizes the "knowledge, innovations and practices of indigenous and local communities" and specifically "encourage[s] the equitable sharing of benefits arising from the utilization of such knowledge, innovations and practices" [Article 8(j) of CBD].

Medicinal folklore over the years has proved to be an invaluable guide for screening and development of drugs. Many important modern drugs like digitoxin, reserpine, tubocurarine, ephedrine, ergometrine, atropine, vinblastine and aspirin have been discovered following the leads from folk uses. In India, the best example of bioprospecting done with the help of ethnobotanical lead is the KANI model or Pushpangadan model which is the pioneer in the field of 'Access and Benefit sharing' and the 1st application of Article 8(j) of CBD in the world. Dr. Pushpangadan and his team of The Tropical Botanic Garden and Research Institute (TBGRI), Thiruvananthapuram have validated the Kani tribe's claim on the anti-fatigue property of Arogyapacha (*Trichopus zeylanicus*) and standardized a herbal formulation 'Jeevani' by the end of 1994 (Pushpangadan, 1994). TBGRI transferred the manufacturing license to a major Ayurvedic drug company in India. The Aryavaidya Pharmacy Ltd., Coimbatore licensed Jeevani as a tonic to bolster the immune system and provide energy for a fee of Rs. 10 lakh (approximately U.S. $25,000). The TGBRI has agreed to share 50% of the license fee and the 2% royalty on profits with the Kani tribe.

The cardiac glycosides digoxin and digitoxin from *Digitalis purpurea* and prostratin, a drug candidate for the treatment of HIV from *Homalanthus nutans* discovered using the ethnobotanical approach. Most of the CNS-active natural products (*Hypericum perforatum*; *Piper methysticum*, *Salvia divinorum*, etc.) have been developed with the help of traditional knowledge. Taking the leads from ancient literature like Susruta Samhita, Charak Samhita, etc. many important drugs have been developed in India such as a hypocholesteraelemic drug GUGULIP from *Commiphora wightii*, a memory enhancer MEMORY PLUS from *Bacopa monnieri*, a hepatoprotective drug PICROLIV from *Picrorrhiza kurrooa* and so on (Mehrotra and Mehrotra, 2005).

Several studies have been focused on selecting prospective plants through the ethnodirected approaches. Active fraction named "Kolaviron" has been patented for commercial exploitation of the fruits of the plant *Garcinia kola* which are traditionally chewed by the African tribes for liver protection (Iwu, 1993; Iwu and Igboko, 1986). The polypeptide "Thaumatin" have been derived from the aril of the seed of red fruit *Thaumatococcus danielli* which is 5000 times sweeter than sucrose on molar basis. From the collaborative work of Nigeria and UK based companies a low-calorie high-intensity sweetener has been developed from the plant (Van der Wel and Loeve, 1972). *Cassia podocarpa* is identified as an alternative of *C. angustifolia* (Senna), a purgative drug and found less toxic than Senna. Leaves of this plant have been formulated into tablets and recommended as substitute for Senna in Nigeria and Ghana, Africa (Elujoba and Iweibo, 1988). A Ghana-base company produces its tea bags on a commercial scale. Michellamines A & B, these two new alkaloids extracted from the plant *Ancistrocladus korupensis*, which have wide range of antiviral activity including anti-HIV. Michellamine B is being developed for use in AIDS treatment. It was characterized by collaborative effort of Cameroon scientists and NCI, USA (Boyd et al., 1994). There are plenty of examples in the field of bioprospecting where ethno-directed leads taken a prominent role in discovery and development of novel natural products of medicinal and nutritional importance.

A minimum percentage of bioresources has come under bioprospecting so far. There is immense scope of bioprospecting with a vast bioresources throughout the world. For this reason, scientists throughout the world are actively engaged in exploring the medicinal potential of plant resources through ethnobotanical research aiming for development of new life saving drug. In this context it has been observed that 'quantitative ethnobotany' can help the scientists to choose right candidate (plant species) for its bioprospection very precisely.

10.3.2 CONSERVATION OF PHYTORESOURCES AND QUANTITATIVE ETHNOBOTANY

It is a management and sustainable use practice of bioresources. Natural resources are being conserved and managed through *in-situ* and *ex-situ* modes of conservation. Traditional knowledge is directly related with the utilization and conservation of bioresources. So detection of threats and adoption of appropriate conservation measures is the best way for management of the bioresources and conservation of related traditional knowledge. Many International and national bodies (WWF, IUCN, CITES, etc.) and NGOs have been working worldwide for the conservation of natural resources and its sustainable utilization. Indigenous people also have their own heritage of conservation practice known as ethno-conservation.

Ethnobiologists are now focusing their research on the conservation of local flora and fauna by estimating their status in a specified area because local flora is greatly influenced by the over-utilization and other anthropogenic activities of the local inhabitants. In this context suitable quantitative indices have been developed combining both ecological as well as ethnobotanical knowledge to understand different utilization pattern and occurrence status of the local plants. Works are being carried out sporadically in different parts of the world employing such quantitative tools to determine the prioritized species which need immediate conservation measure. Researchers who are working in this field of ethnobotany should execute their work in a collaborative way which will help to understand the status of the over-utilized plants in a particular locality and to design conservation measures for those much exploited plant species. A few examples of ethnobotanical research cited below where two unique quantitative methods have been employed for better understanding of conservation status of the local flora.

10.3.2.1 Local Level Conservation of Phytoresources Employing LCPI and CPI

Among 166 native and exotic plants, 11 plant taxa have been identified as prioritized species for conservation employing the quantitative tool of LCPI (Local Conservation Priority Index) from the "Caatinga vegetation" in semi-arid region of northeastern Brazil. The prioritized species identified for their conservation from the "Caatinga vegetation" are *Capparis jacobinae* Moric. ex Eichler, *Cedrela odorata* L., *Schinopsis brasiliensis* Engler, *Croton rhamnifolius* Willd., *Myrciaria cauliflora* (Mart.) O. Berg, *Eugenia uvalha* Cambess, *Ziziphus joazeiro* Mart., *Comiphora leptophloeos* (Mart.) J. B. Gillett, *Clusia* sp., *Manihot dichotoma* Ule, and *Lippia* sp. (Albuquerque et al., 2009).

Later on, Lucena et al. (2013) have identified three plant taxa with the help of CPI, from the "Caatinga vegetation" as species with greater CPI scores which are scarcely found in the region, mainly because of their over extraction. The prioritized species are *Ziziphus joazeiro* Mart., *Schinopsis brasiliensis* Engl. and *Myracrodruon urundeuva* Allemão.

In Paravachasca Valley, Co'rdoba, Argentina, a number of shrubs including a pteridophyte have been identified as most prioritized species employing the CPI method. The prioritized species are namely *Minthostachys mollis*, *Julocroton argenteus*, *Baccharis crispa*, *Trixis divaricata* subsp. *discolor*, *Aloysia gratissima*, *Lippia turbinata* and *Baccahris articulata* and for two herbs, *Hedeoma multiflora* and *Passiflora caerulea*, one lichen *Usnea* spp. and one pteridophyte *Equisetum giganteum* (Martinez et al., 2006).

10.4   PROGRESS IN QUANTITATIVE ETHNOBOTANICAL RESEARCH AND ITS FUTURE PROSPECTS

Ethnobotanical study was initiated by the European scientist long ago and flourishes gradually with the interest of a lot of field botanist, taxonomist, herbarium curator, botanist and many more. The modern approach to the science of ethnobotany and ethnomedicine evolved in United States of America and the foremost center for the botanical aspects is the Botanical Museum of Harvard University in Massachusetts, here the ethnobotanists like Richard Evans Schultes, Richard Gorden Wasson, Siri von Reis Altschul, Timothy Plowman and E. Wade Davis contributed a lot in various fields of ethnobotany. From the end of nineteenth century to the middle of the twentieth century, ethnobotanists were concerned with recording the uses and common names of the plants in a locality and emphasized a utilitarian approach. During the period from 1950s to 1980s, ethnobotany research was concerned with the cognitive and classificatory approaches which dealt with how the people of a region classify and order the plants of their environment. After the 1980s, the focus of ethnobotanical research turned to its socio-ecological aspects, which incorporated ecological tools, techniques and statistical measurements (Clemént, 1998; Oliveira et al., 2010). A lot of books have been published by the eminent scientists describing various quantitative techniques of traditional knowledge (Martin, 1995; Cotton, 1996; Alexiades, 1996; Albuquerque et al., 2014). Methodological tools have been developed to respond to questions about the interrelation between people and plants, both qualitative and quantitative. The criteria for quantitative inferences by ethnobotanists are varied and are presented in a considerable number of published documents (Friedman et al., 1986; Troter and Logan, 1986; Phillips and Gentry, 1993; Heinrich et al., 1998; Bennett and Prance, 2000; Byg and Balslev, 2001; Gomez-Beloz, 2002; Albuquerque et al., 2007; Castañeda and Stepp, 2007). In ethnobotanical research, comparatively lesser number of investigations have been carried out to determine the distribution status of local biological diversity using suitable quantitative tools like CPI and LCPI. More scientists have to come forward from every little part of the world to identify the locally rare, endangered and threatened but culturally important plant species to endure the local tradition associated with them.

Starting from Janaki-Ammal (1955–56), till date Indian ethnobotanists remain uninterested about the quantitative ethnobotanical study and they are engaged mostly in documenting the ethnobotanical knowledge without analysis of the data employing suitable quantitative indices (Jain and Borthakur, 1980; Jain, 1981, 1987, 1991, 1997, 2001; Singh and Pandey, 1998; Rao and Pullaiah, 2007; Maheshwari, 2000; Katewa et al., 2001; Trivedi and Sharma, 2004; Patil and Patil, 2006; Sajem and Gosai, 2006; Rahaman and Pradhan, 2011). Since last five years, this scenario of quantitative ethnobotany in India is gradually being changed and several research articles have been published from different parts of the country analyzing the data with the help of suitable quantitative tools (Ragupathy et al., 2008; Mutheeswaran et al., 2011; Kumar et al., 2012; Bhat et al., 2014; Mandal and Rahaman, 2014; Mootoosamy and Fawzi, 2014; Tarafdar et al., 2014; Shil et al., 2014; Rahaman and Karmakar, 2015; Shah et al., 2015; Francis et al., 2015). Quantitative indices like use value (UV), informant consensus factor (Fic), fidelity level (FL) and relative frequency of citation (RFC) were used by the Indian ethnobotanists for analyzing their ethnobotanical data. In a recent study, Mootoosamy and Fawzi (2014) have used eleven quantitative indices, namely informant consensus factor (FIC), fidelity level (FL), use value (UV), relative frequency of citation (RFC), relative importance (RI), cultural importance index (CII), index of agreement on remedies (IAR), cultural agreement index (CAI), quality use value (QUV), quality use agreement value (QUAV) and ethnobotanicity index (EI) for quantitative analysis of their findings. Statistical analysis such as Pearson correlation and Chi-squared test were also performed to determine any association among the variables taken.

There are about 68 million people belonging to 227 ethnic groups and 573 tribal communities derived from six racial stocks in India (Pushpgandhan, 1994). Nearly 1,75,000 traditional preparations derived from 7500 medicinal species are in use among different ethnic communities of India (AICRPE, Technical Report, 1992–1998). We have a giant volume of data on ethnobotany. In India, there is a vast scope of finding out various promising bioresources through ethnobotanical research employing quantitative indices to measure the authenticity of traditional knowledge and to determine the distribution status of local flora. The quantitative approach in Indian ethnobotanical research will change the dimension of its kind of research which further help in bioprospecting and conservation of its phytoresources. In India, no work has been executed till date on ethnoecology employing the suitable statistical tools like LCPI and CPI to study the conservation status of the ethnobotanical phytoresources. But many phytosociological studies have been carried out in different forest types of India without employing any ethnobotanical quantitative approach (Kala, 2000, 2005; Laloo et al., 2006; Sahu et al., 2007; Joshi, 2012; Pilania et al., 2015; Pradhan and Rahaman, 2015). Researchers, scientists and ethnobiologists engaged in this field of research should adopt quantitative approaches for data analysis to add more objectivity in research and for proper scientific interpretation of the research findings.

10.5 CONCLUSION

Like any scientific research, quantitative approaches make the ethnobotanical research more focused by adding more objectivity to the concern study and it also help to analyze the research findings in a more scientific way. Researchers should be very choosy about the tool selection according to the goal of the study otherwise it will be meaningless.

Ethno-guided bioprospecting of the phytoresources is highly acknowledged by the scientific world as it provides more success rate in discovery of novel drugs. Here in selection of good candidate for bioprospecting, quantitative indices show very positive direction to the scientists. Quantitative ethnobotany has now been recognized globally as an effective tool in the area of bioprospecting research for development of novel natural products which include pharmaceuticals, nutraceuticals and cosmetics. Quantitative ethnobotany is also equally important in identifying the prioritized species for conservation where various consensus and relative importance indices are employed. Then it will be easy to frame the conservation strategy for the prioritized threatened species in a particular region. To set the ethnobotanical research on a solid foundation, scientists from all allied fields should come forward, collaborate themselves and enrich this branch of Ethnobotany by experimenting with more new statistical indices.

KEYWORDS

- future prospects
- global perspective
- Indian scenario
- local conservation priority index
- quantitative ethnobotany

REFERENCES

1. Albuquerque, U. P., Monteiro, J. M., Ramos, M. A., & Amorim, E. L. C. (2007). Medicinal and magic plants from a public market in north-eastern Brazil. *J. Ethnopharmacol. 110*, 76–91.
2. Albuquerque, U. P., Medeiros, P. M., Almeida, A. L. S., Monteiro, J. M., Lins Neto, E. M. F., Melo, J. G., & Santos, J. P. (2007). Medicinal plants of the Caatinga (semi-arid) vegetation of NE Brazil: a quantitative approach. *J. Ethnopharmacol. 114*, 325–354.
3. Albuquerque, U. P., Araujo, T. A. S., Ramos, M. A., Nascimento, V. T., Lucena, R. F. P., Monteiro, J. M., Alencar, N., & Araújo, E. L. (2009). How ethnobotany can aid biodiversity conservation reflections on investigations in the semi-arid region of NE Brazil. *Biodiversity Conservation, 18*, 127–150.
4. Albuquerque, U. P., Cunha, L. V. F. C., Lucena, R. F. P., & Alves, R. R. N. (eds.) (2014). Methods and Techniques in Ethnobiology and Ethnoecology. Humana Press (Springer), New York.

5. Alexiades, M. N. (ed.) (1996). Selected Guidelines for Ethnobotanical Research: a field manual (Advances in Economic Botany. Vol. 10). The New York Botanical Garden, New York.

6. Artuso, A. (2002). Bioprospecting, benefit sharing, and biotechnological capacity building. *World Dev, 30(8)*, 1355–1368.

7. Baker, J. T., Borris, R. P., Carté, B., Cordell, G. A., Soejarto, D. D., Cragg, G. M., Gupta, M. P., Iwu, M. M., Madulid, D. R., & Tyler, V. E. (1995). Natural product drug discovery and development: New perspectives on international collaboration. *J. Nat. Prod. 58(9)*, 1325–1357.

8. Balee, W. (1986). Análise preliminary de inventário florestal e a ethnobotânica ka'apor (Maranhao). *Boletin de Museu Paraense Emilio Goeldi. Botânica, 2(2)*, 141–167.

9. Begossi, A. (1996). Use of ecological methods in ethnobotany: diversity indices. *Economic Botany, 50(3)*, 280–289.

10. Begossi, A., Hanazaki, N., & Tamashiro, J. Y. (2002). Medicinal plants in the Atlantic forest (Brazil) knowledge, use, and conservation. *Human Ecology, 30(3)*, 281–299.

11. Bennett, B. C., & Prance, G. T. (2000). Introduced plants in the indigenous pharmacopoeia of northern South America. *Economic Botany, 54*, 90–102.

12. Bhat, P., Hegde, G. R., Hegde, G., & Mulgund, G. S. (2014). Ethnomedicinal plants to cure skin diseases – an account of the traditional knowledge in the coastal parts of Central Western Ghats, Karnataka, India. *J. Ethnopharmacol. 151(1)*, 493–502. doi: 10.1016/j.jep.2013.10.062.

13. Boyd, M. R., Hallock, Y. F., Cardellina II, J. H., Manfredi, K. P., Blunt, J. W., McMahon, J. B., Buckheit Jr., R. W., Bringmann, G., Schaffer, M., Cragg, G. M., Thomas, D. W., & Jato, J. G. (1994). Anti-HIV michellamines from *Ancistrocladus korupensis*. *J. Medicinal Chem., 37*, 1740–1745.

14. Bruschi, P., Morganti, M., Mancini, M., & Signorini, M. A. (2011). Traditional healers and laypeople: A qualitative and quantitative approach to local knowledge on medicinal plants in Muda (Mozambique). *J. Ethnopharmacol. 138*, 543–563.

15. Byg, A., & Balslev, H. (2001). Diversity and use of palms in Zahamena, eastern Madagascar. *Biodiversity and Conservation, 10*, 951–970.

16. Castañeda, H., & Stepp, J. R. (2007). Ethnoecological importance value (EIV) methodology: assessing the cultural importance of ecosystems as sources of useful plants for the Guaymi people of Costa Rica. *Ethnobotany Research and Applications, 5*, 249–257.

17. Clement, D. (1998). The historical foundations of ethnobiology (1860–1899). *J. Ethnobiology, 18*, 161–187.

18. Cotton, C. (1996). Ethnobotany: Principles and Applications. Wiley & Sons, Chichester.

19. Cox, P. A. (1994). The ethnobotanical approach to drug discovery: Strengths and limitations. In: Chadwick, D. J., & Marsh, J. (eds.), Ethnobotany and the search for new drugs. Wiley, Chichester, UK, pp. 25–41.

20. Dhar, U.; Rawal, R. S., & Upreti, J. (2000). Setting priorities for conservation of medicinal plants – a case study in the Indian Himalaya. *Biological Conservation 95*, 57–65.

21. Elujoba, A. A., & Iweibo, G. O. (1988). *Cassia podocarpa* as substitute for official senna. *Planta Medica, 4,* 372.
22. Etkin, N. (1988). Ethnopharmacology, biobehavioral approaches in the anthropological study of indigenous medicines. *Annual Review of Anthropology, 17,* 23–42.
23. Farnsworth, N. R. (1994). Ethnopharmacology and drug development. In: Chadwick, D. J., & Marsh, J. (eds.), Ethnobotany and the search for new drugs. Wiley, Chichester, UK, pp. 42–59.
24. Francis, X. T., Kannan, M., & Auxilia, A. (2015). Observation on the traditional phytotherapy among the Malayali tribes in Eastern Ghats of Tamil Nadu, South India. *J. Ethnopharmacol., 165,* 198–214. doi: 10.1016/j.jep.2015.02.045.
25. Friedman, J., Yaniv, Z., Dafni, A., & Palewitch, D. (1986). A preliminary classification of the healing potential of medicinal plants, based on a rational analysis of an ethnopharmacological field survey among Bedouins in the Negev desert, Israel. *J. Ethnopharmacol, 16,* 275–287.
26. Gomez-Beloz, A. (2002). Plant knowledge of the Winikina Warao: the case for questionnaires in ethnobotany. *Economic Botany, 56,* 231–241.
27. Hanazaki, N., Tamashiro, J. Y., Leitão-Filho, H. F., & Begossi, A. (2000). Diversity of plant uses in two Caiçara communities from the Atlantic forest coast, Brazil. *Biodiversity Conservation, 9(5),* 597–615.
28. Harshberger, J. W. (1896). The purpose of ethnobotany. *Botanical Gazette, 21,* 146–158.
29. Heinrich, M., Rimpler, H., & Barrera, A. N. (1992). Indigenous phytotherapy of gastrointestinal disorders in a Mixe lowland community. *J. Ethnopharmacol. 36,* 63–80.
30. Heinrich, M., Ankli, A., Frei, B., Weimann, C., & Sticher, O. (1998). Medicinal plants in Mexico: healers' consensus and cultural importance. *Social Science and Medicine, 47(11),* 1859–1871.
31. Hoffman, B., & Gallaher, G. (2007). Importance indices in ethnobotany. *Ethnobotany Research and Applications, 5,* 201–218.
32. Ignacimuthu, S., Ayyanar, M., & Sankarasivaraman, K. (2006). Ethnobotanical investigations among tribes in Madurai district of Tamil Nadu, India. *J. Ethnobiology and Ethnomedicine, 2,* 25. doi: 10.1186/1746-4269-2-25.
33. Iwu, M. M. (1993). Handbook of African medicinal plants. CRC press, Inc Florida.
34. Iwu, M. M., & Igboko, A. O. (1986). The flavonoids of *Garcinia kola. J. Nat. Prod. 45,* 650–651.
35. Jain, A. K., & Patole, S. N. (2001). Less known medicinal values of plants among some tribal and rural communities of Pachmarhi forest (M.P). *Ethnobotany, 13,* 96–100.
36. Jain, S. K. (1981). Glimpses of Indian Ethnobotany. Oxford & IBH Publishing Co., New Delhi.
37. Jain, S. K. (1987). A Mannual of Ethnobotany. Scientific Publishers, Jodhpur, India.
38. Jain, S. K. (1991). Dictionary of Indian Folk Medicine and Ethnobotany. Deep publications, New Delhi.
39. Jain, S. K. (1997). Contribution to Indian Ethnobotany (3rd Edn.). Scientific publishers, Jodhpur.

40. Jain, S. K. (2001). Ethnobotany in modern India, *Phytomorphology*. Goldeen Jublee issue: Trends in Plant Science, pp. 39–54.

41. Jain, S. K. (2004). Credibility of traditional knowledge-The criterion of multilocational and multiethnic use. *Indian J. Trad. Knowl., 3(2)*, 137–153.

42. Jain, S. K., & Borthakur, S. K. (1980). Ethnobotany of the Mikirs of India. *Economic Botany; 34(3)*, 264–272.

43. Joshi, H. G. (2012). Vegetation structure, floristic composition and soil nutrient status in three sites of Tropical dry deciduous forest of West Bengal, India. *Indian J. Fundamental and Applied Life Sciences, 2(2)*, 355–364.

44. Kala, C. P. (2000). Status and Conservation of Rare and Endangered Medicinal plants in the Indian trans-Himalaya. *Conservation Biology, 93*, 371–379.

45. Kala, C. P. (2005). Indigenous Uses, Population Density, and Conservation of Threatened Medicinal Plants in Protected Areas of the Indian Himalayas. *Conservation Biology, 19*, 368–378.

46. Katewa, S. S., Guria, B. D., & Jain, A. (2001). Ethnomedicinal and obnoxious grasses of Rajasthan, India. *J. Ethnopharmacol. 76(3)*, 293–297.

47. Kim, H., & Song, M. J. (2013). Ethnomedicinal practices for treating liver disorders of local communities in the southern regions of Korea. *Evidence Based Complementary and Alternative Medicine, 2013*: 869176. doi: 10.1155/2013/869176.

48. Kumar, A., Pandey, V. C., & Tewari, D. D. (2012). Documentation and determination of consensus about phytotherapeutic veterinary practices among the Tharu tribal community of Uttar Pradesh, India. *Tropical Animal Health and Production, 44*, 863–872.

49. Laloo, R. C., Kharlukhi, L., Jeeva, S., & Mishra, B. P. (2006). Status of medicinal plants in the disturbed and undisturbed sacred forest of Meghalaya. *Current Science, 90(2)*, 225–232.

50. Lucena, R. F. P., Lucena, C. M., Araújo, E. L., Alves, Â. G. C., & Albuquerque, U. P. (2013). Conservation priorities of useful plants from different techniques of collection and analysis of ethnobotanical data. *Annals of the Brazilian Acad. Sci., 85(1)*, 169–186.

51. Lulekal, E., Kelbessa, E., Bekele, T., & Yineger, H. 2008. An ethnobotanical study of medicinal plants in Mana Angetu district, southeastern Ethiopia. *J. Ethnobiology and Ethnomedicine, 4*, 10.

52. Maheshwari, J. K. (2000). Ethnobotany and Medicinal Plants of Indian Subcontinent. Scientific Publishers, Jodhpur.

53. Mandal, S. K., & Rahaman, C. H. (2014). Determination of informants' consensus and documentation of ethnoveterinary practices from Birbhum district of West Bengal, India. *Indian J. Trad. Knowl., 13(4)*, 742–751.

54. Martin, G. J. (2004). Ethnobotany. A Methods Manual (People and Plants Conservation Series). WWF, Earthscan Publications, UK.

55. Martinez, G. J., Planchuelo, A. M., Fuentes, E., & Ojeda, M. (2006). A numeric index to establish conservation priorities for medicinal plants in the Paravachasca valley, Cordoba, Argentina. *Biodiversity Conservation, 15*, 2457–2475.

56. Mathur, M., & Sundaramoorthy, S. (2013). Census of approaches used in quantitative ethnobotany. *Studies on Ethno-Medicine, 7(1)*, 31–58.

57. Medeiros, M. F. T., Silva, P. S., & Albuquerque, U. P. (2011). Quantification in ethnobotanical research: an overview of indices used from 1995 to 2009. *Sientibus-série Ciencias Biológicas, 11(2)*, 211–230.

58. Mehrotra, S., & Mehrotra, B. N. (2005). Role of traditional and folklore herbals in development of new drugs. *Ethnobotany, 17*, 104–111.

59. Melo, J. G. Amorim, E. L. C., & Albuquerque, U. P. (2009). Native medicinal plants commercialized in Brazil priorities for conservation. *Environmental Monitoring and Assessment 156*, 567–580.

60. Moerman, D. E. (1996). An analysis of the food plants and drug plants of native North America. *J. Ethnopharmacol. 52*, 1–22.

61. Mootoosamy, A., & Fawzi, M. M. (2014). Ethnomedicinal application of native remedies used against diabetes and related complications in Mauritius. *J. Ethnopharmacol., 151(1)*, 413–444. doi: 10.1016/j.jep.2013.10.069.

62. Mudgal, V., & Jain, S. K. (1983). Ethnobotany in India. Botanical Survey of India, Culcutta.

63. Mutheeswaran, S., Pandikumar, P., Chellappandian, M., & Ignacimuthu, S. (2011). Documentation and quantitative analysis of the local knowledge on medicinal plants among traditional Siddha healers in Virudhunagar district of Tamil Nadu, India. *J. Ethnopharmacol. 137*, 523–533.

64. Oliveira, R. L. C., Lins Neto, E. M. F., Araújo, E. L., & Albuquerque, U. P. (2007). Conservation priorities and population structure of woody medicinal plants in an area of caatinga vegetation (Pernambuco state, NE Brazil). *Environmental Monitoring and Assessment, 132*, 189–206.

65. Pardo-de-Santayana, M., Tardío, J., Blanco, E., Carvalho, A. M., Lastra, J. J., Miguel, E. S., & Morales, R. (2007). Traditional knowledge of wild edible plants used in the northwest of the Iberian Peninsula (Spain and Portugal): a comparative study. *J. Ethnobiology and Ethnomedicine 3*, 27. doi: 10.1186/1746–4269–3-27

66. Patil, M. V., & Patil, D. A. 2006. Ethnobotany of Nasik district, Maharastra. Daya Publishing house, Delhi.

67. Peroni, N., & Hanazaki, N. (2002). Current and lost diversity of cultivated varieties, especially cassava, under swidden cultivation systems in the Brazilian Atlantic Forest. *Agriculture, Ecosystem and Environment, 92*, 171–183.

68. Phillips, O. (1996). Some quantitative methods for analyzing ethnobotanical knowledge. In: Alexiades, M. (ed.), Selected Guidelines for Ethnobotanical Research: a field manual (Advances in Economic Botany. Vol. 10). The New York Botanical Garden, New York, pp. 171–197.

69. Phillips, O., & Gentry, A. H. (1993). The useful plants of Tambopata, Peru: I. Statistical hypothesis tests with a new quantitative technique. Economic Botany, *47*, 15–32.

70. Pilania, P. K., Gujar, R. V., Joshi, P. M., Shrivastav, S. C., & Panchal N. S. (2015). Phytosociological and Ethnobotanical Study of Trees in a Tropical Dry Deciduous Forest in Panchmahal District of Gujarat, Western India. *The Indian Forester, 141(4)*, 422–427.

71. Pradhan, B., & Rahaman, C. H. (2015). Phytosociological study of plant species in three tropical dry deciduous forests of Birbhum District, West Bengal, India. *J. Biodiversity and Environmental Sciences, 7(2)*, 22–31.

72. Prance, G. T., Balée, W., Boom, B. M., & Carneiro, R. L. (1987). Quantitative ethnobotany and the case for conservation in Amazônia. *Conservation Biology, 1,* 296–310.

73. Pushpangandan, P. (1994). Ethnobiology in India (A status report). Ministry of Enviroment and Forest, Govt. of India, New Delhi.

74. Ragupathy, S., Newmaster, S. G., Murugesan, M., Balasubramaniam, V., & Huda, M. (2008). Consensus of the 'Malasars' traditional aboriginal knowledge of medicinal plants in the Velliangiri holy hills, India. *J. Ethnobiology and Ethnomedicine, 4,* 8. doi: 10.1186/1746-4269-4-8.

75. Rahaman, C. H., & Pradhan, B. (2011). A study on the ethnomedicinal uses of plants by the tribal people of Birbhum district, West Bengal. *J. Econ. Taxon. Bot. 35(3),* 529–534.

76. Rahaman, C. H., & Karmakar, S. (2015). Ethnomedicine of Santal tribe living around Susunia hill of Bankura district, West Bengal, India: The quantitative approach. *J. Applied and Pharmaceutical Science, 5(2),* 127–136.

77. Rao, D. M., & Pullaiah, T. (2007). Ethnobotanical studies on some rare and endemic floristic elements of Eastern Ghats-hill ranges of south-east Asia, India. *Ethnobotanical Leaflets, 11,* 52–70.

78. Rossato, S. C., Leitão Filho, H., & Begossi, A. (1999). Ethnobotany of caiçaras of the Atlantic Forest coast (Brazil). *Economic Botany, 53,* 387–395.

79. Sahu, S. C., Dhal, N. K., Sudhakar Reddy, C., Pattanaik, C., & Brahmam, M. (2007). Phytosociological study of tropical dry deciduous forest of Boudh district, Orissa, India. *Res. J. Forestry, 1,* 66–72.

80. Sajem, A. L., & Gosai, K. (2006). Traditional use of medicinal plants by the Jaintia tribes in North Cachar Hills district of Assam, northeast India. *J. Ethnobiology and Ethnomedicine 2,* 33. doi: 10.1186/1746-4269-2-33.

81. Saqib, Z., Mahmood, A., Malik, N. R., Mahmood, A., Syed, H. J., & Ahmad, T. (2014). Indigenous knowledge of medicinal plants in Kotli Sattian, Rawalpindi district, Pakistan. *J. Ethnopharmacol., 151,* 820–828.

82. Savithramma, N., Sulochana, C. H., & Rao, K. N. (2007). Ethnobotanical survey of plants used to treat asthma in Andhra Pradesh, India. *J. Ethnopharmacol., 113,* 54–61.

83. Schultes, R. E. (1979). Medicinal and toxic uses of *Swartzia* in the northwest Amazon. *J. Ethnopharmacol., 1,* 79–87.

84. Shah, A., Bharati, K. A., Ahmad, J., & Sharma, M. P. (2015). New ethnomedicinal claims from Gujjar and Bakerwals tribes of Rajouri and Poonch districts of Jammu and Kashmir, India. *J. Ethnopharmacol. 166,* 119–28. doi: 10.1016/j.jep.2015.01.056.

85. Shil, S., Dutta Choudhury, M., & Das, S. (2014). Indigenous knowledge of medicinal plants used by the *Reang* tribe of Tripura state of India. *J. Ethnopharmacol., 152(1),* 135–141.

86. Singh, V., & Pandey, R. P. (1998). Ethnobotany of Rajasthan, India. Scientific Publishers, Jodhpur, India.

87. Slish, D. F., Ueda, H., Arvigo, R., & Balick, M. (1999). Ethnobotany in the search for vasoactive herbal medicines. *J. Ethnopharmacol., 66,* 159–165.

88. Tabuti, J. R. S. (2008). Herbal medicines used in the treatment of malaria in Budiopecounty, Uganda. *J. Ethnopharmacol., 116,* 33–42.

89. Tarafdar, R. G., Nath, S., Das Talukdar, A., & Dutta Choudhury, M. (2014). Antidiabetic plants used among the ethnic communities of Unakoti district of Tripura, India. *J. Ethnopharmacol., 160*, 219–226. doi: 10.1016/j.jep.2014.11.019.
90. Trivedi, P. C., & Sharma, N. K. (2004). Ethnomedicinal Plants. Pointer Publishers, Jaipur, India.
91. Troter, R., & Logan, M. (1986). Informant consensus: a new approach for identifying potentially effective medicinal plants. In: Etkin, N. L. (ed.), Indigenous medicine and diet: biobehavioral approaches. Redgrave Bedford Hills, New York, pp. 91–112.
92. Van der Wel, H., & Loeve, K. (1972). Isolation and characterization of thaumatin I and II, the sweet-tasting proteins from *Thaumatococcus daniellii* Benth. *European J. Biochem., 31*, 221–225.
93. Woodward, E., Jackson, S., Finn, M., & McTaggart, P. M. (2012). Utilising indigenous seasonal knowledge to understand aquatic resource use and inform water resource management in northern Australia. *Ecological Management and Restoration, 13(1)*, 58–64.

CHAPTER 11

ETHNOBOTANY OF TURMERIC AND ITS MEDICINAL IMPORTANCE

SUJATHA SAMALA and CIDDI VEERESHAM

University College of Pharmaceutical Sciences, Kakatiya University, Warangal, Telangana–506009, India, E-mail: ciddiveeresham@yahoo.co.in

CONTENTS

Abstract 293

11.1   Introduction 294

11.2   Taxonomy 295

11.3   Ethnobotany of Turmeric 295

11.4   Microscopical Characters of Turmeric Rhizome 298

11.5   Phytochemistry 299

11.6   Uses of Turmeric 301

11.7   Commercial Medicinal Preparations Containing Turmeric 308

11.8   Toxicity 308

Keywords 310

References 310

ABSTRACT

Turmeric is one of the most important and valuable herb spices to humankind. It has been used traditionally, as food flavoring, as a dye, in folk medicine and for religious and ritual ceremonies. In addition to its use as a spice and pigment, turmeric has been used in India for various medicinal purposes for centuries. Turmeric has its origins in Southeast Asia and also can be found growing in India and Tropical Africa. India is the largest producer of turmeric commercially. This chapter includes the ethnobotany of turmeric, different species of the genus curcuma, microscopical characters, phytochemistry, medicinal uses and other various uses of turmeric.

11.1   INTRODUCTION

Turmeric belongs to the genus *Curcuma* and commonly known as haldi or holud. There are around 100–110 species of *Curcuma*, in which *Curcuma longa* is the most important economically, known as turmeric. This genus *Curcuma* belongs to Zingiberaceae family, originated from the Arabic word *kurkum* meaning "yellow," refers to the deep yellow rhizome color of the true turmeric. In India, turmeric is one of the most important spices, which produces nearly the whole world's crop and uses >80% of it. Ayurveda and Unani systems of medicines have used turmeric from time immemorial. In ancient Indian literature, turmeric is referred to as "Haridra" which is being used for cosmetic, coloring, flavoring, food preservative and digestive properties (Patel and Srinivasan, 2004). In India, turmeric is cultivated in the states of Telangana, Andhra Pradesh, Karnataka, Maharashtra, Kerala, Tamilnadu and Orissa. It is also cultivated in Caribbean, Africa, Costa Rica, Australia, Japan, Haiti, Latin America-Jamaica, Peru and Brazil. Among all these turmeric cultivated countries, India is the largest producer, consumer and exporter (Sasikumar, 2005). For cultivation requires a hot and moist climate, a liberal supply of water and a well-drained soil.

   According to the geographical origin of the production of turmeric it is graded in the international market. Alleppey, Madras and West Indian turmeric are the major types in the international trade. In Kerala, Alleppey turmeric comes from the region of Thodupuzha and Muvattupuzha taluks and is characterized by deep yellow to orange yellow in color which has high curcumin content up to 6.5%. Alleppey finger turmeric is preferred as food colorant especially in US (Kurian et al., 2004). The other popular Indian turmeric varieties in trade are Nizamabad turmeric from Telangana, Cuddappah and Duggirala turmeric from Andhra Pradesh, Erode and

Salem turmeric from Tamilnadu and Sangli turmeric from Maharashtra. This chapter summarizes the ethnobotany, phytochemistry and uses of turmeric.

11.2 TAXONOMY

Kingdom: Plantae
Class: Liliospida
Sub class: Commelinids
Order: Zingiberales
Family: Zingiberaceae
Genus: *Curcuma*
Species: *Curcuma longa*

11.3 ETHNOBOTANY OF TURMERIC

India is the largest producer of turmeric in the world (93.7% of the total world production) and its cultivation is done in 150,000 hectares in India (Sasikumar, 2005). In India around 6% of the area is used for turmeric as a spice and 8% of the total production of turmeric is exported annually and the rest is consumed in the domestic purpose (Peter, 1997). Maximum area under turmeric is in Andhra Pradesh, Telangana followed by Maharashtra, Tamil Nadu, Orissa, Karnataka and Kerala. Its production was found throughout the South and South East Asia with a few species extending to China, Australia and South Pacific. In India and Thailand, the highest diversity was concentrated with at least 40 species in each area, followed by Myanmar, Bangladesh, Indonesia and Vietnam. The origin and spread of the *Curcuma* genus initially took place in the Indo-Malayan region.

Around eight tuber bearing, one stolon bearing and 16 non-tuberous species occur in the Western Ghats regions and hence considered as number one hot spot for the genus on par with North eastern region in India. Thus, South Western Peninsular region of India being a center of diversity for the genus in Asia. Turmeric is the main cash crop in the tribal dominated districts of Kandhamal, Gajapati, Ganjam, Mayurbhanj and Koraput of Orissa. In Kerala, turmeric powder, paste and guruthi is still used as offerings to the goddess in the temples and shows how turmeric evolved firstly as an inseparable and important substance of magic, secondly as an integral part of Sakthi worship in Southern India and in other parts of India (Velayudhan et al., 2012). Various names of turmeric in different languages are given in Table 11.1.

The genus *Curcuma* consists of above 100 species (Table 11.2) distributed chiefly in South and Southeast Asia.

From India around 40 *Curcuma* species are reported (Table 11.3). In addition to *C. longa*, the genus includes other economically important species

TABLE 11.1   Various Names of Turmeric in Different Languages

Name in international language	Name in regional language
Spanish: Curcuma	English: Turmeric
French: Curcuma, Saffron des Indes	Hindi: Haldi
German: Kurkumagelbwruzel	Bengali: Holud
Swedish: Gurkmeja	Gujarathi: Haldi
Burmese: Fanwin	Kannada: Arishina
Arabic: Kurkum	Malayalam: Halad
Dutch: Geelwortel	Sindhi: Halda
Thai: Kamin	Punjabi: Haldhor, Haldhar
Indonesian: Kunjit, Kunyit	Tamil: Manjal
Italian: Curcuma	Telugu: Pasupu
Chinese: Yujin	Sanskrit: Haladi, Haridra, Harita

TABLE 11.2   Distribution of the *Curcuma* Species

Geographic Area	*Curcuma* Species (Approximate)
Bangladesh	16–20
China	20–25
India	40–45
Cambodia, Vietnam and Laos	20–25
Malaysia	20–30
Nepal	10–15
The Philippines	12–15
Thailand	30–40
Total	**100–110**

(Reprinted from 74. Ravindran, P. N, Nirmal Babu, K., & Shiva, K. N. (2007). Botany and crop improvement of turmeric. In: P. N. Ravindran, K. Nirmal Babu and K. Sivaraman (eds) Turmeric: The Genus Curcuma. CRC Press, Taylor & Francis Group. New York. Vol. 45; pp. 31. Used with permission of CRC Press/Taylor & Francis.)

TABLE 11.3 *Curcuma* Species Occurring in India and Their Distribution

Species	Distribution
C. longa	All over India
C. aeruginosa	West Bengal
C. amada	All over India
C. decipiens	Kerala, Karnataka
C. albiflora	Kerala
C. amarissima	West Bengal
C. aromatica	South India, Orissa, Bihar
C. caullina	Maharashtra
C. petiolata	West Bengal
C. caesia	West Bengal
C. angustifolia	Uttar Pradesh, Madhya Pradesh, Himachal Pradesh, North East
C. comosa	West Bengal
C. montana	South India
C. oligantha	Kerala
C. ferruginea	West Bengal
C. pseudomontana	South India
C. xanthorrhiza	West Bengal
C. neilgherrensis	South India
C. rubescens	West Bengal
C. reclinata	Madhya Pradesh
C. sylvatica	Kerala
C. zedoaria	All over India
C. inodora	Gujarat, Maharashtra, Karnataka
C. aurantiaca	South India
C. soloensis	West Bengal
C. harita	Kerala
C. sulcata	Maharashtra
C. brog	West Bengal
C. ecalcarata	Kerala
C. raktakanta	Kerala
C. thalakaveriensis	Karnataka
C. cannanorensis	Kerala

TABLE 11.3 (Continued)

Species	Distribution
C. kudagensis	Karnataka
C. malabarica	Kerala, Karnataka
C. vamana	Kerala
C. coriacea	Kerala
C. karnatakensis	Karnataka
C. nilamburensis	Kerala
C. mangga	Andaman
C. lutea	Kerala, Karnataka
C. leucorhiza	West Bengal

(Reprinted from 74. Ravindran, P. N, Nirmal Babu, K., & Shiva, K. N. (2007). Botany and crop improvement of turmeric. In: P. N. Ravindran, K. Nirmal Babu and K. Sivaraman (eds) Turmeric: The Genus Curcuma. CRC Press, Taylor & Francis Group. New York. Vol. 45; pp. 31. Used with permission of CRC Press/Taylor & Francis.)

such as *C. aromatica*, used in medicine and in toiletry articles; *C. kwangsiensis*, *C. ochrorhiza*, *C. pierreana*, *C. zedoaria*, *C. caesia*, etc., used in folk medicines of the Southeast Asian nations; *C. alismatifolia*, *C. roscoeana*, etc., having floricultural importance; *C. amada*, used as a vegetable in a variety of culinary preparations, pickles and salads; and *C. zedoaria*, *C. malabarica*, *C. pseudomontana*, *C. montana*, *C. decipiens*, *C. angustifolia*, *C. aeruginosa*, etc., used in the production of arrow root powder (Ravindran et al., 2006).

11.4 MICROSCOPICAL CHARACTERS OF TURMERIC RHIZOME

The transverse section of cured and uncured turmeric rhizome shows almost similar characters but differing only in the nature of starch. Independent starch grains are present in the uncured rhizome, whereas in the cured rhizome, gelatinized lumps of starch are present. Rhizome consists of an outer zone of cork, followed by a wide zone of cortex, and an endodermoid ring closely covering a discontinuous ring of vascular bundles. A large number of vascular bundles are scattered throughout the section. The parenchyma, cortex and the pith are full of starch grains, the yellow pigment being present at some places only. In the uncured rhizome, the cork is intact throughout, while in the cured rhizome, it is broken at several places. The rhizome cortex is demarcated into two zones. The outer cortex contains a few layers of irregular-shaped to rounded parenchyma with a few starch grains, while the inner cortex, which is large, has parenchyma full of starch grains. In the cured rhizome, these starch grains get gelatinized due to the boiling process and form a compact mass in each of the cells.

The vascular bundles present in the cortex have been called cortical vascular bundles, leaf trace bundles, or cortical meristeles. These bundles are closed types, consisting of phloem and xylem only. These vascular bundles measure 80 to 115 to 124 μm along their major axis. The vascular bundles found towards the outside are smaller, having three to seven xylem elements, while those present towards the inside are bigger, having up to 12 elements. Vascular bundles are arranged as a circle below the endodermoid ring. In unstained sections, a large number of cells having curcumin deposit are found throughout (Ravindran et al., 2007). Comparative rhizome anatomy of different species of *Curcuma* is depicted in Table 11.4.

11.5 PHYTOCHEMISTRY

Rhizomes of turmeric contain pigments that contribute the color, along with the essential and fixed oils, flavonoids, bitter principles, carbohydrates, protein, minerals and vitamins. Different composition of chemicals in turmeric rhizome is presented in Table 11.5.

Curcuminoids are the important compounds found in turmeric, in which curcumin (Curcumin I) is the active constituent and the other curcuminoids in turmeric include demethoxycurcumin (Curcumin II) and bisdemethoxycurcumin (Curcumin III). *Curcuma* species contains various types of plant secondary metabolites, including diphenylheptanoids, monoterpenes and sesquiterpenes, etc. But medicinally important compounds are curcuminoids and its structural analogs, which were found in *C. longa* species. Three major classes of compounds isolated from *Curcuma* species, are diphenylalkanoids, phenylpropene derivatives of cinnamic acid type and terpenoids (Table 11.6).

There are other few types of compounds such as flavonol compound (malvidin-3-rutinoside), acetophenone derivatives (phloracetophenone and myrciaphenone), simple aromatic compounds (3,7- dimethyl-5-indane carboxylic acid, eugenol, vanillic acid and syringic acid) which are also isolated from the different *Curcuma* species (Nakayama et al., 2000; Piyachaturawat et al., 2002).

TABLE 11.4 Comparative Rhizome Anatomy of Some of the *Curcuma* Species (Remashree et al., 2006)

Characters	*C. longa*	*C. aromatica*	*C. amada*	*C. zedoaria*
Rhizome nature	Highly branched finger up to 4th order	Less branched and fingers present	Highly branched and bulbous	Less branched bulbous rhizome
Rhizome color	Yellow	Creamy	Creamy-white	Orange yellow
Trichomes	Absent	Absent	Numerous, uniseriate	Rare, uniseriate
Epidermis	Single layered	Single layered	Single layered	Single layered
Periderm	2–4 layers	8–10 layers	6–8 layers	14–15 layers
Outer zone	Small outer zone contains primary vascular bundles, starch, oil cells and curcumin cells	Small outer zone contains lot of oil cells, few curcumin cells, and primary vascular bundles	Both zones are almost equal in size and contain primary vascular bundles. Starch and oil cells evenly distributed	Both zones are almost of equal size, contain primary vascular bundles, starch, oil cells and curcumin cells
Primary vascular bundles	70–80 vascular bundles evenly distributed	50–60 vascular bundles distributed in inner core of the outer zone	60–70 vascular bundles distributed in inner core of outer zone	90–120 bundles distributed evenly in the outer zone
Endodermoidal layer	Continuous	Discontinuous	Discontinuous	Continuous
Cambium	2 layered	2 layered	2 layered	2–3 layered
Inner zone	Large inner zone; secondary vascular bundles and starch deposition are higher, just below the endodermoidal layer than inner core	Large inner zone; secondary vascular bundles are more, just below the endodermoidal layer than inner core	Both zones are equal sized. Secondary vascular bundles and starch deposition are higher, just below the endodermoidal layer than inner core	Both zones are equal sized. Secondary vascular bundles and starch deposition are higher, just below the endodermoidal layer than inner core

TABLE 11.4 (Continued)

Characters	C. longa	C. aromatica	C. amada	C. zedoaria
Secondary vascular bundles	In groups below the endodermoidal layers and also scattered in the inner core	In groups below the endodermoidal layers and also scattered in the inner core	In groups below the endodermoidal layers and also scattered in the inner core	In groups below the endodermoidal layers and few in the inner core
Xylem tracheids and vessels	Helical and spiral thickening	Helical and spiral thickening	Helical and spiral thickening	Helical and spiral thickening
Fibers	Absent	Absent	Present (rare)	Absent
Phloem	Sieve tube, 1–2 companion cells and phloem parenchyma	Sieve tube, 1–2 companion cells and phloem parenchyma	Sieve tube, 1–2 companion cells and phloem parenchyma	Sieve tube, 1–2 companion cells and phloem parenchyma
Bundle sheath	Absent	Present in the lower side of the bundle	Present in the upper side of the bundle	Absent
Oil cell	Plenty but less than C.aromatica and C. zedoaria	Plenty and more than the other three species	Plenty, small sized compared to the other three	Plenty and large sized
Curcumin cells	Plenty	Few	Rare with smaller size compared to other three	Plenty with large size
Starch grains	Numerous in inner and outer core, triangular shaped. Number varies from 12 to 20/cell	Numerous in inner and outer core, spindle shaped, eccentric; 5–20/cell.	Numerous in inner and outer core, rod shaped; number varies from 8 to 16/cell	Numerous in inner and outer core, large and rod shaped. Number varies from 5 to 20/cell

(Reprinted from 74. Ravindran, P. N, Nirmal Babu, K., & Shiva, K. N. (2007). Botany and crop improvement of turmeric. In: P. N. Ravindran, K. Nirmal Babu and K. Sivaraman (eds) Turmeric: The Genus Curcuma. CRC Press, Taylor & Francis Group. New York. Vol. 45; pp. 31. Used with permission of CRC Press/Taylor & Francis.)

11.6   USES OF TURMERIC

Turmeric and its active constituent's curcuminoids have diverse applications, which can be used as a spice, food colorant and cosmetic and as a drug. Turmeric, which can be used traditionally, medicinally and in preparation of cosmetics.

TABLE 11.5   Different Chemical Composition of Turmeric

Moisture	6–13%
Carbohydrates	60–70%
Protein	6–8%
Fiber	2–7%
Mineral matter	3–7%
Fat	5–10%
Volatile oil	3–7%
Curcuminoids	2–6%

(Reprinted from Balakrishanan, K. V. (2007). Postharvest technology and processing of turmeric. In: P. N. Ravindran, K. Nirmal Babu, & K. Sivaraman (eds.) Turmeric: The Genus Curcuma. CRC Press, Taylor & Francis Group. New York. Vol. 45; pp. 198. Used with permission from CRC Press/Taylor & Francis.)

TABLE 11.6   Compounds Isolated from Various Species of the Genus *Curcuma*

Species	Isolated Compounds	References
C. longa	Curcumin, Demethoxycurcumin, Dihydrocurcumin, Bisdemethoxycurcumin, α-Atlantone, β-Atlantone, Bisacumol, Caffeic acid, Borneol, Camphene, Cinnamic acid, β-Caryophyllene, 1,8-Cineole, α-Curcumene, β-Curcumene, Eugenol, β-Farnesene, Germacrone-4,5-epoxide, Isoborneol, Limonene, Myrcene, α-Pinene, β-Pinene, Turmerone, Zingiberene, etc.	Park and Kim, 2002; Kiuchi et al., 1993; Nakayama et al., 1993; Sastry, 1970; Ravindranath and Satyanarayana, 1980; Roth et al., 1998; Singh et al., 2002; Su et al., 1982; Ohshiro et al., 1990
C. amada	Curcumin, Demethoxycurcumin, Bisdemethoxycurcumin, Calarene, 1,8-Cineole, β-Caryophyllene, Curzerenone, Limonene, Myrcene, α-pinene, β-pinene, Terpinen-4-ol, etc.	Gupta et al., 1999; Singh et al., 2002
C. aromatica	Curcumin, Demethoxycurcumin, Bisdemethoxycurcumin, Acetoxyneocurdione, β-Bisabolene, Bisacumol, Carvacrol, 1,8-Cineole, Curcumadione, Curcumol, *p*-Cymene, *p*-Cymene-8-ol, Germacrone, Linalool, Methylzedoarondiol, Zederone, Xanthorrhizol, Zedoarondiol, Zingiberene, etc.	Kojima et al., 1998; Kuroyanagi et al., 1987; Singh et al., 2002; Pant et al., 2001; Kuroyanagi et al., 1990; Shiobara et al., 1986

TABLE 11.6 (Continued)

Species	Isolated Compounds	References
C. xanthorrhiza	Curcumin, Demethoxycurcumin, Bisdemethoxycurcumin, β-Atlantone, 1,3,5,10-Bisabolapentaen-9-ol, Bisacurone (A, B and C), Curzerenone, Germacrone, Turmerone, Xanthorrhizol, Zingiberene, etc.	Yasni et al., 1993; Itokawa et al., 1985; Uehara et al., 1989, 1990; Ohshiro et al., 1990; Hwang et al., 2000
C. parviflora	Cadalenequinone, 8-Hydroxycadalene, Parviflorene (A, B, C, D, E and F)	Toume et al., 2004
C. zedoaria	Curcumin, Demethoxycurcumin, Bisdemethoxycurcumin, Dihydrocurcumin, Aerugidiol, Alismoxide, Bisacumol, Borneol, Calarene, Curcumadiol, 1,8-Cineole, Curcumalactone (A, B and C), Curcumanolide (A and B), Curdione, β-Dictyopetrol, Ethyl-*p*-methoxycinnamate, Furanodienone, Gajutsulactone (A and B), Nerol, Procurcumenol, Zederone, Zedoarondiol, Zedoarolide (A and B), etc.	Matsuda et al., 2001, 2004; Mau et al., 2003; Jang et al., 2004; Shiobara et al., 1985; Gupta et al., 1976; Pandji et al., 1993; Singh et al., 2002, 2003; Hikino et al., 1968
C. aeruginosa	Aerugidiol, Camphor, 1,8-Cineole, Curcumenol, Curdione, Curzerenone, β-Elemene, Isocurcumenol, Zedoalactone (A and B), Zedoarondiol	Masuda et al., 1991; Jirovetz et al., 2000; Bats et al., 1999; Takano et al., 1995
C. caesia	Borneol, Bornyl acetate, 1,8-Cineole, Camphor, α-Curcumene, γ-Curcumene, β-Elemene, α-Turmerone	Pandey and Chowdhury, 2003; Behura and Srivastava, 2004
C. comosa	(*E*)-5-Acetoxy-1,7-diphenyl-1-heptene, (*E*)-1,7-Diphenyl-1-hepten-5-one, Myrciaphenone A, Phloracetophenone, etc.	Suksamrarn et al., 1997; Jurgens et al., 1994; Claeson et al., 1993

11.6.1 TRADITIONAL USES

Traditionally since 600 B.C. onwards turmeric has been used as a spice, aromatic, stimulant, yellow dye, flavoring agent and medicine. In fact, turmeric has been a traditional remedy in Asian folk medicines for the last 2000 years. In Ayurveda and Chinese medicinal system it has been used as an anti-inflammatory agent. Internally it has been used to treat allergies, diarrhea, fevers, heart burn, stomach problems, chronic cough, wind, colic, bloating, flatulence, bronchial asthma, jaundice (other liver ailments) and externally it has been used for reducing inflammation, swelling due to sprains, cuts and bruises throughout Asia (Khanna, 1999). Traditionally it has been used as cosmetic to impart golden glow to the complexion. The fresh plant juice or a paste is used to treat leprosy and snakebites (Shah, 1997). Turmeric juice with a pinch of salt taken just before breakfast, is believed to be an effective remedy for expelling worms. A teaspoon of raw turmeric juice mixed with honey can be effective in the treatment of anemia. Turmeric with caraway seeds used for the treatment of cold in infants. Turmeric is effective in the treatment of measles and skin diseases. It is also used in traditional medicine as a household remedy for various diseases, including small pox, chicken pox, diabetic wounds, cough, biliary disorders, dyspepsia, rheumatism, conjunctivitis, anorexia, hepatic disorders, elephantiasis, diarrhea, gonorrhea and sinusitis (Chattopadhyay et al., 2004). The people of Ngada have used turmeric for wound healing property (Sachs et al., 2002).

Other uses of turmeric in traditional system are

- Before using gum resin of *Commiphora mukul* (Guggul) in Ayurvedic formulations, it should be purified by using turmeric.
- Turmeric powder coated over the surgical thread by mixing with the latex of *Snuhi* (*Euphorbia nerifolia*) plant. This thread is known as *Ksharasoothra*, which is tied on piles and fistula to cure them effectively.
- In veterinary medicine, turmeric is used to heal wounds or ulcers in animals.
- In "leech therapy," turmeric powder is sprinkled over the leech to detach it from the biting site.
- Turmeric powder is used as an insect and ant repellent and sprinkled around the vessels to be protected.
- Turmeric is included in the group of yellow substances (*Peethavarga*) in *Rasasastra* (Alchemy), used in the processing of Mercury (Shrishail et al., 2013).

11.6.2 SOCIO CULTURAL USES

Turmeric is an auspicious article in all religions of Hindu households and temples. The people in South and Southeast Asia, especially in Bangladesh, India and Indonesia, use turmeric to dye their bodies as part of their wedding rituals. In Bali, rice cooked with turmeric, coconut milk, Indonesian bay leaves, lemongrass and pandanus leaves is considered a "cultic dish" in Hindu culture and sacrificed to the gods (Remadevi and Ravindran, 2005).

11.6.3 MEDICINAL USES

Turmeric has been extensively used in medicine throughout Asia. In Ayurveda, turmeric is administered internally as a tonic, stomachic, blood purifier and topically in the prevention and treatment of skin diseases. The juice of fresh turmeric rhizome is used as an antiparasitic for many skin infections and turmeric with warm milk used in treatment of common cold. Powdered rhizome paste along with lime is used as a remedy for inflamed joints. Traditional healers of India and China used it as a remedy for varied conditions from eye infections to intestinal worms to leprosy. It is reported to be cholagogue, hemostatic, alterative, antiperiodic, depurative, aperient, detergent, astringent, carminative, cordial, diuretic, emmenagogue, maturant and stimulant. In folk medicine, turmeric is used in the treatment of diarrhea, dysmenorrhea, abdominal pain, epistasis, chest pains, flatulence, colic, fever, hematuria, hematemesis and in urinary problems; jaundice, hepatitis and other infections of the liver. It is applied externally for inflammation, itch, indolent ulcers, ringworm, sores, boils, bruises, elephantiasis, leucoderma, scabies, smallpox, snakebite, leech bite and swellings. Turmeric and its active components exhibit a broad spectrum of biological activities viz. antioxidant (Balasubramanyam et al., 2003), antibacterial, antifungal, antiparasitic, antimutagen, anti-inflammatory, hypolipidemic, hepatoprotective, lipoxygenase, cyclooxygenase and protease-inhibitory. Kuttan et al. (1987) reported that an ethanolic extract of turmeric or a curcumin ointment provided symptomatic relief in patients with cancers of oral cavity, breast and skin. Turmeric, curcumin and curcumin analogs are also used in the treatment of patients with HIV infection (Sui et al., 1993; Mazumder, 1997).

Hair tonics that retard hair loss and having antidandruff effects have been developed with curcuminoids as the active components. Herbal mixtures containing turmeric as one of the main ingredients are reported to provide therapeutic weight loss and lipid reduction (Ramirez-Tortosa et al., 1999; Wei and Xu, 2003). Turmeric oil is a powerful anti-inflammatory agent. Both leaf and rhizome oil possesses excellent antimicrobial/antibacterial activity (Iyengar et al., 1995; Singh et al., 2003) and fungicidal activity (Apisariyakul et al., 1995; Jayaprakasha et al., 2001). Turmeric oil given by vapor inhalation is found to have significant effect in removing sputum, relieving coughs and preventing asthma; it is effective for the treatment of respiratory diseases (Ram et al., 2003).

A number of patents have been granted for formulations containing curcumin for human health (Oei, 1992; Ammon et al., 1995; Aggarwal, 1999; Majeed et al., 1999; Santhanam et al., 2001; Graus and Smit, 2002; Saito, 2002; Newmark, 2002; Phan, 2003; Lee et al., 2004; Arbiser, 2004).

Extensive investigation over the last five decades has indicated that curcumin reduces blood cholesterol (Asai and Miyazawa, 2001) prevents LDL oxidation (Naidu and Thippeswamy, 2002), inhibits platelet aggregation (Srivastava et al., 1995), suppresses thrombosis (Srivastava et al., 1985) and myocardial infarction (Venkatesan, 1998), suppresses the symptoms associated with type II diabetes (Arun and Nalini, 2002), rheumatoid arthritis (Deodhar et al., 1980), multiple sclerosis (Natarajan and Bright, 2002), Alzheimer's disease (Lim et al., 2001), inhibits human immunodeficiency virus (HIV) replication (Barthelemy et al., 1998), enhances wound healing (Phan et al., 2001), protects from liver injury (Morikawa et al., 2002), increases bile secretion (Ramprasad and Sirsi, 1956), protects from cataract formation (Awasthi et al., 1996), protects from pulmonary toxicity and fibrosis (Punithavathi et al., 2003), is an antileishmaniasis (Saleheen et al., 2002) and an antiatherosclerotic (Chen and Huang, 1998).

11.6.4 FOOD APPLICATIONS

Turmeric is used in coloring butter, cheese and vanaspati (Kapur et al., 1960). It is also an essential ingredient in curry and curry powders, chutneys and pickles, where it imparts characteristic peppery taste and yellow color. Yellow rice, the sacred dish popular in the eastern islands of

Indonesia, derives its color from fresh or dried turmeric. It is used in fish curry, possibly to mask the fishy odor. Fresh turmeric leaves are used in some regions of Indonesia as flavoring purpose. In Thailand, the fresh rhizome is used as one of the ingredient for the popular yellow curry paste. Turmeric has found application in canned beverages, dairy products, yogurts, baked products, popcorn color, yellow cakes, sauces, biscuits, sweets, cereals, gelatins and in direct compression tablets, etc. Water soluble turmeric can be used to color the dairy foods. For the color shades, combination of turmeric with other natural colorants are used (Freund, 1985). Turmeric is sometimes added to oils as a preservative. In South India, it is added to about every dish, and it is an essential ingredient in all curry masala mixtures. Turmeric is common with baked or fried items especially in the case of deep fried banana chips.

11.6.5   COSMETIC USES

In preparation of cosmetics like lotions, shampoos and sprays, turmeric extract is used as an antibacterial and anti-inflammatory natural dye (Chauhan et al., 2003). To enhance the fairness and complexion of women in India turmeric paste was applied on the face and body. Balms containing turmeric powder or extract are effective in treating acne, rashes, eczema and pimples. Turmeric is said to discourage the growth of facial hair. Hair dye compositions containing turmeric extract are reported to impart golden color to light chestnut hair (Manier and Lutz, 1985).

11.6.6   MISCELLANEOUS USES

Turmeric extract can be used to color the outer coating of pharmaceutical tablets (Woznicki et al., 1984) and also in acrylic dental filling composition (Kemper, 1981). Turmeric produces a yellow dye for fabrics and is used for dyeing wool, silk and cotton. Turmeric is sometimes used in combination with other natural dyes like indigo and safflower to impart different shades (Agrawal et al., 1992). Curcumin can offer protection to photolabile drugs in soft gelatin capsules, thereby replacing synthetic dyes or pigments frequently used (Schranz, 1983).

Curcumin is employed for the purpose of detecting and warning the presence of cyanide in food, drug or oral compositions. Turmeric paper can be used to test the alkalinity and in detection of boric acid. In brown and yellow solutions diluted tincture of turmeric is used as a fluorescence indicator.

11.7 COMMERCIAL MEDICINAL PREPARATIONS CONTAINING TURMERIC

Medicinally turmeric is available in the form of creams, ointments, tinctures, capsules containing powder or extracts. In Malaysia turmeric containing ointment is used as an antiseptic and also in Indian antiseptic creams, an extract of turmeric is used as major ingredient. Ophthacare®, a commercially available eye preparation in India, contains *Carum copticum, Terminalia bellirica, Emblica officinalis, Curcuma longa, Ocimum sanctum, Cinnamomum camphora* and *Rosa damascena* (Biswas et al., 2001). "RA-11 (ARTREX, MENDAR)," a standardized multi plant herbal drug, composed of *Withania somnifera, Boswellia serrata, Zingiber officinale* and *Curcuma longa* extracts and is used in the treatment of arthritis. "Smoke Shield," a formulation composed of the extracts of *Curcuma longa* and green tea, has long been in the market to reduce smoke-related mutagenicity and toxicity in the population. "Hyponidd" is a herbomineral formulation composed of the extracts of *Momordica charantia, Melia azadirachta, Pterocarpus marsupium, Tinospora cordifolia, Gymnema sylvestre, Enicostemma littorale, Emblica officinalis, Eugenia jambolana, Cassia auriculata* and *Curcuma longa*. Some of the commercially available medicinal preparations of turmeric or curcumin are presented in Table 11.7.

11.8 TOXICITY

Turmeric and its active ingredients curcuminoids are considered as safe when taken at the recommended doses. Excessive use of pure curcumin may produce stomach upset and in extreme cases produces ulcers (Ammon and Wahl, 1991). Safety evaluation studies have indicated that

TABLE 11.7 Commercially Available Medicinal Preparations of Turmeric or Curcumin

Products	Supplier/Source
Best Curcumin/Bioperine Capsules, 500 mg	Doctor's Best
Full Spectrum Turmeric Extract Tablets, 450 mg	Planetary Formulas
Curcumin 95 Capsules, 500 mg	Jarrow Formulas
Turmeric Capsules, 250 mg	Paradise Herbs
Ultra Joint Response Tablets, 450 mg	Source Naturals
Turmeric (Standardized 95% Curcuminoids) Tablets, 450 mg	Nature's Way
Turmeric (Curcumin) Extract Tablets, 400 mg	Source Naturals
Curcumin Capsules, 665 mg	Now Foods
Turmeric and Bromelain Capsules, 450 mg	Natural Factors
Turmeric Catechu Extract, 60 ml	Gaia Herbs
Turmeric Extract, 30 ml	Nature's Apothecary
Turmeric Extract Capsules, 500 mg	Turmeric-Curcumin.com

both turmeric and curcumin are well tolerated at a very high dose without any toxic effects (Chattopadhyay et al., 2004). Human clinical trials with curcumin indicated that there was no dose limiting toxicity when administered at doses up to 10 g/d (Aggarwal et al., 2003).

On the basis of the pharmacological and toxicological studies on possible interactions of turmeric or curcumin with other herbs or medicines carried out to date, it can be advised that turmeric or curcumin in medicinal forms should not be used in the following circumstances without prior consultation with a qualified medical practitioner:

- People who are on blood thinning medications, e.g., warfarin, aspirin, etc.
- People using non-steroidal anti-inflammatory drugs, e.g., indomethacin, ibuprofen, etc.
- People who are using hypotensive drug, i.e., reserpine.
- People who are using antidiabetic drugs, e.g., glimepiride and pioglitazone.

In conclusion, the turmeric is an important medicinal plant with a biological diversity of activities.

KEYWORDS

- ethnobotany
- medicinal uses
- phytochemistry
- turmeric

REFERENCES

1. Aggarwal, B. B. (1999). Curcumin (diferuloylmethane) inhibition of NFκB activation. *United States Patent* 5,891,924, April 6, 1999.
2. Aggarwal, B. B., Kumar, A., & Bharti, A. C. (2003). Anticancer potential of curcumin: preclinical and clinical studies. *Anticancer Res 23*, 363–398.
3. Agrawal, A, Goel, A., & Gupta, K. C. (1992). Optimization of dyeing process for wool with natural dye obtained from turmeric (*Curcuma longa*). *Text Dyer Printer 25*, 28–30.
4. Ammon, H. P. T., Safayhi, H., & Okpanyi, S. N. (1995). Use of preparations of curcuma plants. *United States Patent* 5,401,777, March 28, 1995.
5. Ammon, H. P. T., & Wahl, M. A. (1991). Pharmacology of *Curcuma longa*. *Planta Med. 57*, 1–7.
6. Apisariyakul, A., Vanittanakom, N., & Buddhasukh, D. (1995). Antifungal activity of turmeric oil extracted from *Curcuma longa* (Zingiberaceae). *J Ethnopharmacol 49*, 163–169.
7. Arbiser, J. L. (2004). Curcumin and curcuminoid inhibition of angiogenesis. *United States Patent* 6,673,843, January 6, 2004.
8. Arun, N., & Nalini, N. (2002). Efficacy of turmeric on blood sugar and polyol pathway in diabetic albino rats. *Plant Foods Hum. Nutr. 57*, 41–52.
9. Asai, A., & Miyazawa, T. (2001). Dietary curcuminoids prevent high fat diet induced lipid accumulation in rat liver and epididymal adipose tissue. *J. Nutrition 131*, 2932–2935.
10. Awasthi, S., Srivatava, S. K., Piper, J. T., Singhal, S. S., Chaubey, M., & Awasthi, Y. C. (1996). Curcumin protects against 4-hydroxy-2-trans-nonenal-induced cataract formation in rat lenses. *Am. J. Clin. Nutr. 64*, 761–766.
11. Balakrishanan, K. V. (2007). Postharvest technology and processing of turmeric. In: P. N. Ravindran, K. Nirmal Babu, & K. Sivaraman (eds.) *Turmeric: The Genus Curcuma*. CRC Press, Taylor & Francis Group. New York. Vol. 45; pp. 198.
12. Balasubramanyam, M., Koteswari, A. A., Kumar, R. S., Monickaraj, S. F., Maheswari, J. U., & Mohan, V. (2003). Curcumin-induced inhibition of cellular reactive oxygen species generation: Novel therapeutic implications. *J. Biosci. 28*, 715–721.

13. Barthelemy, S., Vergnes, L., Moynier, M., Guyot, D., Labidalle, S., & Bahraoui, E. (1998). Curcumin and curcumin derivatives inhibit Tat-mediated transactivation of type 1 human immunodeficiency virus long terminal repeat. *Res. Virol. 149*, 43–52.

14. Bats, J. W., & Ohlinger, S. H. (1999). Absolute configuration of isocurcumenol. *Acta Crystallographica Section C-Crystal Structure Communications 55*, 1595–1598.

15. Behura, S., & Srivastava, V. K. (2004). Essential oils of leaves of *Curcuma* species. *J. Essential Oil Res. 16*, 109–110.

16. Biswas, N. R., Gupta, S. K., Das, G. K., Kumar, N., Mongre, P. K., Haldar, D., & Beri, S. (2001). Evaluation of ophthacare (R) eye drops – A herbal formulation in the management of various ophthalmic disorders. *Phytotherapy Res. 15*, 618–620.

17. Chattopadhyay, I., Biswas, K., Bandyopadhyay, U., & Banerjee, R. K. (2004). Turmeric and Curcumin: biological actions and medicinal applications. *Curr. Sci. 87*, 44–53.

18. Chauhan, U. K., Soni, P., Shrivastava, R., Mathur, K. C., & Khadikar, P. V. (2003). Antimicrobial activities of the rhizome of *Curcuma longa* Linn. *Oxid. Commun. 26*, 266–270.

19. Chen, H. W., & Huang, H. C. (1998). Effect of curcumin on cell cycle progression and apoptosis in vascular smooth muscle cells. *Br. J. Pharmacol. 124*, 1029–1040.

20. Claeson, P., Panthong, A., Tuchinda, P., Reutrakul, V., Kanjanapothi, D., Taylor, W. C., & Santisuk, T. (1993). 3-Nonphenolic diarylheptanoids with antiinflammatory activity from *Curcuma xanthorrhiza*. *Planta Med. 59*, 451–454.

21. Deodhar, S. D., Sethi, R., & Srimal, R. C. (1980). Preliminary study on antirheumatic activity of curcumin (diferuloyl methane). *Indian J. Med. Res. 71*, 632–634.

22. Freund, P. R. (1985). Natural colors in cereal-based products. *Cereal Foods World 30*, 271–273.

23. Graus, I. M. F., & Smit, H. F. (2002). Composition for the treatment of osteoarthritis. *United States Patent* 6,492,429, December 10, 2002.

24. Gupta, A. P., Gupta, M. M., & Kumar, S. (1999). Simultaneous determination of curcuminoids in *Curcuma* samples using high performance thin layer chromatography. *J. Liq. Chromatog. Related Technol. 22*, 1561–1569.

25. Gupta, S. K., Banerjee, A. B., & Achari, B. (1976). Isolation of Ethyl *p*-methoxycinnamate, the major antifungal principle of *Curcumba zedoaria*. *Lloydia 39*, 218–222.

26. Hikino, H., Takahashi, S., Sakurai, Y., Takemoto, T., & Bhacc, N. S. (1968). Structure of zederone. *Chem. Pharm. Bull. 16*, 1081–1087.

27. Hwang, J. K., Shim, J. S., Baek, N. I., & Pyun, Y. R. (2000). Xanthorrhizol: A potential antibacterial agent from *Curcuma xanthorrhiza* against *Streptococcus mutans*. *Planta Med. 66*, 196–197.

28. Itokawa, H., Hirayama, F., Funakoshi, K., & Takeya, K. (1985). Studies on the antitumor bisabolane sesquiterpenoids isolated from *Curcuma xanthorrhiza*. *Chem. Pharm. Bull. 33*, 3488–3492.

29. Iyengar, M. A., Rama Rao, P. M., Bairy, I., & Kamat, M. S. (1995). Antimicrobial activity of the essential oil of *Curcuma longa* leaves. *Indian Drugs 32*, 249–250.

30. Jang, M. K., Lee, H. J., Kim, J. S., & Ryu, J. H. (2004). A curcuminoid and two sesquiterpenoids from *Curcuma zedoaria* as inhibitors of nitric oxide synthesis in activated macrophages. *Arch. Pharm. Res. 27*, 1220–1225.

31. Jayaprakasha, G. K., Negi, P. S., Anandharamakrishnan, C., & Sakariah, K. K. (2001). Chemical composition of turmeric oil – a byproduct from turmeric oleoresin industry and its inhibitory activity against different fungi. *J. Biosci. 56*, 40–44.

32. Jirovetz, L., Buchbauer, G., Puschmann, C., Shafi, M. P., & Nambiar, M. K. G. (2000). Essential oil analysis of *Curcuma aeruginosa* Roxb. leaves from South India. *J. Essential Oil Res. 12*, 47–49.

33. Jurgens, T. M., Frazier, E. G., Schaeffer, J. M., Jones, T. E., Zink, D. L., Borris, R. P., Nanakorn, W., Beck, H. T., & Balick, M. J. (1994). Novel nematocidal agents from *Curcuma comosa*. *J. Nat. Prod. 57*, 230–235.

34. Kapur, O. P., Srinivasan, M., & Subrahmanyan, V. (1960). Colouring of Vanaspati with Curcumin from turmeric. *Curr. Sci. 29*, 350–351.

35. Kemper, R. N. (1981). Dental filling compositions. *German Patent* 3, 038, 383, 23 Apr 1981. US Appl. 83,896,11 Oct., 1979, 12 pp. (CA Vol 95/1981, 68069w).

36. Khanna, N. M. (1999). Turmeric: Nature's Precious gift. *Curr. Sci. 76*, 1351–1356.

37. Kiuchi, F., Goto, Y., Sugimoto, N., Akao, N., Kondo, K., & Tsuda, Y. (1993). Nematocidal activity of turmeric: synergistic action of curcuminoids. *Chem. Pharm. Bull. 41*, 1640–1641.

38. Kojima, H., Yanai, T., & Toyota, A. (1998). Essential oil constituents from Japanese and Indian *Curcuma aromatica* rhizomes. *Planta Med. 64*, 380–381.

39. Kurian, A., Nybe, E. V., Valsala, P. A., & Sankar, A. (2004). Curcumin rich turmeric varieties from Kerala Agricultural University. *Spice India 14*, 38–39.

40. Kuroyanagi, M., Ueno, A., Ujiie, K., & Sato, S. (1987). Structures of sesquiterpenes from *Curcuma aromatica* Salisb. *Chem. Pharm. Bull. 35*, 53–59.

41. Kuroyanagi, M., Ueno, A., Koyama, K., & Natori, S. (1990). Structures of sesquiterpenes of *Curcuma aromatica* Salisb.2. studies on minor sesquiterpenes. *Chem. Pharm. Bull. 38*, 55–58.

42. Kuttan, R., Sudheeran, P. C., & Joseph, C. D. (1987). Turmeric and curcumin as topical agents in cancer therapy. *Tumori 73*, 29–31.

43. Lee, K. H., Ishida, J., Ohtsu, H., Wang, H. K., Itokawa, H., Chang, C., & Shih, C. C. Y. (2004). Curcumin analogs and uses thereof. *United States Patent* 6,790,979 September 14, 2004.

44. Lim, G. P., Chu, T., Yang, F., Beech, W., Frautschy, S. A, & Cole, G. M. (2001). The curry spice curcumin reduces oxidative damage and amyloid pathology in an Alzheimer transgenic mouse. *J. Neurosci. 21*, 8370–8377.

45. Majeed, M., Badmaev, V., & Rajendran, R. (1999). Bioprotectant composition, method of use and extraction process of curciminoids. *United States Patent* 5,861,415, January 19, 1999.

46. Manier, F., & Lutz, D. (1985). Hair dye compositions containing plant extracts. *Belg.* BE 900, 219, 25 Jan, 1985. Fr. Appl. 83/12,458,28 Jul 1983. (CA Vol. Vol.102/1985, 137585p).

47. Masuda, T., Jitoe, A., & Nakatani, N. (1991). Structure of aerugidiol, a new bridge head oxygenated guaiane sesquiterpene. *Chem. Letts. 9*, 1625–1628.

48. Matsuda, H., Morikawa, T., Ninomiya, K., & Yoshikawa, M. (2001). Absolute stereostructure of carabrane-type sesquiterpenes and vasorelaxant-active sesquiterpenes from Zedoariae Rhizoma *Tetrahedron 57*, 8443–8453.

49. Matsuda, H., Tewtrakul, S., Morikawa, T., Nakamura, A., & Yoshikawa, M. (2004). Anti-allergic principles from Thai zedoary: structural requirements of curcuminoids for inhibition of degranulation and effect on the release of TNF-a and IL-4 in RBL-2H3 cells. *Bioorg. Med. Chem. 12*, 5891–5898.

50. Mau, J. L., Lai, E. Y. C., Wang, N. P., Chen, C. C., Chang, C. H., & Chyau, C. C. (2003). Composition and antioxidant activity of the essential oil from *Curcuma zedoaria*. *Food Chem. 82*, 583–591.

51. Mazumder, A., Neamati, N., Sunder, S., Schulz, J., Pertz, H., Eich, E., & Pommier, Y. (1997). Curcumin analogs with altered potencies against HIV-1 integrase as probes for biochemical mechanisms of drug action. *J. Med. Chem. 40*, 3057–3063.

52. Morikawa, T., Matsuda, H., Ninomiya, K., & Yoshikawa, M. (2002). Medicinal food-stuffs. XXIX. Potent protective effects of sesquiterpenes and curcumin from Zedo-ariae Rhizoma on liver injury induced by D-galactosamine/lipopolysaccharide or tumor necrosis factor-alpha. *Biol. Pharm. Bull. 25*, 627–631.

53. Naidu, K. A, & Thippeswamy, N. B. (2002). Inhibition of human low density lipo-protein oxidation by active principles from spices. *Mol. Cell Biochem. 229*, 19–23.

54. Nakayama, M., Roh, M. S., Uchida, K., Yamaguchi, Y., Takano, K., & Koshioka, M. (2000). Malvidin 3-rutinoside as the pigment responsible for bract color in *Curcuma alismatifolia*. *Biosci. Biotech. Biochem. 64*, 1093–1095.

55. Nakayama, R., Tamura, Y., Yamanaka, H., Kikuzaki, H., & Nakatani, N. (1993). 2-Curcuminoid pigments from *Curcuma domestica*. *Phytochem. 33*, 501–502.

56. Natarajan, C., & Bright, J. J. (2002). Curcumin inhibits experimental allergic encephalomyelitis by blocking IL-12 signaling through Janus kinase-STAT pathway in T lymphocytes. *J. Immunol. 168*, 6506–6513.

57. Newmark, T., & Schulick, P. (2002). Anti-Inflammatory herbal composition and method of use. *United States Patent 6, 387, 416*, May 14, 2002.

58. Oei, B. L. (1992). Combinations of compounds isolated from *Curcuma* spp as anti-inflammatory agents. *United States Patent 5, 120, 538* June 9, 1992.

59. Ohshiro, M., Kuroyanagi, M., & Ueno, A. (1990). Structures of sesquiterpenes from *Curcuma longa*. *Phytochem. 29*, 2201–2205.

60. Pandey, A. K., & Chowdhury, A. R. (2003). Volatile constituents of the rhizome oil of *Curcuma caesia* Roxb. from central India. *Flavour and Fragrance Journal 18*, 463–465.

61. Pandji, C., Grimm, C., Wray, V., Witte, L., & Proksc, P. (1993). Insecticidal constituents from 4 species of the Zingiberaceae. *Phytochem. 34*, 415–419.

62. Pant, N., Jain, D. C., Bhakuni, R. S., Prajapati, V., Tripathi, A. K., & Kumar, S. (2001). Zederone: A sesquiterpenic keto-dioxide from *Curcuma aromatica*. *Indian J. Chem. Sec. B- Org. Chem. Including. Med. Chem. 40*, 87–88.

63. Park, S. Y., & Kim, D. S. H. L. (2002). Discovery of natural products from *Curcuma longa* that protect cells from beta-amyloid insult: A drug discovery effort against Alzheimer's disease. *J. Nat. Prod. 65*, 1227–1231.

64. Patel, K., & Srinivasan, K. (2004). Digestive stimulant action of spices: A myth or reality? *Indian J. Med. Res. 119*, 167–179.

65. Peter, K. V. (1997). Fifty years of research on major spices in India. *Indian Spices 34*, 20–36.

66. Phan, D. (2003). Compositions and methods of treatment for skin conditions using extracts of turmeric. *United States Patent 6,521,271*, February 18, 2003.

67. Phan, T. T., See, P., Lee, S. T., & Chan, S. Y. (2001). Protective effects of curcumin against oxidative damage on skin cells *in vitro*: its implication for wound healing. *J. Trauma 51*, 927–931.

68. Piyachaturawat, P., Srivoraphan, P., Chuncharunee, A., Komaratat, P., & Suksam-ram, A. (2002). Cholesterol lowering effects of a choleretic phloracetophenone in hypercholesterolemic hamsters. *Eur. J. Pharmacol.* 439, 141–147.

69. Punithavathi, D., Venkatesan, N., & Babu, M. (2003). Protective effects of curcumin against amiodarone-induced pulmonary fibrosis in rats. *Br. J. Pharmacol. 139*, 1342–1350.

70. Ram, A., Das, M., & Ghosh, B. (2003). Curcumin attenuates allergen induced airway hyperresponsiveness in sensitized guinea pigs. *Biol. Pharm. Bull. 26*, 1021–1024.

71. Ramirez-Tortosa, M. C., Mesa, M. D., & Aguilera, M. C. (1999). Oral administration of a turmeric extract inhibits LDL oxidation and has hypocholesterolemic effects in rabbits with experimental atherosclerosis. *Atherosclerosis 147*, 371–378.

72. Ramprasad, C., & Sirsi, M. (1956). Studies on Indian medicinal plants: *Curcuma longa* Linn.-effect of curcumin & the essential oils of *C. longa* on bile secretion. *J. Sci. Industr. Res. 15*, 262–265.

73. Ravindran, P. N., Nirmal Babu, K., & Shiva, K. N. (2006). Genetic resources of spices and their conservation. In: P. N. Ravindran, K. Nirmal Babu, K. N. Shiva & A. K. Johny (eds) *Advances in Spices Research*, Agrobios, Jodhpur. pp. 63–91.

74. Ravindran, P. N, Nirmal Babu, K., & Shiva, K. N. (2007). Botany and crop improvement of turmeric. In: P. N. Ravindran, K. Nirmal Babu and K. Sivara-man (eds) *Turmeric: The Genus Curcuma.* CRC Press, Taylor & Francis Group. New York. Vol. 45; pp. 31.

75. Ravindranath, V., & Satyanarayana, M. N. (1980). An unsymmetrical diarylhep-tanoid from *Curcuma longa. Phytochem 19*, 2031–2032.

76. Remadevi, R., & Ravindran, P. N. (2005). Turmeric: Myths and Traditions *Spice India 18*, 11–17.

77. Remashree, A. B., Ravindran, P. N., & Balachandran, I. (2006). Anatomical and histochemical studies on four species of *Curcuma. Phytomorphology 56*, 1–8.

78. Roth, G. N., Chandra, A., & Nair, M. G. (1998). Novel bioactivities of *Curcuma longa* constituents. *J. Nat. Prod. 61*, 542–545.

79. Sachs, M., Eichel, J., & Asskali, F. (2002). Wound treatment with coconut oil in Indonesian natives. *Der Chirurg 73*, 387–392.

80. Saito, K. (2002). Anti-oxidant reducing substance and method of producing the same. *United States Patent* 6,372,265 April 16, 2002.

81. Saleheen, D., Ali, S. A., Ashfaq, K., Siddiqui, A. A., Agha, A., & Yasinzai, M. M. (2002). Latent activity of curcumin against leishmaniasis *in vitro. Biol. Pharm. Bull. 25*, 386–389.

82. Santhanam, U., Weinkauf, R. L., & Palanker, L. R. (2001). Turmeric as an anti-irritant in compositions containing hydroxy acids or retinoids. *United States Patent* 6,277,881 August 21, 2001.

83. Sasikumar, B. (2005). Genetic resources of *Curcuma:* Diversity characterization and utilization. *Plant Genet Res. 3*, 230–251.

84. Sastry, B. S. (1970). Curcumin content of turmeric. *Res. Ind. 15*, 258–260.

85. Schranz, J. L. (1983). Water-soluble curcumin complex. *United States Patent* 4,368,208 January 11, 1983.

86. Shah, N. C. (1997). Traditional uses of turmeric (*Curcuma longa*) in India. *J. Med. Aromatic Plants 19*, 948–954.

87. Shiobara, Y., Asakawa, Y., Kodama, M., & Takemoto, T. (1986). Zedoarol, 13 hydroxygermacrone and curzeone, 3 sesquiterpenoids from *Curcuma zedoaria*. *Phytochem. 25*, 1351–1353.

88. Shiobara, Y., Asakawa, Y., Kodama, M., Yasuda, K., & Takemoto, T. (1985). Curcumenone, curcumanolide-A and curcumanolide – B, 3 sesquiterpenoids from *Curcuma zedoaria*. *Phytochem. 24*, 2629–2633.

89. Shiva, K. N., Suryanarayana, M. A., & Medhi, R. P. (2003). Genetic resources of spices and their conservation in Bay Islands. *Indian J. Plant Genet. Resour. 16*, 91–95.

90. Shrishail, D., Harish K. H., Ravichandra, H., Tulsianand G., & S. D. Shruthi. (2013) Turmeric: Nature's Precious Medicine. *Asian J. Pharm. Clin. Res. 6*, 10–16.

91. Singh, G., Kapoor, I. P. S., Pandey, S. K., & Singh, O. P. (2003). *Curcuma longa* Linn. – Chemical, antifungal and antibacterial investigation on rhizome oil. *Indian Perfum. 47*, 173–178.

92. Singh, G., Singh, O. P., & Maurya, S. (2002). Chemical and biocidal investigations on essential oils of some Indian *Curcuma* species. *Progress in Crystal Growth and Characterization of Materials 45*, 75–81.

93. Singh, G., Singh, O. P., Prasad, Y. R., Lampasona, M. P., & Catalan, C. (2003). Chemical and biocidal investigations on rhizome volatile oil of *Curcuma zedoaria* Rosc – Part 32. *Indian J. Chem. Technol. 10*, 462–465.

94. Srivastava, K. C., Bordia, A., & Verma, S. K. (1995). Curcumin, a major component of food spice turmeric (*Curcuma longa*) inhibits aggregation and alters eicosanoid metabolism in human blood platelets. *Prostaglandins Leukot Essent. Fatty Acids 52*, 223–227.

95. Srivastava, R., Dikshit, M., Srimal, R. C., & Dhawan, B. N. (1985). Anti-thrombotic effect of curcumin. *Thromb. Res. 40*, 413–417.

96. Su, H. C. F., Horvat, R., & Jilani, G. (1982). Isolation, purification, and characterization of insect repellents from *Curcuma longa* L. *J. Agric. Food. Chem. 30*, 290–292.

97. Sui, Z., Salto, R., Li, J., Craik, C., & Ortiz de Montellano, P. R. (1993). Inhibition of the HIV-1 and HIV-2 proteases by curcumin and curcumin boron complexes. *Bioorg. Med. Chem. 1*, 415–422.

98. Suksamrarn, A., Eiamong, S., Piyachaturawat, P., & Byrne, L. T. (1997). A phloracetophenone glucoside with choleretic activity from *Curcuma comosa*. *Phytochem. 45*, 103–105.

99. Takano, I., Yasuda, I., Takeya, K., & Itokawa, H. (1995). Guaiane sesquiterpene lactones from *Curcuma aeruginosa*. *Phytochem. 40*, 1197–1200.

100. Toume, K., Takahashi, M., Yamaguchi, K., Koyano, T., Kowithayakorn, T., Hayashi. M., Komiyama, K., & Ishibashi, M. (2004). Parviflorenes B – F, novel cytotoxic unsymmetrical sesquiterpene-dimers with three backbone skeletons from *Curcuma parviflora*. *Tetrahedron 60*, 10817–10824.

101. Uehara, S., Yasuda, I., Takeya, K., & Itokawa, H. (1989). New bisabolane sesquiterpenoids from the rhizomes of *Curcuma xanthorrhiza* (zingiberaceae). *Chem. Pharm. Bull. 37*, 237–240.

102. Uehara, S., Yasuda, I., Takeya, K., Itokawa, H., & Iitaka, Y. (1990). New bisabolane sesquiterpenoids from the rhizomes of *Curcuma xanthorrhiza* (Zingiberaceae). *Chem. Pharm. Bull. 38*, 261–263.

103. Velayudhan, K. C., Dikshit, N., & Abdul Nizar, M. (2012). Ethnobotany of turmeric (*Curcuma longa* L.). *Indian J Trad. Knowl. 11*, 607–614.

104. Venkatesan, N. (1998). Curcumin attenuation of acute adriamycin myocardial toxicity in rats. *Br. J. Pharmacol. 124*, 425–427.

105. Wei, K., & Xu, X. (2003). Herbal composition and method for controlling body weight and composition. *United States Patent* 6,541,046. April 1, 2003.

106. Woznicki, E. J., Rosani, L. J., & Marshall, K. (1984). Colored medicinal tablet, natural color pigment and method for using the pigment in coloring food, drug and cosmetic products. *United States Patent*, 4,475,919 October 9, 1984.

107. Yasni, S., Imaizumi, K., Sin, K., Sugano, M., Nonaka, G., & Sidik, S. (1993). Identification of an active principle in essential oils and hexane-soluble fractions of *Curcuma xanthorrhiza* Roxb. Showing triglyceride lowering action in rats. *Food Chem Toxicol 32*, 273–278.

CHAPTER 12

TRADITIONAL USE OF HERBAL PLANTS FOR THE TREATMENT OF DIABETES IN INDIA

G. REVATHI,[1] S. ELAVARASI,[2] K. SARAVANAN,[1]
and BIR BAHADUR[3]

[1]P.G. & Research Department of Zoology, Nehru Memorial College (Autonomous), Puthanampatti–621007, Tiruchirappalli, Tamilnadu, India, E-mail: kaliyaperumalsaravanan72@gmail.com

[2]P.G. & Research Department of Zoology, Holy Cross College (Autonomous), Tiruchirappalli, Tamilnadu, India

[3]Department of Botany, Kakatiya University, Warangal–506009, Telangana, India

CONTENTS

Abstract 318
12.1 Introduction 318
12.2 Medicinal Plants 320
12.3 Mangroves as Antidiabetic Plants 344
12.4 Conclusions 344
Acknowledgements 345
Keywords 345
References 345

ABSTRACT

Plants have been used by human beings since time immemorial. Plants are significant and perennial sources of food and medicines that are used for the treatment of various human diseases. Traditional drugs derived from herbal plants are used by about 60% of the world's population, especially in Asia and Africa. The present review focuses on herbal drugs and anti-diabetic plants as traditional practice of Indian people in the treatment of diabetes mellitus. Diabetes mellitus is a major health problem especially in the rural and urban population not only of India but throughout the world. There are several remedies for the treatment of diabetes and its associated secondary complications. Herbal drug formulations are correctly preferred due to low toxicity and no side effects. A list of medicinal plants with proven antidiabetic activity and related beneficial effects has been compiled in this review with their botanical names, common name, family, plant/parts used for the diabetic treatment. We hope that this review would initiate an action plan that would lead to the discovery/development of indigenous antidiabetic plant drugs.

12.1   INTRODUCTION

Plants are the basis of life on earth, central to people's livelihoods, important sources of therapeutic drugs and play a significant role in the survival of human including the tribal/ethnic communities and animals. A number of medicinal plants have been used as important source of traditional medicine for thousands of years. In fact, many of the current drugs either mimic naturally occurring molecules or share structures that are fully or in part derived from natural motifs (Baby and Raj, 2010). The World Health Organization (WHO) has listed 21,000 plants, which are used for medicinal purposes around the world. Among these, 2500 species that occur in India, several hundred species are used commercially on a fairly large scale by Ayurveda, Unani and Siddha systems of medicine. India is rich in cultural and floristic diversity and cradle of ancient ethnobotanical knowledge. The present review focuses on medicinal plants and various herbal drugs commonly used in the treatment of diabetes mellitus called as Sweet urine disease. With growing demands of natural products with antidiabetic activity, investigations on hypoglycemic agents derived from medicinal plants have gained popularity during the last few decades (Pullaiah and Naidu, 2003; Elavarasi et al., 2013). Diabetes mellitus (DM) is the most common metabolic, multifactorial genetic disorder due to a defect in insulin secretion, insulin action gene, or both. Insulin deficiency in turn leads to chronic hyperglycemia with disturbances of carbohydrate, fat and protein metabolism (Lindberg et al., 2004). Diabetes leads to several wide range of heterogeneous complications such as retinopathy (Hove et al., 2004), neuropathy (Moran et al., 2004), nephropathy (Shukla et al., 2003), cardiovascular complications (Saely, 2004) and ulceration (Wallace, 2002). According to World Health Organization (WHO) over 346 million people worldwide suffer with DM which is likely to double by 2030 without any intervention.

Sulphonylureas and few biguanides are valuable treatment for Non Insulin Dependent Diabetes Mellitus (NIDDM), but they are unable to lower blood glucose level within normal range and reinstate a normal pattern of glucose homeostasis permanently and accompanied side effects. Uses of these therapies are restricted by their pharmacokinetic properties, secondary failure rates and accompanying side effects (Bailey et al., 1989). Even insulin therapy does not reinstate a permanent normal pattern of glucose homeostasis and carries an increased risk of atherogenesis and hypoglycemia (Shukla et al., 2000). Based on the recent advances and involvement of oxidative stress in complicating diabetes mellitus, efforts are on to find suitable antidiabetic and antioxidant therapies. Medicinal plants are being tapped as sure cure for the treatment of diabetes. History reveals that medicinal plants have been used in traditional healing around the world over for a long time to treat diabetes; this is because such herbal plants have hypoglycemic properties and other beneficial properties, as reported in the literature (Donga et al., 2011; Elavarasi et al., 2013). Number of review on antidiabetic/hyperglycemic plants have been written in the past (Kaczmar, 1998; Jung et al., 2006; Bhushan et al., 2010; Rao et al., 2010; Manikandan et al., 2011; Elavarasi et al., 2013; Gireesha and Raju, 2013; Sucharitha and Mamidala, 2013). According to Marles and Farnsworth (1994, 1995) more than 1200 species of plants are reported to have been used to treat diabetes and/or investigated for antidiabetic activity, Ayurveda and other systems of medicines have described over 800 traditional plant treatments for diabetes in the Indian sub-continent alone, although only a small number of these have received scientific/medical evaluation for their efficacy. The World Health Organization Expert Committee on diabetes has recommended that the traditional medicinal herbs be intensively investigated. Thus, this review is a timely reminder to identify such plants traditionally used effectively for the treatment of diabetes and for carrying out further studies.

The review deals with the various tribes and other ethnic people of India who have been using several dozen plant species belonging to many families for the treatment of diabetes. A study by Devi et al. (2011) revealed that 73 plant species were used by local practitioners in Manipur for the treatment of diabetes. Devi (2011) recorded 51 plant species used by Meitei community of Manipur for the treatment of Diabetes.

12.2 MEDICINAL PLANTS

The medicinal plants used by the herbalists, tribals and various ethnic people of India for the treatment of diabetes mellitus and their scientific validation are given below.

Abroma angusta (L.) L.f. (Sterculiaceae)
In Sikkim and Darjeeling Himalayas stem bark and leaf decoction (10–20 ml) taken one time each alternate day in empty stomach for 4–6 weeks (Chhetri et al., 2005).

Abrus precatorius L. Wild Liquorice (Fabaceae)
Leaf of this plant is mixed with the leaves of *Andrographis paniculata*, *Gymnema sylvestre* and seeds of *Syzygium cumini*. The mixture is shade dried and ground into powder and given orally along with cow milk for diabetic treatment. About 50 ml of mixture is given twice a day before food for about 120 days (Ayyanar et al., 2008). Tender leaf paste mixed with the seed powder of *Pithecellobium dulce* is given orally in empty stomach to cure diabetes (Manikandan et al., 2006). *A. precatorius* seed has potent antidiabetic property in the diabetic rabbit model (Monago and Alumanah, 2005).

Abutilon indicum (L.) Sw. (Malvaceae)
In Sikkim and Darjeeling Himalayas decoction of stem bark (25–50 ml) given two times daily (after principal meals) for 3–4 weeks (Chhetri et al., 2005).

Acacia nilotica (L.) Delile [Syn.: *Acacia arabica* (Lam.) Willd.]: Indian babool (Fabaceae)

The powder of bark, gum, pods, leaves and seeds are used to treat diabetes mellitus (Elavarasi and Saravanan, 2012). Two teaspoonful of stem bark decoction in water is given twice a day for maintaining normal blood glucose level (Vidyasagar and Murthy, 2013). Over 94% seed diet of *A. arabica* showed hypoglycemic effect in rats by initiating the release of insulin from pancreatic beta cells (Singh, 2011).

Achyranthes aspera L.: Chaff-flower (Amaranthaceae)

In Rewa district of Madhya Pradesh, ash of this plant (about 10 g) with equal quantity of sugar and milk is practiced after meal for 7 days to cure of diabetes (Yadav et al., 2012). Further, *A. aspera* serves as a good adjuvant in the present armamentarium of antidiabetic drug (Sivanesan and Anand, 2014).

Aconitum palmatum D. Don. (Ranunculaceae)

Root decoction (10–15 ml) taken with a cup of milk one time daily (after lunch) for 7–10 days (Chhetri et al., 2005).

Adhatoda vasica Nees: Vasaka (Acanthaceae)

Leaves, flowers and root are used for treatment of diabetes by Meitei community of Manipur (Devi, 2011).

Adhatoda zeylanica Medik.: Malabar Nut (Acanthaceae)

Leaves of *A. zeylanica* are used as the main ingredient in the polyherbal antidiabetic drug formulation. The herbal healers of Kolli hills prepare a polyherbal drug formulation by mixing equal combination of six plants *viz.*, *A. zeylanica* leaves, *Syzygium cumini* bark, *Terminalia arjuna* bark, leaves of *Andrographis paniculata*, flower of *Cassia auriculata* and leaves of *Aegle marmelos* for the effective treatment of diabetes (Elavarasi and Saravanan, 2012). The leaf juice *viz.* vasaka is often taken with ginger or honey at a dose of 15 to 30 ml to reduce blood glucose level (Kumar et al., 2010). Chloroform and ethanol extracts of leaves of this plant favorably reduced the blood glucose level in the alloxan induced diabetic rats (Ilango et al., 2009).

Aegle marmelos (L.) Correa: Bael (Rutaceae)

Dried leaf powder of *A. marmelos*, *Azadirachta indica* and *Ocimum sanctum* is given thrice a day for 15 days to cure diabetes (Vijayalakshmi et al., 2014). Leaves of *A.marmelos* are used as an important ingredient in the polyherbal drug formulations to treat diabetes (Elavarasi and Saravanan, 2012). Regular eating of few leaves of *A. marmelos* daily at morning half an hour before breakfast would reduce blood glucose level (Vidyasagar and Murthy, 2013). Leaves are used for the treatment of diabetes by the ethnic tribes of Manipur (Devi, 2011; Devi et al., 2011).

Alangium salvifolium (L.f.) Wangerin: Sage leaved alangium (Alangiaceae)

The fruit juice is used to treat diabetes (Raghavendra et al., 2015). The root powder is given orally in tablet form for 1 month to treat diabetes (Rekka et al., 2014). Vineet et al. (2010) reported that methanolic extract of *A. salvifolium* decreased serum glucose, triglyceride and total cholesterol concentrations and increased serum insulin level in dexamethasone-administered rats. *A. salvifolium* leaves were found to contain flavonoids, terpenoids, alkaloids and steroids which are known to be bioactive antidiabetic principles and its antioxidant properties.

Allium sativum L.: Garlic (Liliaceae)

Bulb is used for the treatment of diabetes by the ethnic tribes of Manipur (Devi, 2011; Devi et al., 2011).

Alocasia indica Roxb.: Giant taro (Araceae)

Rhizome is used for the treatment of diabetes by the ethnic tribes of Manipur (Devi, 2011; Devi et al., 2011).

Aloe barbadensis Mill.: *Aloe vera* (Aloeaceae)

In Sikkim and Darjeeling Himalayas fresh leaf pulp (40–50 g) taken once a day in empty stomach for 10–12 weeks (Chhetri et al., 2005). In Thirumoorthi hills of Western Ghats, the fresh leaf pulp (40 to 50 g) given once a day on empty stomach for 12 weeks to the diabetic patients to reduce the blood glucose level (Vijayalakshmi et al., 2014). Treatment of exudates of *A. barbadensis* leaves gel showed hypoglycemic effect in alloxanized diabetic rats. Bitter principle of *Aloe vera* is through stimulation of synthesis and/or release of insulin from pancreatic beta cells (Ajabnoor, 1990).

Ananas comosus L.: Pineapple (Bromeliaceae)

Whole plant is used for the treatment of diabetes by the ethnic tribes of Manipur (Devi et al., 2011).

Andrographis paniculata **Wall. ex Nees: The Creat (Acanthaceae)**

The leaves of *A. paniculata* in combination with *Polygala elongata* and *Gymnema sylvestre* leaves is given in powder form before food for one week to the patients which effectively controls the blood glucose level (Elavarasi and Saravanan, 2012). Decoction of the leaves (50 ml) is prescribed thrice a day after food or fresh raw leaves eaten every day for diabetic treatment (Rajendren and Manian, 2011). Whole plant is used for the treatment of diabetes by the ethnic tribes of Manipur (Devi, 2011; Devi et al., 2011). *A. paniculata* or its active compound andrographolide is known to show hypoglycemic and hypolipidemic effects in high-fat-fructose-fed rat (Nugroho et al., 2012).

Annona squamosa **L.: Custard apple (Annonaceae)**

In Assam, the Dimasa villagers use this plant for various medicinal purposes especially diabetes. Plant bark decoction is given orally once a day on empty stomach to cure the diabetes (Naui et al., 2011). In Bodoland, in Northeast India, raw bark or/and leaf were ground and the extracts were obtained by squishing, the extract is then filtered and used 2 to 3 teaspoon full of extract every morning (Swargiary et al., 2013).

Antidesma acidum **Retz.: Rohitaka (Euphorbiaceae)**

Leaves and seeds are used for the treatment of diabetes by the ethnic tribes of Manipur (Devi et al., 2011).

Ardisia colorata **Roxb.: Uthum (Myrsinaceae)**

Leaves are used for the treatment of diabetes by the ethnic tribes of Manipur (Devi et al., 2011).

Areca catechu **L.: Betel palm (Arecaceae)**

Nut is used for the treatment of diabetes by the ethnic tribes of Manipur (Devi, 2011; Devi et al., 2011).

Aristolochia indica **L.: Birthwort (Aristolochiaceae)**

In Rewa district of Madhya Pradesh, the Baiga tribes use the seeds of this plant mixed with black pepper and made into a paste and taken orally thrice a day for about 15 days to cure diabetes (Yadav et al., 2012).

Artemisia maritima **L.: Sea wormwood (Asteraceae)**

Whole plant is used for the treatment of diabetes by the ethnic tribes of Manipur (Devi et al., 2011).

Artocarpus heterophyllus **Lamk.: Jack fruit (Moraceae)**
Leaves are used for the treatment of diabetes by the ethnic tribes of Manipur (Devi, 2011; Devi et al., 2011).

Artocarpus lakoocha **Lamk.: Money jack (Moraceae)**
Bark and fruit are used for the treatment of diabetes by the ethnic tribes of Manipur (Devi et al., 2011).

Asparagus racemosus **Willd.: Climbing Asparagus (Asparagaceae)**
In Sikkim and Darjeeling Himalayas decoction of tender shoots (25 ml) taken once a day for 6–8 weeks (Chhetri et al., 2005). Root powder of *A. racemosus* made into pills and one pill is prescribed to take twice a day for 21 days to complete cure of diabetes (Malek et al., 2012). The ethanolic extract of *A. racemosus* showed significant antidiabetic activity, antihyperlipidemic and antioxidant properties against STZ induced diabetic rats (Vadivelan et al., 2011).

Azadirachta indica **A.Juss.: Neem (Meliaceae)**
Palliyar tribe of Sirumalai hills use raw leaf juice mixed with honey, cow milk, butter and ghee and taken twice a day for 45 days to treat diabetes (Ayyanar, 2008; Maruthapandian et al., 2011; Dey and Dey, 2013). 30 ml of juice prepared from the tender leaves with an unripe fruit of *Terminalia chebula* is taken along with a teaspoon of castor oil (oil obtained from the seeds of *Ricinus communis*) to treat diabetes (Maruthupandiyan et al., 2011). In Bodoaland raw leaf extracts mixed with little water is taken at a dose of 2–3 teaspoons daily in empty stomach (Swargiary et al., 2013). Leaves and seeds are used for the treatment of diabetes by the ethnic tribes of Manipur (Devi, 2011; Devi et al., 2011).

Hydroalcoholic extracts of *A. indica* showed antihyperglycemic activity in streptozotocin treated rats and this effect is because of increase in glucose uptake and glycogen deposition in isolated rat hemidiaphragm (Chattopadhyay et al., 1987).

Benincasa hispida **(Thunb.) Cogn.: Pani-kakharu (Cucurbitaceae)**
In coastal district of Odisha, the fruit juice (20 ml) with seed powder (1 g) of *Syzygium cumini* is given twice a day for one month for controlling diabetes (Sahu, 2015). Fruit is used for the treatment of diabetes by the ethnic tribes of Manipur (Devi, 2011; Devi et al., 2011). Mishra and Barik (2009) have reported that *B. hispida* produced better hypoglycemic action in animal model.

Berberis aristata DC. (Berberidaceae)

In Sikkim and Darjeeling Himalayas root bark extract (5–10 ml) taken twice daily (after breakfast and dinner) for 1–2 weeks (Chhetri et al., 2005).

Biophytum sensitivum (L.) DC.: Sikerpud (Oxalidaceae)

Leaf juice is taken early morning on empty stomach to treat diabetes (Basha et al., 2011). The leaves are diuretic and relieve strangury and commonly known as "Nagbeli," a folk medicine against "Madhumeha" (Diabetes mellitus), particularly in Eastern Nepal (Pant and Joshi, 1993; Puri et al., 1997). The ethanol and ethylacetate extract of the whole plant has significant hypoglycemic effect, which is possibly due to pancreatic beta-cell stimulating action of the fractions of plant extracts (Renuka, 2012).

Boenninghausenia albiflora (Hook. f.) Reich ex Meissn. (Rutaceae)

In Sikkim and Darjeeling Himalayas the whole plant is crushed without water and the juice (5–10 ml) taken one to two times daily for 3–4 weeks (Chhetri et al., 2005).

Bombax ceiba L.: Silk cotton tree (Bombacaceae)

Bark, flower and fruit are used for the treatment of diabetes by the ethnic tribes of Manipur (Devi, 2011; Devi et al., 2011).

Brassica juncea (L.) Czern: Mustard (Brassicaceae)

Seed decoction is given daily to cure diabetes (Thirumalai et al., 2012). It is a traditional medicinal plant and its seed extract possess hypoglycemic activity (Arumugam et al., 2013). Oral feeding of *B. juncea* diet (10% w/w) for 60 days to normal rats led to significant hypoglycemic effect. This effect was attributed to stimulation of glycogen synthetase (leading to increase in hepatic glycogen content) and suppression of glycogen phosphorylase and other gluconeogenic enzymes (Mukesh and Namita, 2013).

Brucia javanica L.: Macassar Kernels (Simaroubaceae)

Fruits and seeds are used for treatment of diabetes by the Meitei tribe of Manipur (Davi, 2011).

Butea monosperma (Lam.) Taub.: Bastard teak (Fabaceae)

Leaf juice (10 ml) of this plant is administered once a day for 5 to 10 days on empty stomach by villagers in coastal districts of Odisha. It helps in reducing blood sugar favorably (Sahu, 2015). Whole plant is useful for the treatment of diabetes by the ethnic tribes of Manipur (Devi et al., 2011).

Caesalpinia bonducella **(L.) Fleming: Bonduc nut (Cesalpinaceae)**
Roasted seed powder (20 g) is orally given twice a day for diabetic patients (Pushpakarani and Natarajan, 2014). Oral administration of the seed extract (300 mg/kg) of *C. bonducella* produced significant antihyperglycemic action as well as it lowered the Blood Urea Nitrogen (BUN) levels significantly. The antihyperglycemic action of the extract may be due to the blocking of glucose absorption. The drug has the potential to act as antidiabetic as well as antihyperlipidemic (Kannur et al., 2006).

Calamus rotang **(L.), (Arecaceae)**
In Sikkim and Darjeeling Himalayas raw fruit (1–2) taken as masticatory two times daily (after breakfast and lunch) for 6–8 weeks (Chhetri et al., 2005).

Calotropis procera **(Aiton) Dryand: Giant Milkweed (Asclepiadaceae)**
The latex of this plant is used to treat diabetes (Saravanan and Karuppannan, 2013). *C. procera* dried leaves extract (300 and 600 mg/kg) significantly reduced the blood glucose level in the STZ induced diabetic rats and improved metabolic status of the animals and ameliorate the oral tolerance glucose test (Neto et al., 2013).

Campylandra aurantiaca **Baker, (Liliaceae)**
In Sikkim and Darjeeling Himalayas flowers are made into curry and taken with staple food two times per week for 4–6 weeks (Chhetri et al., 2005).

Canna indica **L.: Indian shot (Cannaceae)**
Leaves and aerial parts are used for the treatment of diabetes by the ethnic tribes of Manipur (Devi, 2011; Devi et al., 2011).

Cannabis sativa **L.: Marijuana (Cannabinaceae)**
Leaves, flower and resins are used for the treatment of diabetes by the ethnic tribes of Manipur (Devi, 2011; Devi et al., 2011). In Sikkim and Darjeeling Himalayas leaf extract (5–10 ml) taken two times daily for 3–4 weeks (Chhetri et al., 2005).

Canthium parviflorum **Lam.: Carray cheddile (Rubiaceae)**
Shade dried leaf powder is mixed with cup of water or goat or cow milk or boiled rice are taken orally. One or two teaspoon is taken regularly in the early morning until cure (Ayyanar et al., 2008).

Carica papaya **L.: Papaya (Caricaceae)**
Fruit is used for the treatment of diabetes by the ethnic tribes of Manipur (Devi, 2011; Devi et al., 2011).

Cassia alata L.: Candle bush (Fabaceae)

Leaf and flower are used for the treatment of diabetes by the ethnic tribes of Manipur (Devi et al., 2011).

Cassia auriculata L.: Tanner's Cassia (Fabaceae)

Flowers of *C. auriculata* are used as an important ingredient in the poly-herbal drug formulations. It is widely used in Indian folk medicine for the treatment of diabetes mellitus (Elavarasi and Saravanan, 2012). Flowers, stem, bark and seeds are used to treat diabetes by the Meitei community of Manipur (Devi, 2011). 30 ml of the boiled water extract of the roots is taken twice a day for a period of one month to treat diabetes (Maruthupandian et al., 2011). Methanol extract of *C. auriculata* bark has been found to have potent antidiabetic activity that reduces blood sugar level in strepto-zotocin (STZ) induced diabetic rats (Daisy et al., 2012).

Cassia bicapsularis L.: Butterfly bush (Fabaceae)

Tender shoot is used for the treatment of diabetes by the ethnic tribes of Manipur (Devi et al., 2011).

Cassia fistula L.: Golden shower (Fabaceae)

About 20 ml of the boiled water extract of the flowers is taken regularly twice a day by diabetic patients to reduce the blood glucose level (Maruthupandian et al., 2011). One teaspoon powder of seeds is given once in the morning for about 15 days or more for diabetic treatment (Yadav et al., 2012; Vijayalakshmi et al., 2014). Bark and seeds are used to treat diabetes by the Meitei commu-nity of Manipur (Devi, 2011).

Catharanthus roseus (L.) G.Don: Periwinkle (Apocyanaceae)

A thick extract is made from 250 g crushed root or leaf in 2.5 liters or even more water. It is strained and evaporated on gentle heat. When the volume is reduced to about ½ liter, 1–2 teaspoonful is administered orally twice a day or whole plant is powdered and mixed with cow's milk and given orally to the diabetic patients (Vijayalakshmi et al., 2014; Maruthapandian et al., 2011). In Bodoland in North-East India fresh leaf extracts or fresh leaf may be chewed in empty stomach (Swargiary et al., 2013). Tender leaves are used for the treatment of diabetes by the ethnic tribes of Manipur (Devi et al., 2011). In Sikkim and Darjeeling Himalayas raw leaf (1–2) chewed daily for 2 weeks for curing diabetes (Chhetri et al., 2005).

Methanol extract of leaves at a dose 500 mg/kg given orally for 15 days showed 57.6% hypoglycemic activity in the STZ induced diabetic rats (Singh et al., 2001) and increased plasma insulin level (Elavarasi et al., 2013).

Celosia argentea L.: Cockscomb (Amaranthaceae)
Tender shoots are used for the treatment of diabetes by the ethnic tribes of Manipur (Devi et al., 2011).

Centella asiatica (L.) Urb.: Brahmi (Apiaceae)
The whole plant (5 ml of expressed juice) is taken daily once for 21 days for effective treatment of diabetes by villagers of Bhatiya district of Madhya Pradesh (Ahirwar, 2014). In Bodoland, in North-east India fresh leaf extracts 2–3 teaspoon in empty stomach nearly 21 days in the early diabetic conditions (Swargiary et al., 2013).

Cinnamomum tamala (Buch.-Ham.) Nees & Eberm.: Indian bay leaf (Lauraceae)
Bark, stem, root and seeds are used for the treatment of diabetes by the ethnic tribes of Manipur (Devi, 2011; Devi et al., 2011). In Sikkim and Darjeeling Himalayas decoction of stem bark taken three times daily for 3–4 weeks to cure diabetes (Chhetri et al., 29005).

Cinnamomum zeylanicum Breyn.: Cinnamon (Lauraceae)
In Thirumoorthy hills, local people used (3 times/day) decoction of the stem bark for the treatment of diabetes (Elavarasi et al., 2013). About 5 g of stem bark powder is taken with water daily once for 2–3 weeks for reducing blood glucose (Vidyasagar and Murthy, 2013). Bark, flower, fruit and root are used for the treatment of diabetes by the ethnic tribes of Manipur (Devi, 2011; Devi et al., 2011).

Cissampelos pareira L. var.*hirsuta* (Buch.-Ham ex DC) Forman (Menispermaceae)
In Sikkim and Darjeeling Himalayas Root bark extract (5–10 ml) taken one to two times daily for 2–3 weeks to cure diabetes (Chhetri et al., 2005).

Citrullus colocynthis (L.) Schrad.: Bitter apple (Cucurbitaceae)
In Bodoland, North-East India the bark of the red ripened fruit is dried and powdered. Powder is taken 5–10 g with water in empty stomach (Swargiary et al., 2013).

Citrullus vulgaris Schrad.: Watermelon (Cucurbitaceae)
Fruits are used for the treatment of diabetes by the ethnic tribes of Manipur (Devi et al., 2011).

Citrus aurantifolia L.: Common lime (Rutaceae)

Meitei community of Manipur treat diabetes with fruits of *Citrus aurantifolia* (Devi, 2011).

Citrus limon L.: Lemon (Rutaceae)

Stem and fruit are used for the treatment of diabetes by the ethnic tribes of Manipur (Devi et al., 2011).

Citrus medica L.: Citron (Rutaceae)

Peels of three fruits are boiled in 1 liter of water for 10 minutes and filtered and the decoction is cooled and taken daily for permanent cure of diabetes (Vijayalakshmi et al., 2014). Seeds of *C. medica* are potent antihyperglycemic and hypolipidemic agent (Archana et al., 2011).

Citrus reticulata Blanco (Rutaceae)

Root and fruit are used for the treatment of diabetes by the ethnic tribes of Manipur (Devi, 2011; Devi et al., 2011).

Clerodendrum viscosum Vent. (Verbenaceae)

Tender leaves are used for the treatment of diabetes by the ethnic tribes of Manipur (Devi et al., 2011).

Coccinia grandis (L.) Voigt (Syn.: *Coccinia indica* Wight & Arn): Ivy gourd (Cucurbitaceae)

In Sikkim and Darjeeling Himalayas fresh root extract (5–10 ml) taken two times daily (before principal meals) for 3–4 weeks for curing diabetes (Chhetri et al., 2005). Leaf juice and mucilage from immature fruits (2 teaspoon) are given twice or thrice a day after food (Rajendren and Manian, 2013). Two fresh fruits are taken regularly to prevent diabetes (Maruthapandian et al., 2011). The leaves in the form of curry or as decoction are taken orally to cure diabetes (Vijayalakshmi et al., 2014). Oral administration of dried (powder) extract for 6–8 weeks significantly increases insulin concentration in a clinical study. The plant extract exert beneficial hypoglycemic effect in experimental animals as well as human diabetic subject possibly through an insulin secreting effect or through influence of enzymes involved in glucose metabolism (Singh, 2011).

Coix lacryma-jobi L.: Jobs tears (Poaceae)

Flower, fruit and root are used for the treatment of diabetes by the ethnic tribes of Manipur (Devi, 2011; Devi et al., 2011).

Coriandrum sativum L.: Coriander (Apiaceae)

C. sativum has been documented as a traditional treatment of diabetes. Coriander seeds (5 g) are boiled, filtered and given orally for a month to treat diabetes. Gray and Flatt (1999) demonstrated the presence of anti-hyperglycaemic, insulin-releasing and insulin-like activity in *C. sativum*.

Costus igneus N. E.Br.: Insulin plant (Costaceae)

Consumption of 2 to 3 fresh leaves per day is found to lower blood glucose levels (Elavarasi and Saravanan, 2012; Kumudhavalli and Jayakar, 2012). Oral administration of ethanolic extract of *C. igneus* leaves significantly increased the body weight and decreased blood glucose level in diabetic rats (Vishnu et al., 2010).

Costus speciosus (J. Konig) Sm.: Crepe ginger (Costaceae)

In Sikkim and Darjeeling Himalayas decoction of rhizome (10–20 ml) taken two to three times daily for 2–4 weeks to cure diabetes (Chhetri et al., 2005). About 20 to 25 g of fresh rhizome is ground into a paste and given orally after food thrice a day for 2 months to treat diabetes (Ayyanar et al., 2008). The powdered leaves are taken internally with cow milk (Ignacimuthu et al., 2006; Vijayalakshmi et al., 2014).

Crateva magna (Lour.) DC.: Tree leaved caper (Capparaceae)

In coastal district of Odisha, the decoction of bark (5 g) of this plant and juice of the leaves (19 g) of *Gymnema sylvestre* is mixed and given to the diabetic patients for permanent cure (Sahu, 2015). The major constituents present in this herbal mixture are alkaloids, minor flavonoids, sterols, triterpines and the isothiocyanate glucosides which are responsible for various medicinal activities. *Crateva magna* is beneficial in lowering the blood sugar concentration and in management of other diabetic complications without any doubt (Das et al., 2010).

Cuminum cyminum L.: Cumin seeds (Apiaceae)

Seeds of the plant used for the treatment of diabetes by the local people of Javathu Hills, Tamilnadu (Thirumalai et al., 2012). The Leaves consumed as decoction, juice or infusion to treat diabetics (Kadhirvel et al., 2010).

Curcuma longa L.: Turmeric (Zingiberaceae)

Fresh juice (15 ml) of the rhizome with equal amount of fresh juice of *Phyllanthus emblica* leaves given (3 times/day) to reduce glucose level in urine (Dixit and Sudurshan, 2011; Thirumalai et al., 2012). In Bodoland,

Northeast India about 8 g of raw turmeric grind with water and ½ spoon of honey and given for 1 month after meal to cure diabetes (Swargiary et al., 2013). The aqueous extract of *C. longa* rhizome possesses antidiabetic activity and used for the management of diabetes and associated metabolic alterations (Olatunde et al., 2014).

Cyanotis cristata **D. Don: Nabhali (Commelinaceae)**

Leaves are used for the treatment of diabetes by the ethnic tribes of Manipur (Devi et al., 2011).

*Cyathea nilgiriensis***: Tree Fern (Cyatheaceae)**

The pith of the plant is given to diabetic patients and it also given with milk of *Pterocarpus marsupium* for 3 months (Saravanan and Karuppannan, 2013; Elavarasi, 2015).

Cynodon dactylon **(L.) Pers.: Bermuda grass (Poaceae)**

Whole plant is used for the treatment of diabetes by the ethnic tribes of Manipur (Devi, 2011; Devi et al., 2011).

Cyperus esculentus **L.: Tiger nut (Cyperaceae)**

Fruit and root are used for the treatment of diabetes by the ethnic tribes of Manipur (Devi, 2011; Devi et al., 2011).

Cyperus rotundus **L.: Coco-grass (Cyperaceae)**

Roots are used for the treatment of diabetes by the ethnic tribes of Manipur (Devi, 2011; Devi et al., 2011).

Dioscorea alata **L.: Purple yam (Dioscoreaceae)**

Tubers are used for the treatment of diabetes by the ethnic tribes of Manipur (Devi, 2011; Devi et al., 2011).

Eleusine coracana **(L.) Gaertn.: Finger millet (Poaceae)**

Boiled ragi rice (chodi kangi) with buttermilk in the morning is a good diet for diabetes to maintain normal blood glucose level (Singh and Panda, 2005). The grains are used for the various medical treatments especially to diabetic patients for reducing the blood glucose level (Elavarasi and Saravanan, 2012). Phenolic compounds from the millet seed coat showed strong inhibition towards α-glucosidase and pancreatic amylase and the IC_{50} values were 16.9 and 23.5 µg of phenolics, respectively. It indicated the therapeutic potentiality of millet phenolics in the management of post-prandial hyperglycemia (Shobana et al., 2009).

Emblica officinalis **Gaertn.: (Syn.:** *Phyllanthus emblica* **L.) Indian Goose berry (Euphorbiaceae)**
About 10 ml of fresh fruit juice is taken twice daily to control diabetes. Five-gram powder of fruit and seed is taken daily with luke warm water controls blood sugar (Mall and Sahani, 2013). In Bodoland, North-east India, about 10 numbers of fruits were grounded and juice was mixed with honey and taken every day (Swargiary et al., 2013). Oral administration of ethanolic extract of seed powder of *E. officinalis* decreased the blood glucose level and serum cholesterol level in alloxan induced diabetic rats (Saravanan, 2008).

Equisetum debile **Roxb.: Horse tail (Equisetaceae)**
Rhizomes are used for the treatment of diabetes by the ethnic tribes of Manipur (Devi, 2011; Devi et al., 2011).

Erythrina variegata **L.: Indian coral tree (Fabaceae)**
In Bodoland, North-east India, fresh roots were grounded for obtaining juice. 25 ml of juice were taken for one week without water (Swargiay et al., 2013).

Euphorbia neriifolia **L.: Common milk Hedge (Euphorbiaceae)**
In Kolli hills, the leaf juice of this plant is given to diabetic patients to manage blood glucose level (Elavarasi and Saravanan, 2012). Ethanolic extract of *E. neriifolia* (400 mg/kg) exhibited anti diabetic potential along with antihyperlipidemic activity after repeated oral administration in the STZ induced diabetic rat model (Mansuri and Patel, 2013).

Euryale ferox **Salisb.: Prickly water lily (Nymphaeaceae)**
Raw fruit is used for the treatment of diabetes by the ethnic tribes of Manipur (Devi et al., 2011).

Ficus benghalensis **L.: Banyan tree (Moraceae)**
Stem bark of *F. benghalensis* and root bark of *F. religiosa* are mixed with equal proportions and crushed into a paste. Five gram of the preparation is eaten with honey or milk at every morning and evening to cure diabetes (Devi et al., 2011; Vijayalakshmi et al., 2014). The alcoholic extract of fruits of *F. benghalensis* was found to exert a more pronounced antidiabetic activity than the other parts of the tree (Sharma et al., 2007).

Ficus glomerata **Roxb.: Cluster fig (Moraceae)**
Root and fruits are used for the treatment of diabetes by the ethnic tribes of Manipur (Devi, 2011; Devi et al., 2011).

Ficus hispida L.: **Hairy fig (Moraceae)**
Fruit is used for the treatment of diabetes by the ethnic tribes of Manipur (Devi, 2011; Devi et al., 2011).

Ficus racemosa L.: **Fig tree (Moraceae)**
In Sikkim and Darjeeling Himalayas fruit juice (20–25 ml) taken two times daily (before meals) for 4–8 weeks to cure diabetes (Chhetri et al., 2005). In Kolli hills, the Malayali tribes practiced the bark of this plant as main ingredient in the polyherbal antidiabetic drug formulation. This drug is given to the diabetic patients as one teaspoon before food in the morning and after food in the evening for the effective treatment of diabetes (Saravanan and Karuppannan, 2013; Elavarasi, 2015). The methanol extract of the bark of *F. racemosa* acted in a similar fashion to glibenclamide (standard drug) and it can be suggested that these results provide pharmacological evidence for its folklore claim as an antidiabetic agent (Rao et al., 2002).

Flacourtia jangomas (Lour.) **Raeusch.: Indian plum (Flacourtiaceae)**
Raw fruit is used for the treatment of diabetes by the ethnic tribes of Manipur (Devi et al., 2011).

Garuga pinnata Roxb.: **Garuga (Burseraceae)**
A handful of fresh stem bark boiled in 100 ml of water with few dried leaves of *Gymnema sylvestre*. The decoction so obtained is taken twice a day for seven weeks to treat diabetes (Maruthapandian et al., 2011).

Girardiana heterophylla Decne. **(Urticaceae)**
In Darjeeling Himalayas root decoction (25–50 ml) taken two times daily for 4–8 weeks to cure diabetes (Chhetri et al., 2005).

Glycine max Merril: **Wild soybean (Fabaceae)**
Fruits are used for the treatment of diabetes by the ethnic tribes of Manipur (Devi, 2011; Devi et al., 2011).

Glycosmis pentaphylla (Retz.) **Correa: Ban nimbu (Rutaceae)**
Leaves are used for the treatment of diabetes by the ethnic tribes of Manipur (Devi et al., 2011).

Gymnema sylvestre (Retz.) **Schult.: Gymnema (Ascelpiadaceae)**
Before meal, two leaves are given to the diabetic patients for 48 days for complete cure of diabetes. This is the most common practice of the local herbal

healers of Kolli hills (Elavarasi and Saravanan, 2012). The Powdered leaves are mixed with cow milk and boiled rice, kept over night and taken internally twice a day (Ignacimuthu et al., 2006). The fasting blood glucose, cholesterol and serum triglyceride content were found to be reduced in aqueous leaf extract of *G. sylvestre* treated diabetic rats and the extract also showed the potent elevation in the level of serum HDL-cholesterol (Mall et al., 2009).

Gynocardia odorata R. Br. (Flacourtiaceae)
In Sikkim and Darjeeling Himalayas fruit juice (10–15 ml) taken one time daily for 2 weeks to cure diabetes (Chhetri et al., 2005).

Helicteres isora L.: East Indian Screw tree (Sterculiaceae)
Decoction or juice of root bark given in diabetes to reduce of glucose level in the blood (Kapoor, 2000). The butanol extracts the root of *Helicteres isora* at 250 mg/kg, possess antihyperglyceic activity in glucose loaded rats acts through insulin-sensitizing activity (Ayodhya et al., 2010).

Heliotropium indicum L.: Indian Heliotrope (Boraginaceae)
Leaves are used for the treatment of diabetes by the ethnic tribes of Manipur (Devi et al., 2011).

Hemidesmus indicus (L.) R.Br. ex Schult.: Indian Sarsaparilla (Asclepidaceae)
The root infusion is taken twice a day for a period of six weeks to treat diabetes (Manikandan et al., 2006). Four weeks treatment of diabetic rats with *H. indicus* root extract (40 mg/g body weight/day) showed significant hypoglycemic effect (Sowmia and Kokilavani, 2007).

Hibiscus rosa-sinensis L.: Shoe flower (Malvaceae)
Two teaspoonful of root paste is given twice a day to treat diabetes (Vidyasagar and Murthy, 2013). The flower powder is used for the control of blood glucose level (Elavarasi et al., 2013). Ethanolic extract of *H. rosa-sinensis* flowers showed a maximal diminution in blood glucose (41–46%) and an increased insulin level (14%) in STZ induced diabetic rats. Further, the extract lowered the total cholesterol and serum triglycerides by 22 and 30%, respectively (Sachdewa and Khemani, 2003).

Hodgsonia heteroclita Roxb.: Chinese lard seed (Cucurbitaceae)
In Bodoland, Northeast India, fresh or dry extracts of the fruit juice is taken 2–3 teaspoons in empty stomach (Swargiary et al., 2013).

Hybanthus enneaspermus (L.) F. Muell.: Spade flower (Violaceae)

20 ml juice of the whole plant is taken with cow milk for a period of four to five months to treat diabetes (Manikandan et al., 2006). The whole plant mixtures along with cow milk two times a day for 60 days also a good ailment for the disease (Vijayalakshmi et al., 2014). Aqueous extract of *H. enneaspermus* reduce blood glucose level in STZ-induced diabetic model. The drug also shows significant hypoglycemic activity but the effect is dose independent (Patel et al., 2011).

Imperata cylindrica L.: Blady grass (Poaceae)

Rhizome is used for the treatment of diabetes by the ethnic tribes of Manipur (Devi, 2011; Devi et al., 2011).

Ipomoea aquatica Forssk.: Swamp morning glory (Convolvulaceae)

Whole plant is used for the treatment of diabetes by the ethnic tribes of Manipur (Devi, 2011; Devi et al., 2011).

Ipomoea batatas (L.) Poir.: Sweet potato (Convolvulaceae)

The pericarp of fruit is obtained and dried for 4 to 5 days. Then they are ground to make a paste. From the paste, about half teaspoon is mixed in a glass of water and taken at every morning for one month to cure diabetes (Vijayalakshmi et al., 2014). *I. batatas* can be recommended to be used as an antidiabetic agent for patients living with diabetes due to the fact that it is cheap and also a natural agent (Ijaola et al., 2014). In Sikkim and Darjeeling Himalayas the juice of the aerial part of the plant (25–30 ml) taken two times daily for 3–4 weeks to cure diabetes (Chhetri et al., 2005).

Jatropha curcas L.: Barbados nut (Euphorbiaceae)

Whole plant is used for the treatment of diabetes by the ethnic tribes of Manipur (Devi, 2011; Devi et al., 2011).

Justicia tranquebarienis L.f.: Justicia (Acanthaceae)

The leaf powder of the *J. tranquebarienis* is given orally to the diabetic patients to control the blood sugar level (Elavarasi and Saravanan, 2012). Pre-treatment with aqueous leaf extract of *J. tranquebariensis* reduced the enhanced level of SGOT and SGPT, ACP, ALP which seems to offer the protection and maintain the functional integrity of hepatic cells (Shabanan Begum et al., 2011).

Kaempferia galanga L.: Aromatic ginger (Zingiberaceae)

Rhizome is used for the treatment of diabetes by the ethnic tribes of Manipur (Devi et al., 2011).

Kalanchoe pinnata (Lam.) Pers.: Cathedral bells (Crassulaceae)

In Bodoland, North-east India 1 g of raw leaves grinded with 100 ml of water. Leaf extract, 2–3 teaspoons early in the morning (Swargiary et al., 2013).

Lagenaria siceraria (Molina) Standley: Bottle gourd (Cucurbitaceae)

Fruit and seeds are used for the treatment of diabetes by the ethnic tribes of Manipur (Devi et al., 2011).

Lawsonia inermis L.: Henna (Lythraceae)

In rural/local people all over India particularly south India practiced decoction of flowers and seeds taken once in a day for 10 to 15 days for reducing blood glucose level (Yadav et al., 2012). An ethanolic extract of *L. inermis* leaves showed a significant fall in fasting blood glucose (Chikkareddy et al., 2012).

Litsea cubeba Pers. (Lauraceae)

In Sikkim and Darjeeling Himalayas one raw fruit chewed as masticatory two times daily for 4–6 weeks to cure diabetes (Chhetri et al., 2005).

Lysimachia obovata Buch.-Ham. ex Wall.: (Primulaceae)

Fruit is used for the treatment of diabetes by the ethnic tribes of Manipur (Devi et al., 2011).

Mangifera indica L.: Mango tree (Anacardiaceae)

Two to three seeds are powdered with same number of seeds of *Syzygium cumini* (L.) Skeels and given thrice a day (Vidyasagar and Murthy, 2013). Fruit and tender leaves are used for the treatment of diabetes by the ethnic tribes of Manipur (Devi, 2011; Devi et al., 2011).

Memecylon umbellatum Burm. f.: Iron wood tree (Melastomataceae)

Shade dried leaf powder is mixed with cup of water and boiled rice and kept overnight and taken orally. One teaspoon is taken early in the morning for 45 days or until cure (Ayyanar et al., 2008). The administration of methanolic extract of the plant resulted in significant reduction of blood glucose level, urea, creatinine, SGOT and SGPT ($p<0.001$) in diabetic rats (Puttaswamy et al., 2013).

Momordica charantia L.: Bitter gourd (Cucurbitaceae)

About 5 g of fruit powder is mixed with equal quantity of seed powder of *Syzygium cumini* (L.) Skeels and this mixture is prescribed for the treatment of diabetes. One teaspoon of this powder is taken with a cup of butter milk twice a day for curing diabetes (Vidyasagar and Murthy, 2013). Further, the Palliyar tribals in Sirumali hills, Western Ghats, Tamilnadu used 30 ml of fresh juice of unripe fruit and few fresh leaves with pieces of stem bark of *Syzygium cumini* once in a day to treat diabetes (Maruthupandian et al., 2011). In Bodoland, Northeast India, fresh extracts of fruit juice one ounce to be taken in empty stomach (Swargiary et al., 2013). In Sikkim and Darjeeling Himalayas fruit extract (25 ml) taken two times daily for 12–14 weeks to cure diabetes (Chhetri et al., 2005). Administration of ethanolic extract of *Momordica charantia* suppressed gluconeogenesis in normal and streptozotocin (STZ) induced diabetic rats by depressing the hepatic gluconeogenic enzymes fructose-1, 6-bisphosphatase and glucose-6-phosphatse (Chowdhury et al., 2012).

Momordica dioica L. Kakroon: Spine gourd (Cucurbitaceae)

In Hamirpur district of Himachal Pradesh the local people use fruit as vegetable and 20 ml of fruit juice is taken once a day to control diabetes (Kumar et al., 2014). This is commonly used as vegetable in many parts of India.

Moringa oleifera Lam.: Drumstick tree (Moringaceae)

The fruit juice (15–20 ml) along with little old jaggery is given once daily for 15 days (Pavani et al., 2012). The leaves extract of *Moringa oleifera* revealed anti-hyperglycemic activity in diabetic mice and improved the glucose tolerance impairment in mildly diabetic mice. Thus, *Moringa oleifera* Lam. may be introduced as an antidiabetic herb (Luangpiom et al., 2013).

Murraya koenigii (L.) Spreng.: Curry leaf plant (Rutaceae)

About 2 to 3 teaspoon of fresh leaves extract is taken in the early morning results reduced blood glucose (Swargiary et al., 2013). In Bodoland, Northeast India leaf extract, 2–3 teaspoon early in the morning (Swargiary et al., 2013). *M. koenigii* leaf extract showed hypoglycemic activity and may also reverse dyslipidemia associated with diabetes, and prevent the cardio vascular complications which are very prevalent in diabetic patients (Kesari et al., 2007).

Musa paradisiaca L.: **Banana (Musaceae)**
Leaves, flowers and unripe fruits are used for the treatment of diabetes by the ethnic tribes of Manipur (Devi, 2011; Devi et al., 2011).

Nardostachys jatamansi DC. **(Valerianaceae)**
In Sikkim and Darjeeling Himalayas decoction of rootstock (30–50 ml) taken once daily for 2–3 weeks to cure diabetes (Chhetri et al., 2005).

Nelumbo nucifera Gaertn.: **Holy Lotus (Nymphaeaceae)**
Flowers are made into juice and taken orally for about 15 days to cure diabetes mellitus (Yadav et al., 2012). Extract of flowers at a dosage of 250 mg/kg is a good choice for controlling the blood glucose level in diabetic rats (Sakuljaitrong et al., 2013).

Nigella sativa L.: **Black cumin (Ranunculaceae)**
One spoon of the powdered seeds is taken orally before meal for curing diabetes (Andaloussi et al., 2008). Significant decreases in blood glucose level, and increase in serum insulin level were observed on treatment with *N. sativa* oil for 4 weeks. Immunohistochemical staining of pancreas from *N. sativa* oil-treated group showed large areas with positive immunoreactivity for the presence of insulin (Fararh et al., 2002; Meddah et al., 2009).

Nyctanthes arbor-tristis L.: **Har Singar (Oleaceae)**
Flowers and leaves are used for the treatment of diabetes by the ethnic tribes of Manipur (Devi, 2011; Devi et al., 2011).

Ocimum tenuiflorum L. (Syn.: *O. sanctum* L.): **Holy basil (Lamiaceae)**
Leaves are dried under shade and ground to make powder. 21 g of powdered leaves is taken twice a day to cure diabetes (Vijayalakshmi et al., 2014). The consumption of fresh leaves is also used to reduce the blood glucose level (Elavarasi and Saravanan, 2012; Gireesha and Raju, 2013). Ethanolic extract of *O. sanctum* has significant and sustained oral hypoglycemic activity, comparable with the hypoglycemic effect of glibenclamide, a sulfonylurea (Rao et al., 2013).

Oreocnide integrifolia Miq.: **Wild Rhea (Ulmaceae)**
Whole plant is used for the treatment of diabetes by the ethnic tribes of Manipur (Devi et al., 2011).

Oroxylum indicum (L.) Vent. **(Bignoniaceae)**
In Sikkim and Darjeeling Himalayas stem bark decoction (15–20 ml) or juice (5–10 ml) taken two to three times daily to cure diabetes (Chhetri et al., 2005).

Oxalis corniculata L.: Yellow wood sorrel (Oxalidaceae)
Fruits and leaves are used for the treatment of diabetes by the ethnic tribes of Manipur (Devi, 2011; Devi et al., 2011).

Paederia foetida L. (Rubiaceae)
In Sikkim and Darjeeling Himalayas leaf infusion (50–60 ml) taken one time in the morning for 2–3 weeks to cure diabetes (Chhetri et al., 2005).

Panax pseudoginseng Wall. (Araliaceae)
In Sikkim and Darjeeling Himalayas dried rhizome powder (0.5–1 g) taken one time daily with warm milk to cure diabetes (Chhetri et al., 2005).

Parkia roxburghii G.Don: Yongchak (Fabaceae)
Inflorescence and bark are used for the treatment of diabetes by the ethnic tribes of Manipur (Devi, 2011; Devi et al., 2011).

Passiflora edulis Sims.: Passion fruit (Passifloraceae)
Leaves are used for the treatment of diabetes by the ethnic tribes of Manipur (Devi, 2011; Devi et al., 2011).

Phlogocanthus thyrsiflorus Nees: Nongmancha (Acanthaceae)
In Bodoland, North-east India, fresh extract of the leaf, 2–3 teaspoons early in the morning (Swargiary et al., 2013).

Phyllanthus niruri L.: Stone breaker (Euphorbiaceae)

Whole plant is used for the treatment of diabetes by the ethnic tribes of Manipur (Devi, 2011; Devi et al., 2011). *Phyllanthus simplex* Retz.: Kaya-am (Euphorbiaceae)
Fruits and leaves are used for the treatment of diabetes by the ethnic tribes of Manipur (Devi et al., 2011).

Picrorhiza kurrooa Royle ex Benth. (Scrophulariaceae)
In Sikkim and Darjeeling Himalayas dry rhizome powder (0.5 g) taken with two tablespoon of curd and a pinch of pepper power one time daily for 1–2 weeks to cure diabetes (Chhetri et al., 2005).

Plumbago rosea L.: Laurel (Plumbaginaceae)
Stem is used for the treatment of diabetes by the Meitei tribe of Manipur (Devi, 2011).

Pongamia pinnata (L.) Pierre: Indian beech (Fabaceae)
The flowers are fried in ghee/butter and taken with honey thrice a day to treat diabetes (Maruthupandian et al., 2011). Ethanolic and aqueous

extract of *P. pinnata* leaves showed significant antidiabetic activity in alloxan induced diabetic rats (Sikarwar and Patil, 2010).

Potentilla fulgens Wall. (Rosaceae)
In Sikkim and Darjeeling Himalayas decoction of root (20–25 ml) taken two times daily for 4–8 weeks to cure diabetes (Chhetri et al., 2005).

Psidium guajava L.: Guava (Myrtaceae)
Hot water extract of dried leaves or the fresh juice of leaves (2 teaspoon) and fruits are taken orally thrice a day to reduce blood glucose level of diabetic patients (Elavarasi and Saravanan, 2012; Gireesha and Raju, 2013).

The extract showed significant hypolipidemic activity in addition to its hypoglycemic and antidiabetic activity. In view of its relative non-toxic nature *P. guajava* raw fruit peel may be a potential antidiabetic agent (Rai et al., 2010).

Pterocarpus marsupium Roxb.: Indian Kino tree (Fabaceae)
In Sirumalai of Western Ghats, hot water extract of the stem bark (20 ml in twice a day) is used by the Palliyar tribes as household remedy to treat diabetes (Marudhapandian, 2011). It is scientifically proved by the study of Mishra et al. (2013) in which, the ethanolic extract and hexane and n-butanol fractions of heartwood of this plant administered in diabetic model and results showed marked decline in blood glucose level and significant increase in insulin level.

Punica granatum L.: Pomegranate (Punicaceae)
Seeds are used for the treatment of diabetes by the ethnic tribes of Manipur (Devi et al., 2011).

Quercus lanata Sm. (Fagaceae)
In Sikkim and Darjeeling Himalayas decoction of stem bark (20–25 ml) taken one or two times daily for 2–3 week to cure diabetes (Chhetri et al., 2005).

Rubus fruticosus L.: Blackberry (Rosaceae)
In Bodoland, Northeast India, dried barks of the plant is soaked into water for 12 hours and filtered; the filtrate (approximately 30 ml) is taken every day in empty stomach for 1 month (Swargiary et al., 2013).

Salacia oblonga Wall.: Saptrangi (Celastraceae)
About 50 g leaves are mixed with sufficient amount of ghritkumari (*Aloe vera*) gel and tablets are formed. One tablet is taken twice daily with honey, which cure diabetes (Mall and Sahani, 2013).

Salvia officinalis **L.: Garden sage (Lamiaceae)**
Consumption of fresh leaves on an empty stomach control the blood sugar level (Manikandan et al., 2006). The *S. officinalis* extract revealed significant hypoglycemic activity in STZ-induced diabetic rats (Khattab et al., 2012).

Saraca asoca **(Roxb.) De Wilde (Caesalpiniaceae)**
In Sikkim and Darjeeling Himalayas infusion of the dry flower (50–100 ml) taken two times daily (before principal meals) for 4–5 weeks to cure diabetes (Chhetri et al., 2005).

Sesbania sesban **L.: Egyptian pea (Fabaceae)**
Bark and seeds are used for the treatment of diabetes by the ethnic tribes of Manipur (Devi et al., 2011).

Solanum nigrum **L.: Black night shade (Solanaceae)**
Fruit and leaves are used for the treatment of diabetes by the ethnic tribes of Manipur (Devi et al., 2011).

Solanum xanthocarpum **Schrad & H.Wendl.: Yellow berried nightshade (Solanaceae)**
In Bodoland, North-east India the juice extract of the fresh fruits (1–3 no.) is taken as a remedy to the high blood glucose in the body (Swargiary et al., 2013).

Spinacia oleracea **L.: Spinach (Amaranthaceae)**
In Bodoland, North-east India, about 200 g of *S. oleracea* mixed with a most equal amount of fresh carrot and grounded to obtain juice which is taken every day in empty stomach (Swargiary et al., 2013).

Spondias pinnata **(L.f.) Kurz.: Wild mango (Anacardiaceae)**
Bark and seeds are used for the treatment of diabetes by the ethnic tribes of Manipur (Devi et al., 2011).

Stellaria media **(L.) Vill.: Chickweed (Caryophyllaceae)**
In Bodoland, North-East India aqueous extracts of the whole plant at a dose of 2–3 teaspoon in empty stomach is believed to help reduce the glucose concentration in blood (Swargiary et al., 2013).

Stephania glabra **(Roxb.) Miers (Menispermaceae)**
In Sikkim and Darjeeling Himalayas root decoction (20–25 ml) taken with milk two to three times daily for 1–2 weeks to cure diabetes (Chhetri et al., 2005).

Swertia angustifolia **Buch.-Ham. ex D. Don (Gentianaceae)**
In Sikkim and Darjeeling Himalayas infusion of whole plant (40–50 ml) taken two times daily (before principal meals for 3–4 weeks to cure diabetes (Chhetri et al., 2005).

Swertia chirayita **(Roxb. ex Flem.) Karst. (Gentianaceae)**
In Sikkim and Darjeeling Himalayas infusion of the whole plant (50–60 ml) taken one time daily in empty stomach for 2 weeks to cure diabetes (Chhetri et al., 2005).

Swertia pedicellata **Banerji (Gentianaceae)**
In Sikkim and Darjeeling Himalayas decoction of shoot (20–25 ml) taken two times daily (before meals) for 4–6 weeks to cure diabetes (Chhetri et al., 2005).

Syzygium cumini **(L.) Skeels: Java plum (Myrtaceae)**
The decoction of stem bark (50 ml) is taken orally twice a day till cure and the mature fruits are eaten as raw (Rajendren and Manian, 2011). The seed powder reduces the blood glucose level and reported to possess hypoglycemic effect (Elavarasi et al., 2013). Fruits, bark and seeds are used for the treatment of diabetes by the ethnic tribes of Manipur (Devi, 2011; Devi et al., 2011). In Sikkim and Darjeeling Himalayas decoction of stem bark (25–30 ml) taken three times daily for 2–3 weeks to cure diabetes (Chhetri et al., 2005).

Syzygium fruticosum **DC.: Taw-thybe (Myrtaceae)**
Leaves are used for the treatment of diabetes by the ethnic tribes of Manipur (Devi et al., 2011).

Tamarindus indica **L.: Tamarind (Fabaceae)**
The seeds of *T. indica* are made into pills. One pill is taken twice daily for 21 days to cure diabetes (Malek et al., 2012). Leaf decoction is given to diabetic patients (Dey and Dey, 2013). Aqueous extract of seed of *T. indica* has potent antidiabetogenic activity that reduces blood sugar level in streptozotocin (STZ) induced diabetic male rat (Maiti et al., 2004).

Terminalia arjuna **(Roxb. ex DC.) Wight & Arn.: Arjuna (Combretaceae)**
Bark of Arjuna tree is used as an important ingredient in the poly herbal antidiabetic drug formulation (Kumar and Prabhakar, 1987). Oral administration of ethanolic extract of *T. arjuna* bark (250 and 500 mg/kg body weight) in alloxan induced diabetic rats resulted in significant decrease of blood glucose and decrease in the activities of glucose-6-phosphatase,

fructose-1,6-disphosphatase, aldolase and an increase in the activity of phosphoglucoisomerase and hexokinase in tissues (Ragavan and Krishnakumari, 2006).

Tinospora cordifolia Willd.: Guduchi (Menispermaceae)
Whole plant, stem, bark and leaves are used for the treatment of diabetes by the ethnic tribes of Manipur (Devi, 2011; Devi et al., 2011).

Tinospora crispa (L.) Hook.f. & Thoms.: Indian tinospora (Menispermaceae)
An infusion of the stem is to treat diabetes mellitus. *T. crispa* extract possesses an antihyperglycaemic effect which is probably due to the stimulation of insulin release *via* modulation of beta-cell Ca^{2+} concentration (Noor et al., 1998).

Trichosanthes dioica Roxb.: Pointed gourd (Cucurbitaceae)
Fruit and seeds are used for the treatment of diabetes by the Meitei community of Manipur (Devi, 2011).

Trigonella foenum-graecum L.: Fenugreek (Fabaceae)
It is a common antidiabetic plant used all over India. The seeds are commonly used to treat diabetes as powder, roasted seeds or seeds soaked in water overnight and the decoction is taken in the morning. About 5 to 10 gram of powdered seed is taken daily with cold water is an easy remedy for diabetes (Renuka et al., 2009; Kumar et al., 2014). About 25 g seeds are given daily for 21 days with water. The inhabitants claimed that it is one of the effective treatments to reduce blood glucose in diabetic patients (Ahmad et al., 2009). The administration of seed extract of fenugreek reduced the glucose level of not only blood but also other tissue like liver and pancreas (Sarasa et al., 2012). The leaves both dried and fresh are also used as powder or made into curries, commonly called as Methi. Leaves and seeds are used for the treatment of diabetes by the Meitei community of Manipur (Davi, 2011). In Sikkim and Darjeeling Himalayas sprouted seeds mixed with chilly, salt and garlic and ground into a paste. 5–10 g of the paste taken with two principal meals daily to cure diabetes (Chhetri et al., 2005).

Urtica dioica L. (Urticaceae)
In Sikkim and Darjeeling Himalayas decoction of young leaves and shoots (50–100 ml) taken as curry one or two times daily with meals for 4–8 weeks to cure diabetes (Chhetri et al., 2005).

Vigna mungo L.: Black gram (Fabaceae)

In Bodoland, North-east India about 50 g of raw seeds grounded and soaked in 1 cup of milk overnight and taken for 20 days (Swargiary et al., 2013).

Wattakaka volubilis (L.f.) Stapf: Green milk weed (Asclepiadaceae)

About 50 to 75 ml of leaf powder is taken orally along with cow milk twice a day after food for 90 days (Ayyanar et al., 2008) to complete cure of diabetes.

Withania somnifera (L.) Dunal: Winter cherry (Solanaceae)

Leaf powder in one cup of water is taken once a day for the treatment of diabetes and its allied complications (Thirumalai et al., 2012). It decreases blood glucose level, prevents hyperinsulinemia and improved glucose tolerance in NIDDM rats and it can improve insulin sensitivity (Anwer et al., 2008).

Zanthoxylum alatum Roxb.: Prickly ash (Rutaceae)

Leaves and roots are used for the treatment of diabetes by the ethnic tribes of Manipur (Devi, 2011; Devi et al., 2011).

Zingiber officinale Rosc. (Zingigeraceae)

In Sikkim and Darjeeling Himalayas decoction of rhizome (25–50 ml) taken as herbal tea with a pinch of salt two to three times daily for 8–12 weeks to cure diabetes (Chhetri et al., 2005).

12.3   MANGROVES AS ANTIDIABETIC PLANTS

Walters et al. (2008) in their review mention the wide range medicinal properties of several mangroves for teeth problems and diabetes. According to Govindasamy and Kannan (2012) several mangroves species are used to treat range of ailments including diabetes. Prabhakaran and Kavitha (2012) stated that *Rhizophora mucronata* Lamk. (Rhizophoraceae) bark is a powerful astringent is useful in diabetes. Its bark used to treat diabetes, leprosy hemorrhage and dysentery (Sathe et al., 2014).

12.4   CONCLUSIONS

To conclude many different Indian plants described above have been traditionally used individually or in various formulations for treatment of diabetes and its complications. This review hopefully will help to find out the safe drug for the treatment of diabetes. However, the active ingredients in the herbal formulations are not well defined. It is therefore important to know the active component and their molecular interactions, which will help to analyze the therapeutic efficacy of the product and also to standardize the product. In this regard the observations of Marles and Farnsworth (1995) are relevant. A scientific investigation of traditional herbal remedies for diabetes may provide valuable leads for the development of alternative drugs and therapeutic strategies. Alternatives are clearly needed because of the inability of current therapies to control all of the pathological aspects of diabetes, and the high cost and poor availability of current therapies for many rural populations. Considering the rich cultural ethnotraditions of plant use and the high prevalence of diabetes mellitus in India, more *in vivo* investigations should be encouraged in order to validate the antidiabetic activity of the identified plants as claimed by the traditional healers.

ACKNOWLEDGEMENTS

The authors (GR, SE & KS) thank the University Grants Commission, New Delhi, for financial assistance and also thank the management, Principal and Head of the Department of Zoology, Nehru Memorial College (Autonomous) Puthanampatti for encouragement and financial assistance.

KEYWORDS

- antidiabetic activity
- diabetes mellitus
- ethnomedicinal plants
- traditional medicine

REFERENCES

1. Ahmad, M., Qureshi, R., Arshad, M., Khan, M. A., & Zafar, M. (2009). Traditional herbal remedies used for the treatment of diabetes from district Attock (Pakistan). *Pakistan J. Bot., 41*, 2777–2782.

2. Ahirwar, K. (2014). Utilization of medicinal plants by the tribes of Bhatiya, Shahdol district, Madhya Pradesh. *Int. J. Sci. Res. 3(9)*, 149–151.

3. Ajabnoor, M. A. (1990). Effect of aloes on blood glucose levels in normal and alloxan diabetic mice. *J. Ethnopharmacol., 8*, 215–220.

4. Andaloussi, A. B., Martineau, L. C., Spoor, D., Vuong, T., Leduc, C., Joly, E., Burt, A., Meddah, B., Settaf, A., Arnason, J. T., Prentki, M., & Haddad, P. S. (2008). Antidiabetic activity of *Nigella sativa* seed extract in cultured pancreatic β-cells, skeletal muscle cells, and adipocytess. *Pharmaceutical Biol., 46*, 96–104.

5. Anwer, T., Sharma, M., Pillai, K. K., & Iqbal, M. (2008). Effect of *Withania somnifera* on insulin sensitivity in Non-Insulin-Dependent Diabetes Mellitus rats. *J. Pharmacol. Soc. Basic & Clin. Pharmacol. & Toxicol., 102*, 498–503.

6. Archana, N., Joshi, S. A., Juyal1, V., & Kumar, T. (2011). Antidiabetic and hypolipidemic activity of *Citrus medica* Linn. seed extract in Streptozotocin induced diabetic rats. *Pharmacogn Jour., 3(23)*, 187–194.

7. Arumugam, G., Manjula, P., & Paari, N. A. (2013). Review: anti diabetic medicinal plants used for diabetes mellitus. *J. Acute Dis., 2(3)*, 196–200.

8. Ayyanar, M., Sankarasivaraman, K., & Ignacimuthu, S. (2008). Traditional herbal medicines used for the treatment of diabetes among two major tribal groups in South Tamilnadu, India. *Ethnobot. Leaflets, 12*, 276–280.

9. Ayodhya, S., Kusum, S., & Anjali, S. (2010). Hypoglycemic activity of different extracts of various herbal plants. *Int. J. Ayurveda Res. Pharm., 1(1)*, 212–224.

10. Baby, J., & Raj, S. J. 2010. Pharmacognostic and phytochemical properties of *Aloe vera* Linn.–an overview. *Int. J. Pharmaceutical Sci. Rev. Res., 4(2)*, 106–110.

11. Bailey, C. J., Flatt, P. R., & Marks, V. (1989). Drugs inducing hypoglycemia. *Pharmacol. Ther., 42*, 361–384.

12. Basha, S. K, Sudarsanam, G., Silar Mohammad, M., & Niaz Parveen, D. (2011). Investigations on anti-diabetic medicinal plants used by Sugali tribal inhabitants of Yerramalais of Kurnool district, Andhra Pradesh, India. *J. Pharm. Sci., 4(2)*, 19–24.

13. Bhushan, M. S., Rao, C. H. V., Ojha, S. K., Vijayakumar, M., & Verma, A. (2010). An analytical review of plants for anti diabetic activity with their phytoconstituent & mechanism of action. *Int. J. Pharm. Sci. Res., 1(1)*, 29–46.

14. Chattopadhyay, R. R., Chattopadhyay, R. N., Nandy, A. K., Poddar, G & Maitra, S. K. (1987). The effect of fresh leaves of *Azadirachta indica* on glucose uptake and glycogen content in the isolated rat hemi diaphragm. *Bull. Calcutta Sch. Trop. Med., 35*, 8–12.

15. Chhetri, D. R., Parajuli, P., Subba, G. C. (2005). Antidiabetic plants used by Sikkim and Darjeeling Himalayan tribes, India. *J. Ethnopharmacol. 99*, 199–202

16. Chikaraddy, A., Maniyar, Y., & Mannapur, B. (2012). Hypoglycemic activity of ethanolic extract of *Lawsonia inermis* Linn., (Henna) in alloxan induced diabetic albino rats. *Int. J. Pharma. Biosci., 2(4)*, 287–292.

17. Chowdhury, Md. A. Z., Hossain, M. I., Hossain, Md. S., Ahmed, S., Afrin, T., & Karim, N. (2012). Antidiabetic Effects of *Momordica charantia* (Karela) in Male long Evans Rat. *J. Advanced Laboratory Res. Biol., 3, 3.*

18. Daisy, P., & Saipriya, K. (2012). Biochemical analysis of *Cassia fistula* aqueous extract and phytochemically synthesized gold nanoparticles as hypoglycemic treatment for diabetes mellitus. *Int. J. Nanomed., 7*, 1189–1202.

19. Das, P., Mekap, R. S., & Pani, S. (2010). Phytochemical and pharmacological screening of the plant *Crateva magna* against alloxan induced diabetes in rats. *J. Pharm. Sci. & Res. 2(4)*, 257–263.

20. Devi, A. P. (2011). Plants used by Meitei community of Manipur for the treatment of diabetes. *Assam Univ. J. Sci. &Tech.:Biol. Environ. Sci. 7*, 63–66.

21. Devi, W. I., Devi, G. S., & Singh, C. B. (2011). Traditional herbal medicina used for the treatment of diabetes in Manipur, India. *Res. J. Pharmaceut. Biol. Chem. Sci. 2(4)*, 709–715.

22. Dey, A., & Dey, A. (2013). Tribal way to treat diabetes: Potentials of traditional phototherapy in the ethnic belts of Purulia district, India and socio-economic relevance. *Int. J. Med. Plants. Res., 2(1)*, 198 – 203.

23. Dixit, A. K., & Sudurshan, M. (2011). Review of flora of anti-diabetic plants of Puducherry. *Intern. J. Appl. Biol. Pharma Technol., 2(4)*, 455–462.

24. Donga, J. J., Surani, V. S., Sailor, G. U., Chauhan, S. P., & Seth, A. K. (2011). A systematic review on natural medicine used for therapy of diabetes mellitus of some Indian medicinal plants, *Int. J. Pharm. Sci., 2*, 36.

25. Elavarasi, S. (2015). Evaluation of antidiabetic potential of traditionally used medicinal plants, *Cyathea nilgiriensis* (Holttum) and *Pterocarpus marsupium* Roxb. in Streptozotocin (STZ) induced diabetic rat model. PhD thesis submitted to the Bharathidasan University, Tiruchirappalli, India.

26. Elavarasi, S., & Saravanan, K. (2012). Ethnobotanical study of plants used to treat diabetes by tribal people of Kolli hills, Nammakkal District, Tamilnadu, Southern India. *Int. J. PharmTech Res., 4(1)*, 404–411.

27. Elavarasi, S., Saravanan, K., & Renuka, C. (2013). A systematic review on medicinal plants used to treat diabetes mellitus. *Int. J. Phramacuet., Chem and Biol. Sci., 3(3)*, 983–992.

28. Fararh, K. M., Atoji, Y., Shimizu, Y., & Takewaki, T. (2002). Insulinotropic properties of *Nigella sativa* oil in streptozotocin plus nicotinamide diabetic hamster. *Res. Ve. Sci., 73(3)*, 279–282

29. Gireesha, J., & Raju, N. S. (2013). Ethnobotanical study of medicinal plants in BR Hills region of Western Ghats, Karnataka. *Asian J. Plant Sc. Res., 3(5)*, 36–40.

30. Govindasamy, C., & Kannan, R. (2012). Pharmacognosy of mangrove plants in the system of Unani medicine. *Asian Pacific J. Trop. Disease 2*, S38–S41.

31. Gray, A. M., & Flatt, P. R. (1999). Insulin-releasing and insulin-like activity of the traditional anti-diabetic plant, *Coriandrum sativum* (coriander). *Brit. J. Nutr., 81*, 203–209.

32. Hove, M. N., Kristensen. J. K., Lauritzen, T., & Bek. T. (2004). The prevalence of retinopathy in an unselected population of type 2 diabetes patients from Arhus County, Denmark. *Acta. Ophthalmol. Scand., 82*, 443–448.

33. Ignacimuthu, S., Ayyanar, M., & Sankarasivaraman, K. (2006). Ethnobotanical investigations among tribes in Madurai district of Tamil Nadu, India. *J. Ethnobiol. Ethnomed., 2*, 25–34.

34. Ijaola, T. O., Osunkiyesi, A. A., Taiwo, A. A., Oseni, O. A., LanreIyanda, Y. A., Ajayi J. O., & Oyede, R. T. (2014). Antidiabetic effect of *Ipomoea batatas* in normal and alloxan-induced diabetic rats. *I O S R J. Appl. Chem., 7(5)*, 16–25.

35. Ilango, K., Chitra, V., Kanimozhi, P., & Balaji1, G. (2009). Antidiabetic, antioxidant and antibacterial activities of leaf extracts of *Adhatoda zeylanica* (Acanthaceae). *J. Pharm. Sci. & Res., 1(2)*, 67–73.

36. Jafri, M. A., Aslam, M., Javed, K., & Singh, S. (2000). Effect of *Punica granatum* L. flowers on blood glucose levels in normal and alloxan induced diabetic rats. *J. Ethnopharmacol.*, *70*, 309–314.

37. Jung, M., Park, M., Lee, H. C., Kang, Y. H., Kang, E. S., & Kim S. K. (2006). Antidiabetic agents from medicinal plants. *Curr Med Chem.*, *13(10)*, 1203–1218.

38. Kaczmar, T. (1998). Herbal support for diabetes management. *Clin. Nutr. Insights.*, *6(8)*, 1–4.

39. Kadhirvel, K., Ramya, S., Sudha, T. P. S., Ravi, A. V., Rajasekaran, C., Vanitha Selvi, R., & Jayakumararaj, R. (2010). Ethnomedicinal survey on plants used by tribals in Chitteri hills. *Eviron. We Int. J. Sci. Tech.*, *5*, 35–46.

40. Kannur, D. M., Hukkeri, V. I., & Akki, K. S. (2006). Antidiabetic activity of *Caesalpinia bonducella* seed extracts in rats. *Fitoterapia 77*, 546–549.

41. Kapoor, L. D. (2000). Handbook of Ayurvedic medicinal plants. CRC Press, Boca Raton, USA.

42. Kesari, A. N., Kesari, S., Singh, S. K., Gupta, R. K., & Geeta, W. (2007). Studies on the glycemic and lipidemic effect of *Murraya koenigii* in experimental animals. *J. Ethnopharmacol.*, *112*, 305–311.

43. Khattab, H. A., Mohamed, R. A., & Hashemi, J. M. (2012). Evaluation of hypoglycemic activity of *Salvia officinalis* L. (Sage) infusion on streptozotocin induced diabetic rats. *J. Amer. Sci.*, *8(11)*, 411–416.

44. Kumar, D. S., & Prabhakar, V. S. (1987). On the ethnomedical significance of the arjuna tree, *Terminalia arjuna* Roxb. *J. Ethnopharmacol.*, *20*, 173–190.

45. Kumar, N., Jakhar, A & Choyal, R. (2014). Traditional uses of some medicinal plants of Hamirpur district of Himachal Pradesh for the treatment of diabetes. *Int. J. Adv. Res, 2(2)*, 131–138.

46. Kumudhavalli, M. V., & Jaykar, B. (2012). Evaluation of antidiabetic activity of *Costus igneus* (L.) leaves on STZ induced diabetic rats. *Der Pharmacia Sinica.*, *3 (1)*, 1–4.

47. Lindberg, G., Lindblad, U., & Melander, A. (2004). Sulfonylureas for treating type 2 diabetes mellitus. *Cochrane Database Systemic Reviews*, 3, 254.

48. Luangpiom, A., Kourjampa, W., & Junaimaung, T. (2013). Anti-hyperglycemic properties of *Moringa oleifera* Lam. Aqueous leaf extract in normal and mildly diabetic mice. *British J. Pharmacol. Toxicol.*, *4 (3)*, 106–109.

49. Maiti, R., Jana, D., Das, U. K & Ghosh, D. (2004). Antidiabetic effect of aqueous extract of seed of *Tamarindus indica* in streptozotocin-induced diabetic rats. *J Ethnopharmacol.*, *92 (1)*, 85–91.

50. Malek, I., Islam, T., Hasan, E., Akter, S., Rana, M., Das, P., Samarrai, W., & Rahmatullah, M. (2012). Medicinal plants used by the mandais – a little known tribe of Bangladesh. *Afr. J. Trad. Complement. Altern. Med.*, *9(4)*, 536–541.

51. Mall, G. K., Mishra, P. K., & Prakash, V. (2009). Antidiabetic and hypolipidemic activity of *Gymnema sylvestre* in alloxan induced diabetic Rats. *Global J. Biotech. & Biochem.*, *4 (1)*, 37–42.

52. Mall, T. P., & Sahani, S. (2013). Diversity of ethnomedicinal plants for diabetes from Bahraich (U. P.) India. *Int. J. Interdiscipl and Multidiscipl Stud.*, *1(1)*, 13–23.

53. Manikandan, P. N. A., Jayendran, M., & Rajasekaran, C. (2006). Study of plants used as antidiabetic agents by the Nilgiri aborigines. *Ancient Science Life*, *3*, 101–103.

54. Manikandan, P. N. A., Dixit, A., & Sudurshan, M. (2011). Review of flora of antidiabetic plants of Puducherry YT. *Int. J. Appl. Pharmaceut. Technol.*, *2*, 455–462.

55. Mansuri, M. I., & Patel, V. M. (2013). Evalution of anti-diabetic and anti-hyperlipidemic activity of *Euphorbia neriifolia* Linn. in high fat diet Streptozotocin induced type-2 diabetic model. *Int. J. Pharmaceutical Res Scholars, 2(1)*, 83–89.

56. Marles, R., & Farnsworth, N. R. (1994). Plants as sources of antidiabetic agents. In: Wagner H., & Farnsworth N. R. (eds.). Economic and Medicinal Plant Research. vol. 6. Academic Press Ltd., UK, pp. 149–187.

57. Marles, R. J., & Farnsworth, N. R. (1995). Antidiabetic plants and their active constituent. *Phytomedicine, 2*, 137–189.

58. Maruthupandian, A., Mohan, V. R., & Kottaimuthu, R. (2011). Ethnomedicinal plants used for the treatment of diabetes and jaundice by Palliyar tribals in Sirumalai hills, Western Ghats, Tamil Nadu, India. *Indian J. Nat. Prod. & Resou., 2(4)*, 493–497.

59. Meddah, B., Ducroc, R., Faouzi, M. E., Eto, B., Mahraoui, L., Benhaddou-Andaloussi A., Martineau, L. C., Cherrah, Y., & Haddad, P. (2009). *Nigella sativa* inhibits intestinal glucose absorption and improves glucose tolerance in rats. *J. Ethnopharmacol., 121*, 419–24.

60. Mishra, A., Srivastava, R., Srivastava, S. P., Gautam, S., Tamrakar, A. K., Maurya, R., & Srivastava, A. K. (2013). Antidiabetic activity of heart wood of *Pterocarpus marsupium* Roxb. and analysis of phytoconstituents. *Indian J. Exp. Biol., 51(5)*, 363–374.

61. Mishra, M. K., & Barik, B. B. (2009). Antidiabetic activity of *Benincasa hispida* (Thunb.) Cogn. fruit peels on alloxan induced diabetic rats. *Indian Drugs 46(10)*, 66–69.

62. Monago, C. C., & Alumanah, E. O. (2005). Antidiabetic effect of chloroform-methanol extract of *Abrus precatorius* Linn. seed in alloxan diabetic rabbit. *J. Appl. Sci. Environ. Mgt. 9(1)*, 85–88.

63. Moran, A., Palmas, W., & Field, L. (2004). Cardiovascular autonomic neuropathy is associated with microalbuminuria in older patients with type 2 diabetes. *Diabetes care, 27*, 972–977.

64. Mukesh, R., Namita, P. (2013). Medicinal plants with antidiabetic potential – A review. *American-Eurasian J. Agric. & Environ. Sci. 13(1)*, 81–94.

65. Naui, M., Dutta, B. K., & Hajra P. K. (2011). Medicinal plants used in major diseases by Dimasa tribe of Barak Valley. *J. Sci. & Tec., 7(1)*, 18–26.

66. Neto, M. C. L., de Vasconcelos, C. F. B., Thijana, G. F. R., Araújo, C. A. V., Costa-Silvac, J. H., Amorima, E. L. C., Ferreira, F., de Oliveirad, A. F. M., & Wanderley, A. G. (2013). Evaluation of antihyperglycaemic activity of *Calotropis procera* leaves extract on streptozotocin-induced diabetes in Wistar rats. *Rev. Bras. Farmacogn., 23*, 913–919.

67. Noor, H., & Ashcroft, S. J. H. (1998). Pharmacological characterisation of the antihyper- glycaemic properties of *Tinospora crispa* extract. *J Ethnopharmacol., 62(1)*, 7–13.

68. Nugroho, A. E., Andrie, M., Warditiani, N. K., Siswanto, E., Pramono, S., & Lukitaningsih, E. (2012). Antidiabetic and antihiperlipidemic effect of *Andrographis paniculata* (Burm. f.) Nees and andrographolide in high-fructose-fat-fed rats. *Indian J. Pharmacol., 44(3)*, 377–381.

69. Olatunde, A., Joel, E. B., Tijjani H., Obidola. S. M., & Luka. C. D. (2014). Anti-diabetic activity of aqueous extract of *Curcuma longa* Linn. rhizome in normal and alloxan-induced diabetic rats. *Researcher, 6(7)*, 58–65.

70. Pant, P. C., & Joshi, M. C. (1993). Studies on some controversial indigenous herbal drugs based on ethnobotanical research: A review. *J. Res. Edu. Indian Med., 12*, 19–29.

71. Patel, D. K., Kumar, R., Prasad, S. K., Sairam, K., & Hemalatha. S. (2011). Antidiabetic and *in vitro* antioxidant potential of *Hybanthus enneaspermus* (Linn.) F. Muell in Streptozotocin-induced diabetic rats. *Asian Pacific J. Trop. Biomed., 1*(4), 316–322.

72. Pavani, M., Sankara Rao, M., Mahendra Nath, M., & Appa Rao, Ch. (2012). Ethnobotanical explorations on anti-diabetic plants used by tribal inhabitants of Seshachalam forest of Andhra Pradesh, India. *Indian J. Fundamental and Applied Life Sci., 2(3),* 100–105.

73. Prabhakaran, J., & Kavitha, D. (2012). Ethnomedicinal importance of mangroves of Pichavaram. *Int. J. Res. Pharmaceut. Biomedical Sci., 3,* 611–614.

74. Pullaiah, T., & Naidu, K. C. (2003). Antidiabetic plants in India and Herbal based Antidiabetic research. Regency Publications, New Delhi, India.

75. Puri, D., Baral, N., & Upadhyaya, B. P. (1997). Indigenous plant remedies in Nepal used in heart diseases. *J. Nepal Med. Assoc., 36,* 334 –337.

76. Pushpakarani, R., & Natarajan, S. (2014). Ethnomedicines used by Kaniyakaran tribes in Kaniyakumari district: Southern Western Ghats of Tamil Nadu, India. *J. Appl. Pharmaceut. Sci., 4(2),* 056–060.

77. Puttaswamy, R., Peethambar, S. K., & Rajeshwara, N. (2013). Achur hypoglycemic activity of *Memecylon umbellatum* leaves methanolic extract world. *J. Pharm. Pharmaceut. Sci., 2(6),* 6202–6211.

78. Ragavan, B., & Krishnakumari, S. (2006). Antidiabetic effect of *Terminalia arjuna* bark extract in alloxan induced diabetic rats. *Indian J. Clinical Biochem., 21 (2),* 123–128.

79. Raghavendra, M. P., Devi Prasad, A. G., & Shyma, T. B. (2015). Investigations on anti-diabetic medicinal plants used by tribes of Wayanad district, Kerala. *Intern. J. Pharmaceut. Sci. Res., 6(8),* 3617–3625.

80. Rai, P. K., Mehta, S., & Watal, G. (2010). Hypolipidaemic and hepatoprotective effects of *Psidium guajava* raw fruit peel in experimental diabetes. *Indian J. Med. Res., 131,* 820–824.

81. Rajendran, A., & Manian, S. (2011). Herbal remedies for diabetes from Kolli hills, Eastern Ghats, India. *J. Nat. Prod. Resour., 2(3),* 383–386.

82. Raju, P., & Mamidala, E. (2015). Anti-diabetic activity of compound isolated from *Physalis angulata* fruit extracts in alloxan induced diabetic rats. *Amer. J. Sci. & Med. Res., 1(1),* 40–43.

83. Rao, B., Murugesan, R., Sanghamitra Sinha, T., Saha, B. P., Pal, M., & Mandal, S. C. (2002). Glucose lowering efficacy of *Ficus racemosa* bark extract in normal and alloxan diabetic rats. *Phytother. Res., 16,* 590–592.

84. Rao, M. U., Sreenivasulu, M., Chengaiah, B., Reddy, K. J., & Chetty, C. M. (2010). Herbal medicines for diabetes mellitus: a review. *Int. J. Pharm. Tech. Res., 2(3),* 1883–1892.

85. Rao, S. A., Vijay, Y., Deepthi, T., Sri Lakshmi, C., Rani, V., Rani, S., Bhuvaneswara Reddy, Y., Swaroop, P. R., Laxmi V. S., Chakravarthy, K. N., & Arun, P. (2013). Anti diabetic effect of ethanolic extract of leaves of *Ocimum sanctum* in alloxan induced diabetes in rats. *Int. J. Basic Clin Pharmacol., 2(5),* 613–616.

86. Rekka, R. Murugesh, S., & Prabakaran, R. (2014). Ethnomedicinal study of plants used for the treatment of diabetetes and antidote for poisonous bite by Malayali tribes of Yercaud hills, southern Eastern Ghats, Salem district, Tamilnadu. *Life Sci. Leaflets, 49,* 89–96.

87. Renuka, C. (2012). Effect of *Biophhytum sensitivum* extracts in the treatment of diabetic albino rats. PhD Thesis submitted to the Bharathidasan University, Tiruchirappalli., India.

88. Renuka, C., Ramesh, N., & K. Saravanan. (2009). Evaluation of the antidiabetic effect of *Trigonella foenum-graecum* seed powder on alloxan-induced diabetic albino rats. *Intern. J. Pharm. Tech. Res. 1(4)*, 1580–1584.

89. Sachdewa, A., & Khemani, L. D. (2003). Effect of *Hibiscus rosa-sinensis* Linn. Ethanol flower extract on blood glucose and lipid profile in streptozotocin induced diabetes in rats. *J. Ethnopharmacol., 89*, 61–66.

90. Saely, C. H., Aczel, S., Marte, T., Lnger, P., & Drexel, H. (2004). Cardiovascular complications in Type 2 diabetes mellitus depend on the coronary angiographic state rather than on the diabetic state. *Diabetologia 47(1)*, 145–146.

91. Sahu, S. (2015). Medico botany of some anti diabetics plants used in sculptures and rituals in Coastal districts of Odisha. *Int. J. Multidiscipl. Res. Develp, 2(3)*, 75–85.

92. Sakuljaitrong, S., Buddhakala, N., Chomko, S., & Talubmook, C. (2013). Effects of flower extract from lotus (*Nelumbo nucifera*) on hypoglycemic and andhypolipidemic in streptozotocin-induced diabetic rats. *IJSRET., 4*, 1441–1446.

93. Saravanan. K. (2008). Evaluation of antidiabetic effect of herbal extract mixture on alloxan induced diabetic rats. *J. Ecotoxicol. Environ. Monit*, 18, 489–494.

94. Saravanan, K., & Karuppannan, P. (2013). Isolation, characterization and evaluation of antidiabetict compounds of traditionally used herbal plants on STZ induced diabetic rats. Annual Report, UGC major research Project, New Delhi. India

95. Sarasa, D., Sridhar, S., & Prabakaran, E. (2012). Effect of an antidiabetic extract of *Trigonella foenum – graecum* on normal and alloxan induced diabetic mice. *Int. J. Pharm. Pharmaceut. Sci., 4(1)*,

96. Sathe, S. S., Lavate, R. A., & Patil, S. B. (2014). Ethnobotanical and medicinal aspects of mangroves from southern Kokan (Maharashtra). *Int. J. Emerging Trends Pharmaceut. Sci., 3(4)*, 12–17.

97. Shabana Begum. M., Muhammad Ilyas. M. H., & Burkanudeen, A.(2011). Protective and curative effects of *Justicia tranquebariensis* (Linn.) leaves in Acetamenophen induced hepatotoxicity. *Int. J. Pharmaceut. & Biol. Arch., 2(3)*, 989–995.

98. Sharma, S., Chaturvedi, M., Edwin, E., Shukla, S., & Sagarwat, H. (2007). Evaluation of the phytochemicals and antidiabetic activity of *Ficus benghalensis*. *Int. J. Diabetes Dev. Ctries.*, 27, 56–59.

99. Shobana, S., Sreerama, Y. N., & Malleshi, N. G. (2009). Composition and enzyme inhibitory properties of finger millet (*Eleusine coracana* L.) seed coat phenolics: mode of inhibition of α-glucosidase and pancreatic amylase. *Food Chem., 115*, 1268–1273.

100. Shukla, N., Angelini, G. D., & Jeremy, J. Y. (2003). Homocysteine as a risk factor for nephropathy and retinopathy in type 2 diabetes. *Diabetologia, 46*, 766–777.

101. Shukla, R., Sharma, S. B., Puri, D., Prabhu, K. M., & Murthy, P. S. (2000). Medicinal plants for treatment of diabetes mellitus. *Indian J. Clin. Biochem., 15*, 169–177.

102. Sikarwar, M. S., & Patil, M. B. (2010). Antidiabetic activity of *Pongamia pinnata* leaf extracts in alloxan-induced diabetic rats. *Int. J. Ayurveda Res., 1*, 199–204.

103. Singh, M. P., & Panda, H. (2005). Medicinal herbs with their formulations. Handbook of Ayurvedic medicinal plants: Herbal Reference Library, Daya Books.

104. Singh, L. W. (2011). Traditional medicinal plants of Manipur as anti-diabetics. *J. Med. Plant Res., 5*, 677–68.

105. Singh, S. N., Vats, P., Suri, S., Shyam, R., Kumria, M. M. L., Ranganathan, S., & Sridharan, K. (2001). Effect of an antidiabetic extract of *Catharanthus roseus* on enzymic activities in streptozotocin induced diabetic rats. *J. Ethnopharmacol., 76*, 269–277.

106. Sivanesan, D., & Anand, V. (2014). Biochemcial antidiabetic and characterization of medicinal plant. *Achyranthes aspera. Int. J. Curr. Res. Chem. Pharmaceut. Sci. 1(1)*, 75–92.

107. Sowmia, C., & Kokilavani, R. (2007). Antidiabetic and antihyperglycolesterolemic effect of *Hemidesmus indicus* Linn. root in alloxan induced diabetic rats. *Ancient Sci. Life, 36*, 4–10.

108. Sucharitha, S., & Mamidala, E. (2013). Evaulation of antidiabetic activity of medicinal plant extracts used by tribal communities in rural areas of Warangal, Andhra Pradesh. *Biol. & Med., 5*, 20–25.

109. Swargiary, A., Boro, H., Brahma, B. K., & Rahman, S. (2013). Ethno-botanical study of anti-diabetic medicinal plants used by the local people of Kokrajhar district of Bodoland Territorial Council, India. *J. Med. Plants Stud., 1(5)*, 51–58.

110. Thirumalai, T., David, B. C., Sathiyaraj, K., Senthilkumar, B., & David, E. (2012). Ethnobotanical study of anti-diabetic medicinal plants used by the local people in Javadhu hills Tamilnadu, India. *Asian Pacific J. Trop. Biomed., 2(2)*, 910–913.

111. Vadivelan, R., Dipanjan, M., Umasankar, M., Sangai, P. D., Satishkumar, M. N., Antony. S., & Elango, K. (2011). Hypoglycemic, antioxidant and hypolipidemic activity of *Asparagus racemosus* on Streptozotocin-induced diabetic in rats. *Adv. Appl. Sci Res., 2*, 179–185.

112. Vidysagar, G. M., & Murthy, S. M. S. (2013). Medicinal plants used in the treatment of Diabetes mellitus in Bellary district, Karnataka. *Indian J. Trad. Knowl., 12(4)*, 747–751.

113. Vineet, C. J., Patel, N. M., & Dhiren, P. (2010). Antioxidant and antimicrobial activities of *Alangium salvifolium* (L. f.) Wang. root. *Global J. Pharmacol., 4*, 13–18.

114. Vijayalakshmi, N., Anbazhagan, M., & Arumugam, K. (2014). Medicinal plants for Diabetes used by the people of Thirumoorthy hills region of Western Ghats, Tamil Nadu, India. *Int. J. Curr. Microbiol. App. Sci., 3(7)*, 405–410.

115. Vishnu, B., Naveen, A., Akshay, K., Mukesh, S., & Patil, M. B. (2010). Antidiabetic activity of insulin plant (*Costus igneus*) leaf extract in diabetic rats. *J. Pharm Res., 3*, 608–611.

116. Wallace, C., Reiber, G. E., & Le Master, J. (2002). Incidence of falls, risk factors for falls, and fall-related factures in individuals with diabetes and a prior foot ulcer. *Diabetes Care, 25*, 1983–1986.

117. Walters, B. B., Ronnback, Kovacs, J. M., Crona, B., Hussain, S. A., Badola, R., Primvera, J. H., Barbier, E., & Dahdouh-Guebas, F. (2008). Ethnobiology, socioeconomics and management of mangrove forests: A review. *Aquatic Bot. 89*, 220–236.

118. Yadav, M., Khan, K. K., & Beg, M. Z. (2012). Medicinal Plants used for the treatment of diabetes by the Baiga tribe living in Rewa District M. P. *Indian J. L. Sci., 2(1)*, 99–102.

CHAPTER 13

ETHNOBOTANY OF ORAL AND DENTAL PROBLEMS IN INDIA

K. V. KRISHNAMURTHY,[1] BIR BAHADUR,[2] S. JOHN ADAMS,[3] and GAUTAM SRIVASTAVA[4]

[1]*Consultant, R&D, Sami Labs Ltd., Peenya Industrial Area, Bangalore, Karnataka, India*

[2]*Department of Botany, Kakatiya University, Warangal–505009, Telangana, India*

[3]*Department of Pharmacognosy, R&D, The Himalaya Drug Company, Makali, Bangalore, Karnataka, India*

[4]*Government Dental College and Hospital, Vijayawada, Andhra Pradesh, India*

CONTENTS

Abstract 354

13.1   Introduction 354

13.2   Teeth Cleaning 355

13.3   Plant-Based Toothbrushes 356

13.4   Toothpastes and Tooth Powders 358

13.5   Oral Diseases and Problems 358

13.6   Discussion 368

Keywords 369

References 369

ABSTRACT

Oral hygiene and dental care has been the subject of different traditional medicinal systems for a very long time in different parts of the world including India. The ethnic tribals living in different parts of India have been using different plants to up keep their oral hygiene and dentition. They used different parts of these plants to brush their teeth and clean them as well as to prevent various types of oral and dental diseases using powders, pastes or extracts of these plants. This review gives a detailed list of such plants used by tribals in different parts of India. However, it is sad that the chemical basis of such uses as well as the therapeutic efficiency of these plants have not been adequately validated till date. These aspects are discussed in this communication.

13.1 INTRODUCTION

Oral hygiene involves the keeping the oral cavity, gingival and the teeth clean and in healthy condition so as to prevent gingival, periodontal and dental problems due to bacteria (mostly commonly, gingivitis, periodontitis and caries) and halitosis (bad breath). Poor dental health can also adversely affect speech and self-esteem (Bairwa et al., 2012) as well as impose financial and social burdens (Jenkinson and Lamont, 2005). Oral and dental problems form one of the most common health hazards among the people of the world and many children and adults are affected by them (Peterson et al., 2005; Muhammad and Lawal, 2010; Szyszkowska et al., 2010). These problems are also prevalent in India in the last 50 to 100 years since there was a major shift among people from the traditional methods of maintaining oral hygiene to more westernized methods. People have almost forgotten the traditional methods of keeping away the oral and dental problems. People losing their teeth at an earlier age (around 40 to 45 years of age) have substantially increased in number in the last four to five decades and more and more people are subjecting themselves to root-canal treatment, bridges and implants.

In addition, western culture has led to improper brushing habits leading to dental caries, gingivitis and periodontitis. This is also partly due to the drastic change in the type of food taken and due to change in dietary habits mostly western. More people now suffer from plaque-forming bacteria and yeasts such as species of *Actinomyces*, *Actinobacillus* and *Candida* (Van Ooster et al., 1987). Dental treatment has also become very expensive and out of reach for the common man, moreover, various chemical agents have been introduced to maintain oral hygiene, which include bisgranide antiseptics, quaternary ammonium antiseptics, phenolic antiseptics, a number of oxygenating agents and even metal ions (Bairwa et al., 2012), which produce many side-effects such as vomiting, diarrhea and discoloration of teeth.

Many antibiotics are being used to treat or prevent gingivitis, periodontitis and infections due to dental caries and this has also have resulted in antibiotic-resistance microbial strains. It is therefore, very essential now to review the traditional methods of oral and dental care that are in existence among the ancient ethnic communities of India. These are not only preventive but are also curative and inexpensive. Many plants have been reported in the various pharmacopoeias of the world that have efficacy to treat oral problems (Cowan, 1999; Kalemba and Kunicka, 2003; Lewis, 1990; Bairwa et al., 2012). India is very rich in traditional medical knowledge, both codified and non-codified, as there are several ancient ethnic tribes living in various parts of India and exploiting the very rich flora around them. This review summarizes the available information on the ethnobotany of oral and dental problems in India.

13.2   TEETH CLEANING

Teeth cleaning refer to the removal of dental plaque formed by microbes and calculus (tartar) so as to prevent the formation of caries, gingivitis and periodontitis. Gingivitis, periodontitis and dental caries causes tooth loss. Caries invariably are formed inside pits and fissures on occlusal surfaces where the toothbrush normally does not easily reach to remove food particles. Sticky film that forms on teeth is well-evident at gingival margins. The bacteria present in the plaque converts the carbohydrate component of the food into organic acids which in turn demineralize the teeth and form caries. Brushing and flossing are used to remove plaque and prevent calculus formation. Good oral hygiene results in preventing plaque and calculus formation and its associated problems.

Flossing removes food particles and plaque at and below the gingival margin and in-between the teeth and the actual method of flossing is described in Bairwa et al. (2012). Gums and resins obtained from some plant species are used in forming chewing gums/resins for maintaining teeth cleanliness. These plants include *Croton* species, *Ficus* species, *Acacia* species, some species of Sapotaceae, etc. Although some of these are of bitter taste and unpleasant flavor they reduce, prevent dental caries and mask halitosis. The leaves of the following three plants are chewed to clean teeth: *Anacardium occidentale*, *Mangifera indica* and *Pongamia pinnata* (Jose et al., 2011); also used are the pericarps of coconut fruit or Areca nut fruit. Chewing sponges are used in Ghana and are made from *Acacia pennata*, *Hibiscus rostellatus* and *Lasianthera africana.* The stems or vines of these plants are collected from the forest, bark removed and beaten on rocks till they become fibrous. This is washed and made into sponges that are about five inches in diameter. To clean the teeth, a small portion of the sponge is placed in the mouth and vigorously chewed for 20–30 minutes.This activity produces foam and stimulates saliva flow. In addition, charcoal, burnt rice bran mixed with salt, soot formed by burning wood, etc. are used by tribes for cleaning their teeth.

13.3   PLANT-BASED TOOTHBRUSHES

Normally plant-based, toothbrushes are used to clean the teeth and the gingiva (Lewis, 1990). Usually one end of these toothbrushes are chewed by the teeth and the extracted juice is allowed to act on the teeth and gingiva where cleaning is needed. This chewing also makes the twig end to look like a brush. Normally tender to semi-mature stem twigs are used, although in some cases the root is also used (for example root of *Senna*). A list of plants of India whose twigs are used as toothbrushes are given in Table 13.1. The juice emanating from these brushes are often antimicrobial, antiseptic and aromatic/flavor so that dental caries, halitosis, etc. are prevented and controlled. Chewed toothbrush sticks impart different tastes such as sweet, bitter, sour, peppery, etc. The twigs used must be smooth, easily chewable, and should not harm. Toothbrush is that there is no need to use toothpaste or tooth powder under normal circumstances. A list of ethnobotanically important toothbrushes is given in Table 13.1.

TABLE 13.1   Stem Twigs Used As Toothbrush

Sl. No	Plant name	Family name	References
1.	*Acacia nilotica*	Mimosaceae	Punjani, 1998; Pratap et al., 2007; Jadhav, 2009; Singh et al., 2013
2.	*Achyranthes aspera*	Amaranthaceae	Punjani, 1998; Pratap et al., 2007; Badgujar et al., 2008; Jadhav, 2009
3.	*Anacardium occidentale*	Anacardiaceae	Jose et al., 2011
4.	*Azadirachta indica*	Meliaceae	Punjani, 1998; Pratap et al., 2007; Jadhav, 2009; Singh et al., 2013
5.	*Bauhinia variegata*	Caesalpiniaceae	Kadhirvel et al., 2010
6.	*Buchanania cochinchinensis*	Anacardiaceae	Singh et al., 2013
7.	*Dicoma tomentosa*	Asteraceae	Katewa and Galav, 2005
8.	*Ehretia laevis*	Boraginaceae	Jagtap et al., 2009
9.	*Ficus benghalensis*	Moraceae	Badgujar et al., 2008
10.	*Flemingia chappar*	Fabaceae	Singh et al., 2013
11.	*Haldina cordifolia*	Rubiaceae	Jagtap et al., 2009
12.	*Jatropha curcas*	Euphorbiaceae	Dinesh, 2006; Natarajan et al., 2010; Singh et al., 2013
13.	*Jatropha gossypifolia*	Euphorbiaceae	Achuta et al., 2010; Pratap et al., 2007; Jose et al., 2011
14.	*Madhuca longifolia*	Sapotaceae	Punjani, 1998; Badgnjar et al., 2008; Singh et al., 2013
15.	*Mangifera indica*	Anacardiaceae	Achuta et al., 2010, Jose et al., 2011
16.	*Miliusa velutina*	Annonaceae	Singh et al., 2013
17.	*Mimusops elengi*	Sapotaceae	Singh et al., 2013
18.	*Phyllanthus reticulatus*	Euphorbiaceae	Singh et al., 2013
19.	*Salvadora persica*	Salvadoraceae	Jose et al., 2011
20.	*Senna sulfurea*	Caesalpiniaceae	Singh et al., 2013
21.	*Shorea robusta*	Dipterocarpaceae	Mohanty, 2003; Singh et al., 2013
22.	*Sida acuta*	Malvaceae	Singh et al., 2013
23.	*Smilax ovalifolia*	Smilacaceae	Mohanty, 2003; Singh et al., 2013
24.	*Smilax zeylanica*	Smilacaceae	Achuta et al., 2010
25.	*Vitex negundo*	Verbenaceae	Punjani, 1998; Singh et al., 2013

13.4   TOOTHPASTES AND TOOTH POWDERS

Traditionally a number of plants were used to prepare toothpastes, powders and gels. A list of plants from which toothpastes and powders are made is given in Table 13.2. Even in artificially made toothpastes and powders many plant extracts/essences are often mixed, e.g., Oils of Eucalyptus, tea, clove, cinnamon, cardamom, betel leaf, etc. A number of chemicals found in these plant materials such as tannins and other phenolics, alkaloids, terpenoids, glycosides, etc., are important not only to clean the teeth and oral cavity but also to prevent/cure oral and dental problems which are mainly caused by different microbes.

13.5   ORAL DISEASES AND PROBLEMS

Ayurveda recognizes the following oral and dental diseases (rogas): Diseases of lips, gums, teeth, tongue, palate and throat (Amruthesh, 2015) with each one labeled differently. Siddha, another traditional codified Indian medical system, recognizes the same diseases although naming them in a different

TABLE 13.2   Plants Used As Tooth Powders and Toothpaste Formulation

Sl. No	Plant	Family	Plant Part	References
1.	*Acacia arabica*	Mimosaceae	Bark tooth powder	Jose et al., 2011
2.	*Achyranthes aspera*	Amaranthaceae	Whole plant ash used as tooth powder	Badgujar et al., 2008
3.	*Albizia lebbeck*	Mimosaceae	Dried bark powder used as tooth powder	Munisamy and Padmavathy, 2010
4.	*Azadirachta indica*	Meliaceae	Whole Plant powder	Bairwa et al., 2012
5.	*Calotropis gigantea*	Asclepiadaceae	Paste of root used as toothpaste	Badgujar et al., 2008
6.	*Elephantopus scaber*	Asteraceae	Root paste with pepper powder	Katewa and Galav, 2005
7.	*Salvadora persica*	Salvadoraceae	Whole Plant	Bairwa et al., 2012
8.	*Tamarindus indica*	Caesalpiniaceae	Bark powder as tooth powder	Natarajan et al., 2010

way. However, as per allopathy dental caries and periodontal diseases are the two most common dental pathologies of the humans. Both caries and gingivitis emerge at an early stage, i.e., even in childhood. Caries is due to excess use of sweets and chocolates and is almost non-reversible and sometimes difficult to treat. On the contrary, gingivitis at an early stage is curable if teeth brushing are done regularly and effectively. The oral diseases in adults are invariably the result of diseases not properly treated or cured in the childhood and are due to age changes in gingiva. Susceptibility to dental carries varies between individuals and between different teeth in the same individual. The configuration of jaw and oral cavity, tooth structure and quantity and quality of saliva produced are all equally important. The other important factor is the type and number of caries-causing bacteria present in the mouth. All these bacteria convert carbohydrates into acids but some species are very powerful acid-producers; the latter's presence in plaque increases the risk of tooth decay. Eating habits and composition of food eaten also play a vital role in dental caries, especially sweets and confectionary carbohydrates, pasta, rice, potato, fruits and bread. On the other hand, milk and milk products especially cheese induce less caries.

Traditional codified and non-codified Indian medical systems employ wide variety of plant materials to prevent and cure the different types of oral/dental diseases and these are mentioned in Table 13.3. A number of plants are also used as mouth fresheners for removing bad breath and to prevent/cure ulcers on lips, tongue and gingiva and these are listed in Table 13.4.

TABLE 13.3 Plants Used Against Tooth Ache and Decay and Gum Problems (Including Pyorrhea)

Sl. No	Plant	Family	Plant Part	References
1.	*Abrus precatorius*	Fabaceae	Leaf	Pandi et al., 2007 Umapriya et al., 2010 Jose et al., 2011
2.	*Abutilon indicum*	Malvaceae	Juice	Chellaiah et al., 2006
3.	*Acacia arabica*	Mimosaceae	Bark, leaves	Jain et al., 2010; Jose et al. 2011
4.	*Acacia arabica*	Mimosaceae	Bark decoction	Amruthesh, 2015
5.	*Acacia catechu*	Mimosaceae	Bark	Jose et al., 2011

TABLE 13.3   (Continued)

Sl. No	Plant	Family	Plant Part	References
6.	*Acalypha indica*	Euphorbiaceae	Whole plant decoction	Shanmugam et al., 2009
7.	*Achillea millefolium*	Asteraceae	Leaves	Khan et al., 2004
8.	*Achyranthes aspera*	Amaranthaceae	Ash of plant Root decoction	Badgujar et al., 2008 Singh et al., 2013
9.	*Agave americana*	Agavaceae	Whole plant	Vanila et al., 2008
10.	*Amaranthus viridis*	Amaranthaceae	Whole plant	Vanila et al., 2008
11.	*Ampelocissus latifolia*	Vitaceae	Tender leaf juice	Achuta et al., 2010
12.	*Annona squamosa*	Annonaceae	Leaf decoction gargled	Singh et al., 2013
13.	*Arnebia euchroma*	Boraginaceae	Roots	Praveen et al., 2006
14.	*Barleria prionitis*	Acanthaceae	Root and leaves chewed	Meena and Yadav, 2010; Achuta et al., 2010
15.	*Basella alba*	Basellaceae	Leaf, seed	Jose et al., 2011
16.	*Berberis aristata*	Berberidaceae	Wood	Amruthesh, 2015
17.	*Bombax ceiba*	Bombacaceae	Bark	Dowlathabad et al., 2006
18.	*Borreria articularis*	Rubiaceae	Whole plant vapor	Kambaska, 2006
19.	*Bridelia scandens*	Euphorbiaceae	Leaf	Jose et al., 2011
20.	*Buchanania lanzan*	Anacardiaceae	Gum	Badgujar et al., 2008
21.	*Caesalpinia sappan*	Caesalpiniaceae	Wood/bark	Amruthesh, 2015
22.	*Cajanus cajan*	Fabaceae	Fruit	Dowlathabad et al., 2006
23.	*Callicarpa macrophylla*	Verbenaceae	Leaf	Amruthesh, 2015
24.	*Calotropis gigantea*	Asclepiadaceae	Latex	Jose et al., 2011
25.	*Calotropis procera*	Asclepiadaceae	Latex	Jadhav, 2009; Singh et al., 2013

TABLE 13.3   (Continued)

Sl. No	Plant	Family	Plant Part	References
26.	*Canarium bengalense*	Burseraceae	Resin	Ganesan et al., 2006
27.	*Carica papaya*	Caricaceae	Latex	Achuta et al., 2010
28.	*Cassia alata*	Caesalpiniaceae	Leaf decoction	Jose et al., 2011
29.	*Cassia occidentalis*	Caesalpiniaceae	Root Paste	Reddy et al., 2008
30.	*Cassia tora*	Caesalpiniaceae	Leaf decoction	Jose et al., 2011
31.	*Centipeda minima*	Asteraceae	Whole plant	Achuta et al., 2010
32.	*Cleistanthus collinus*	Euphorbiaceae	Leaf	Dowlathabad et al., 2006
33.	*Cyperus rotundus*	Cyperaceae	Rhizome	Amruthesh, 2015
34.	*Datura stramonium*	Solanaceae	Seed paste	Phondani et al., 2010
35.	*Desmodium gangeticum*	Fabaceae	Root	Badgujar et al., 2008
36.	*Desmodium triflorum*	Fabaceae	Whole plant	Achuta et al., 2010
37.	*Desmodium velutinum*	Fabaceae	Young stem	Jagtap et al., 2009
38.	*Desmostachya* sp.	Poaceae	Root powder	Badgujar et al., 2008
39.	*Dipterocarpus alatus*	Dipterocarpaceae	Bark	Amruthesh, 2015
40.	*Drosera peltata*	Droseraceae	Whole plant	Bairwa et al., 2012
41.	*Embelia ribes*	Myrsinaceae	Fruit/seed	Amruthesh, 2015
42.	*Emilia sonchifolia*	Asteraceae	Leaf juice	Badgujar et al., 2008
43.	*Erythrina indica*	Fabaceae	Leaf decoction	Jose et al., 2011
44.	*Erythrina variegata*	Fabaceae	Leaf	Jose et al., 2011
45.	*Ferula asafoetida*	Apiaceae	Root extract	Dinesh, 2006
46.	*Ficus benghalensis*	Moraceae	Latex	Jain et al., 2010; DeBritto and Mahesh, 2007
	Ficus benghalensis	Moraceae	Latex	Jose et al., 2011

TABLE 13.3 (Continued)

Sl. No	Plant	Family	Plant Part	References
47.	*Ficus religiosa*	Moraceae	Tender twigs	Badgujar et al., 2008
48.	*Glycosmis pentaphylla*	Rutaceae	Leaf, Seed	Animesh et al., 2010
49.	*Gossypium herbaceum*	Malvaceae	Seed ash	Koche et al., 2008
50.	*Gynocardia odorata*	Achariaceae	Leaf	Pranjiv et al., 2009
51.	*Hemidesmus indicus*	Asclepiadaceae	Root	Amruthesh, 2015
52.	*Hugonia mystax*	Linaceae	Root	Dowlathbad et al., 2006
53.	*Hyoscyamus niger*	Solanaceae	Seed smoke	Dolui et al., 2004
54.	*Indigofera aspalathoides*	Fabaceae	Powdered root	Pandi et al., 2007
55.	*Jatropha curcas*	Euphorbiaceae	Root decoction, Leaf, Stem twig	Rao et al., 1996; Pratap et al., 2007; Jose et al., 2011
56.	*Jatropha glandulifera*	Euphorbiaceae	Latex	Sivaperumal et al., 2010
57.	*Jatropha gossypifolia*	Euphorbiaceae	Latex	Jadhav, 2009
58.	*Justicia diffusa*	Acanthaceae	Leaves boiled in gingelly oil	Meena and Yadav, 2010; Pandi et al., 2007
59.	*Lavandula bipinnata*	Lamiaceae	Leaf paste	Shubangi and Patil, 2004
60.	*Lawsonia alba*	Lythraceae	Stem bark	Badgujar et al., 2008
61.	*Leucas aspera*	Lamiaceae	Leaf	Sivaperumal et al., 2010
62.	*Madhuca longifolia*	Sapotaceae	Stem bark	Rao et al., 1996; Singh et al., 2013
63.	*Mangifera indica*	Anacardiaceae	Leaf decoction	Jose et al., 2011
64.	*Melastoma malabathricum*	Melastomataceae	Root	Rethy et al., 2010
65.	*Mikania* sp.	Asteraceae	Whole plant	Bairwa et al., 2012

TABLE 13.3   (Continued)

Sl. No	Plant	Family	Plant Part	References
66.	*Mimusops elengi*	Sapotaceae	Fruit and bark juice	Rao et al., 1996; Pratap et al., 2007; Rout and Panda 2010; Dolui et al., 2004
67.	*Mollugo cerviana*	Molluginaceae	Seed	Amruthesh, 2015
68.	*Moringa oleifera*	Moringaceae	Root bark fresh juice	Jose et al., 2011
69.	*Mukia maderaspatana*	Cucurbitaceae	Root decoction & Root	Shanmugan et al., 2009; Badgujar et al., 2008
70.	*Murraya paniculata*	Rutaceae	Stem	Badgujar et al., 2008
71.	*Myrica nagi*	Myricaceae	Nut	Amruthesh, 2015
72.	*Onosma bracteatum*	Boraginaceae	Leaf	Amruthesh, 2015
73.	*Pedalium murex*	Pedaliaceae	Leaf	Achuta et al., 2010
74.	*Phyllanthus emblica*	Euphorbiaceae	Fruit	Udhayam et al., 2005; Murthy et al., 2008
75.	*Phyllanthus reticulatus*	Euphorbiaceae	Stem	Rao et al., 1996; Singh et al., 2013
76.	*Piper betle*	Piperaceae	Leaf decoction	Jose et al., 2011
77.	*Piper cubeba*	Piperaceae	Whole plant	Bairwa et al., 2012
78.	*Piper longum*	Piperaceae	Fruit	Amruthesh, 2015
79.	*Piper nigrum*	Piperaceae	Seed	Amruthesh, 2015
80.	*Plantago major*	Plantaginaceae	Leaf extract	Jagtap et al., 2009
81.	*Plumeria alba*	Apocynaceae	Bark paste	Singh et al., 2013
82.	*Pongamia pinnata*	Fabaceae	Tender twigs	Badgujar et al., 2008
83.	*Potentilla fulgens*	Rosaceae	Root and leaf decoction	Semwal et al., 2010
84.	*Potentilla lineata*	Rosaceae	Root paste	Phondani et al., 2010
85.	*Psidium guajava*	Myrtaceae	Leaf decoction	Jose et al., 2011
86.	*Pterocarpus marsupium*	Fabaceae	Stem powder	Singh et al., 2013
87.	*Pterocarpus santalinus*	Fabaceae	Wood	Amruthesh, 2015

TABLE 13.3   (Continued)

Sl. No	Plant	Family	Plant Part	References
88.	*Pueraria tuberosa*	Fabaceae	Root oil	Amruthesh, 2015
89.	*Punica granatum*	Punicaceae	Bark	Amruthesh, 2015
90.	*Ricinus communis*	Euphorbiaceae	Fried cotyledon (in mustard oil) smoke	Badgujar et al., 2008
91.	*Rubia cordifolia*	Rubiaceae	Leaf paste	Udhayan et al., 2005
92.	*Salix caprea*	Salicaceae	-	Amruthesh, 2015
93.	*Santalum album*	Santalaceae	Heart wood paste	Amruthesh, 2015
94.	*Sapindus trifoliatus*	Sapindaceae	Seed exudates	Singh et al., 2013
95.	*Saussurea costus*	Asteraceae	Tuber decoction	Phondani et al., 2010
96.	*Saussurea lappa*	Asteraceae	-	Amruthesh, 2015
97.	*Scoparia dulcis*	Scrophulariaceae	Whole plant	Achuta et al., 2010
98.	*Semecarpus anacardium*	Anacardiaceae	Leaf	Dowlathabad et al., 2006
99.	*Shorea robusta*	Dipterocarpaceae	Resin	Pratap et al., 2007
100.	*Solanum ferox*	Solanaceae	Smoke of fruit	Veeramuthu et al., 2006
101.	*Solanum surattense*	Solanaceae	Dried fruit smoke	Meena and Yadav 2010; Kadhirvel et al., 2010; Sivaperumal et al., 2010
102.	*Solanum torvum*	Solanaceae	Seed	Rethy et al., 2010
103.	*Solanum viarum*	Solanaceae	Smoked seed	Singh et al., 2013
104.	*Solanum virginianum*	Solanaceae	Burnt fruit/ seed	Singh et al., 2013; Jadhav, 2009
105.	*Solanum xanthocarpum*	Solanaceae	Smoke of fruit	Veeramuthu et al., 2006
106.	*Solanum xanthocarpum*	Solanaceae	Leaf/Fruit	Amruthesh, 2015
107.	*Spilanthes acmella*	Asteraceae	Flower	Revathi and Parimelazhagan, 2010
108.	*Spilanthes aromaticum*	Asteraceae	Flowers	Jose et al., 2011

TABLE 13.3 (Continued)

Sl. No	Plant	Family	Plant Part	References
109.	*Spilanthes calva*	Asteraceae	Root and inflorescence	Pratap et al., 2007; Badgujar et al., 2008 Ganesan et al., 2006; Singh et al., 2013
110.	*Spilanthes paniculata*	Asteraceae	Root and leaf	Prusti and Behera, 2007
111.	*Symplocos racemosa*	Symplocaceae	Stem bark or its decoction	Rao et al., 1996; Singh et al., 2013
112.	*Syzygium cumini*	Myrtaceae	Nut	Amruthesh, 2015
113.	*Tabernaemontana divaricata*	Apocynaceae	Latex	Albert and Kuldip, 2010
114.	*Tectona grandis*	Verbenaceae	Wood	Jose et al., 2011
115.	*Terminalia alata*	Combretaceae	Stem bark	Pratap et al., 2007
116.	*Terminalia arjuna*	Combretaceae	Bark	Amruthesh, 2015
117.	*Thevetia peruviana*	Apocynaceae	Latex	Achuta et al., 2010
118.	*Toddalia asiatica*	Rutaceae	Seed	Igacimuthu et al., 2006; Bipul et al., 2010
119.	*Tragia involucrata*	Euphorbiaceae	Bark paste	Singh et al., 2013
120.	*Trapa bispinosa*	Trapaceae	Fruit	Amruthesh, 2015
121.	*Trewia nudiflora*	Euphorbiaceae	Bark Paste	Singh et al., 2013
122.	*Vitex negundo*	Verbenaceae	Leaf Paste	Singh et al., 2013
123.	*Wrightia tinctoria*	Apocynaceae	Leaf paste	Kottaimuthu, 2008
124.	*Wrightia tinctoria*	Apocynaceae	Stem Bark	Singh et al., 2013
125.	*Zanthoxylum alatum*	Rutaceae	Seed	Prasanna et al., 2010
126.	*Zingiber officinale*	Zingiberaceae	Rhizome	Amruthesh, 2015
127.	*Ziziphus rugosa*	Rhamnaceae	Bark decoction	Singh et al., 2013

TABLE 13.4   Mouth Fresheners, Mouth Washes and Mouth Ulcers (Stomatitis)

Sl. No	Plant	Family	Parts used	References
1.	*Abrus precatorius*	Fabaceae	Juice of tender leaf for ulcers	Jose et al., 2011
2.	*Acacia arabica*	Mimosaceae	Bark for mouth ulcers	Jain et al., 2010
3.	*Achillea millefolium*	Asteraceae	Leaf as mouth freshener	Khan et al., 2004
4.	*Ageratum conyzoides*	Asteraceae	Leaf for mouth ulcer	Rout and Panda, 2010
5.	*Albizia amara*	Mimosaceae	Leaf, bark, fruit for mouth ulcers	Kadaval and Dixit, 2009
6.	*Artocarpus heterophyllus*	Moraceae	Ash of fruit spines for mouth ulcers	Patil and Patil, 2005
7.	*Azadirachta indica*	Meliaceae	Flowers for mouth infections	Natarajan et al. 2010; Chellaiah et al., 2006; Munisamy and Padmavathy, 2010
8.	*Caesulia axillaris*	Asteraceae	Roots	Achuta et al., 2010
9.	*Calotropis gigantea*	Asclepiadaceae	Latex for mouth ulcers	Jose et al., 2011
10.	*Carica papaya*	Caricaceae	Mouth ulcers	Jose et al., 2011
11.	*Cassia alata*	Caesalpiniaceae	Leaf and flowers for ulcers	Jose et al., 2011
12.	*Cassia javanica*	Caesalpiniaceae	Young leaf to remove bad breath	Ganesan et al., 2006
13.	*Cedrus deodora*	Coniferae	Resin	Amruthesh, 2015
14.	*Commiphora mukul*	Burseraceae	Resin	Amruthesh, 2015
15.	*Crotalaria retusa*	Fabaceae	Whole plant	Revathi and Parimelazhagan, 2010
16.	*Cuminum cymimum*	Apiaceae	Seed for mouth ulcer	Prusti and Behera, 2007
17.	*Ficus virens*	Moraceae	Decoction for mouth ulcers	Achuta et al., 2010

TABLE 13.4 (Continued)

Sl. No	Plant	Family	Parts used	References
18.	*Garcinia indica*	Clusiaceae	Fruit as mouth wash material	Bairwa et al., 2012; Almas, 1999
19.	*Glycyrrhiza glabra*	Fabaceae	Root	Amruthesh, 2015
20.	*Hemidesmus indicus*	Periplocaceae	Root paste for mouth ulcers	Udhayan et al., 2005
21.	*Indigofera tinctoria*	Fabaceae	Young branches for ulcers	Jose et al., 2011
22.	*Jatropha villosa*	Euphorbiaceae	Latex for mouth ulcer	Kottaimuthu, 2008
23.	*Lawsonia inermis*	Lythraceae	Fresh leaf for mouth ulcers	Rout and Panda, 2010; Revathi and Parimezhagan, 2010
24.	*Momordica charantia*	Cucurbitaceae	Fruit	Jose et al., 2011
25.	*Nelumbium speciosum*	Nymphaeaceae	Flower	Amruthesh, 2015
26.	*Ocimum basilicum*	Lamiaceae	Fresh leaf for mouth ulcers	Rout and Panda, 2010; Revathi and Parimezhagan, 2010
27.	*Plumeria obtusa*	Apocynaceae	Latex to cure mouth ulcers	Kadhirvel et al., 2010
28.	*Piper betle*	Piperaceae	Leaf for removing floul smell of mouth	Praveen et al. 2006; Jose et al., 2011
29.	*Plumeria acutifolia*	Apocynaceae	Latex to cure mouth ulcers	Sivaperumal et al., 2010
30.	*Psidium guajava*	Myrtaceae	Leaf for mouth ulcers	Prasanna et al., 2010
31.	*Ricinus communis*	Euphorbiaceae	Seed oil (external application)	Amruthesh, 2015
32.	*Sesamum indicum*	Pedaliaceae	Seed oil (external application)	Amruthesh, 2015
33.	*Sesbania grandiflora*	Fabaceae	Boiled leaf for mouth ulcers	Natarajan et al., 2010

TABLE 13.4   (Continued)

Sl. No	Plant	Family	Parts used	References
34.	*Solanum nigrum*	Solanaceae	Cooked leaf/ fruit for mouth ulcers	Mohana et al., 2008; Kingston et al., 2007
35.	*Solanum nigrum*	Solanaceae	Leaf and Fruit	Amruthesh, 2015
36.	*Sphaeranthus indicus*	Asteraceae	Inflorescence	Amruthesh, 2015
37.	*Symplocos racemosa*	Symplocaceae	Leaf	Amruthesh, 2015
38.	*Syzygium cumini*	Myrtaceae	Bark decoction as mouth wash, flower buds	Jose et al., 2011
39.	*Tamarindus indica*	Caesalpiniaceae	Fruit to treat ulcers	Jose et al., 2011
40.	*Terminalia chebula*	Combretaceae	Fruit to treat ulcers	Jose et al., 2011
41.	*Thysanolaena maxima*	Poaceae	Root decoction for mouth ulcers	Udhayan et al., 2005
42.	*Trichosanthes dioica*	Cucurbitaceae	Root ulcer	Amruthesh, 2015

13.6   DISCUSSION

It is sad to note that there is no baseline catalog available for listing and describing the plants used for the ethnomedical treatments of dental and oral diseases (Colvard et al., 2006). There is also a significant lack of published research work on the ethnography, ethnomedicine, ethnopharmacology and clinical application of plant-based medicines that are specifically used for dental and oral diseases. Most publications on hand merely describe anecdotal dental therapeutic applications of the current medical uses of ethnobotanicals. These papers at best provide various descriptive dental therapies attributed to traditional herbs (Yatsu, 1985; Boisyvon, 1986; Jacobsen and Cohan, 1998; Ocasio et al., 1999; see also Colvard et al., 2006; Szyszkowska et al., 2010). There are also research papers that deal with individual plants that are used for dental and oral healthcare (see detailed literature in Colvard et al., 2006). There are also reference books that describe the possible medical applications of ethnobotanicals (Johnson, 1999; Gage and Pickett, 2005). From the foregoing review it is evident that:

1. There is the lack of proper recording/database of the ethnographic component within dental and oral and medicine.
2. There is a lack of clinical documentation of the ethnomedical treatment for the dental/oral diseases experienced by ethnic people in their actual cultural and socio-ecological settings.
3. There are no details on the phytochemical basis of why these plants are used against oral and dental diseases.

To conclude there is thus an urgent need to establish the chemical basis for all the ethnobotanical plants listed in this paper so as to prove the veracity of the claims made on them by various researchers.

KEYWORDS

- caries
- dental care
- gingival
- mouth ulcers
- oral hygiene
- tooth paste
- tooth powders

REFERENCES

1. Achuta, N. S., Sharad, S., & Rawat, A. K. S. (2010). An ethnobotanical study of medicinal plants of Rewa districts, Madhya Pradesh. *Indian J. Trad. Knowl. 9*, 191–202.
2. Albert, L. S., & Kuldip, G. (2010). Ethnobotanical investigations among the Lushai tribes in North Cachar hills district of Assam, northeast India. *Indian J. Trad. Knowl. 9*, 108–113.
3. Almas, K. (1999). The antimicrobial effects of extracts of *Azadirachta indica* (Neem) and *Salvadora persica* (Arak) chewing sticks. *Indian J. Dental Research 10*, 23–26.

4. Amruthesh, S. (2011). Dentistry & Ayurveda V: An Evidence based approach. *Intern. J. Clinical Dental Sci. 2*, 3–9.

5. Amruthesh, S. (2015). Dentistry and Ayurveda-IV: Classification and Management of Common oral diseases. *Indian J. Dental Res. 19*, 52–61.

6. Animesh, B., Moheshweta, B. R. M. A., & Bhadra, S. K. (2010). Inherited folk pharmaceutical knowledge of tribal people in the Chittagong hill tracts, Bangladesh. *Indian J. Trad. Knowl. 9*, 77–89.

7. Badgujar, S. B., Maharajan, R. T., & Kosalge, S. B. (2008). Traditional practice for oral health care in Nandurbar district of Maharashtra, India. *Ethnobot. Leaflets. 12*, 1137–44.

8. Bairwa, R. Gupta, P., Gupta, V. K., & Strivastava, B. (2012). Traditional medicinal plants: Use in oral hygiene. *Internal J. Pharmaceut. Chem. Sci. 1*, 1529–1538.

9. Bipul, S., Borthakar, S. K., & Saikia, N. (2010). Medico-ethnobotany of Bodo trials in Gohpur of Sonitpur district, Assam, *Indian J. Trad. Knowl. 9*, 52–54.

10. Boisyvon, M. F. (1986). Use of plants in dental therapeutics and current oral medicine. *L'Formation Dentaire. 68*, 3309–3314.

11. Chellaiah, M., Muniappan, A. Nagappan, R., & Savarimuthu, I. (2006). Medicinal plants used by traditional healers in Kancheepuram District of Tamil Nadu, India. *J. Ethnobiol. Ethnomed. 2*, 43.

12. Colvard, M. D., Cordell, G. A., Villalobos, R., Sancho, G., Soejarto, D. D., Pestle, W., Echeverri, T. L., Perkowitz, K. M., & Michel, J. (2006). Survey of medical ethnobotanicals for dental and oral medicine conditions and pathologies. *J. Ethnopharmacol. 107*, 134–142.

13. Cowan, M. M. (1999). Plant Products as antimicrobial Agent. *Clin. Micro. Rev. 12*, 564–582.

14. De Britto, J., & Mahesh. (2007). Evolutionary medicine of Kani Tribal's botanical knowledge in Agasthiyamalai Biosphere Reserve, South India. *Ethnobotanical Leaflets 11*, 280–290.

15. Dinesh, J. (2006). Ethnomedicinal plants used by Bhil tribe of bidbod, Madhya Pradesh. *Indian J. Trad. Knowl. 5*, 263–267.

16. Dolui, A. K., Sharma, H. K., Theresia, B. M., & Lalhriatpuii, T. C. (2004). Folk herbal remedies from Meghalaya. *Indian J. Trad. Knowl. 3*, 358–364.

17. Dowlathabad, M. R., Buvu, R., & Sudharshanam, G. (2006). Ethnomedico-botanical studies from Rayalaseema region of Southern Eastern Ghats, Andhra Pradesh, India. *Ethnobotanical Leaflets 10*, 198–207.

18. Gage, T., & Pickett, F. (2005). Mosby's Dental Drug Reference, 7th ed. Mosby, St. Louis. 858–897.

19. Ganesan, S., Venkatesan, G., & Bhanumathi, N. (2006). Medicinal plants used by ethnic group Thottinaickkans of Semmali (Reserved forest), Thiruchirapalli district, Tamil nadu. *Indian J. Trad. Knowl. 5*, 245–252.

20. Ignacimuthu, S., Ayyanar, M., & Sankara, S. K. (2006). Ethnobotanical investigations among tribes in Madurai District of Tamil Nadu (India). *J. Ethnobiol Ethnomed. 2*, 1–7.

21. Jacobsen, P. L., & Cohan, R. P. (1998). Alternative dental products. *J. California Dental Association. 26*, 191–198.

22. Jadhav, D. (2009). Ethno-Medicinal Plants used for dental troubles by the Bhill tribes of Ratlam district (M.), India. *Indian For. 135*, 140–142.

23. Jagtap, S. D., Deokule, S., Pawar, P. K., & Harsulkar, A. M. (2009). Traditional Ethnomedicinal knowledge confined to the Pawra tribe of Satpura hills, Maharashtra, India. *Ethnobotanical Leaflets. 13*, 98–115.

24. Jain, D. L., Baheti, A. M., Jain, S. R., & Khandelwal, K. R. (2010). Use of medicinal plants among tribes in Satpuda region of Dhule and Jalgaon districts of Maharashtra: A ethno botanical survey. *Indian J. Trad. Knowl. 9*, 152–157.

25. Jenkinson, H. F., & Lamont, R. J. (2005). Oral microbial communities in sickness and in health. *Trends in Microbiol. 13*, 589–595.

26. Johnson, T. (1999). CRC Ethnobotany Desk Reference. CRC Press, Boca Raton: Florida.

27. Jose, M. Bhagya, B., & Shantaram, M. (2011). Ethnomedicinal herbs used in oral health and hygiene in coastal Dakshina Kannada. *J. Oral health Community Dentistry 5*, 119–123.

28. Kadaval, K., & Dixit, A. K. (2009). Ethno medical studies of the woody species of Kalrayan and Shervarayan hills, Eastern Ghats, Tamil Nadu. *Indian J. Trad. Knowl. 8*, 592–597.

29. Kadhirvel, K., Ramya, S., Palin, S. S. T., Veera, R. A., & Rajasekaran. C. (2010). Ethnomedicinal Survey of Plants used by tribals in Chitteri Hills. *Environ. We. Int. J. Sci. Tech. 5*, 35–46.

30. Kalemba, D., & Kunicka, A. (2003). Antibacterial and antifungal properties of essential oils. *Current Medicinal Chem. 10*, 813–829.

31. Kambaska, K. B. (2006). Ethnomedicinal plants used by the tribals of Similipal Bioreserve, Orissa, India: A pilot study. *Ethnobot Leaflets 10*, 149–173.

32. Katewa, S. S., & Galav, P. K. (2005). Traditional herbal medicines from Shekhawati Region of Rajasthan. *Indian J. Trad. Knowl. 4*, 237–245.

33. Khan, Z. S., Khuroo, A. A., & Dar, G. H. (2004). Ethnomedicinal survey of Uri, Kashmir Himalaya. *Indian J. Trad. Knowl. 3*, 351–57.

34. Kingston, C., Nisha, B. S., Kiruba, S., & Jeeva, S. (2007). Ethnomedicinal plants used by Indigenous community in a traditional healthcare system. *Ethnobot Leaflets 11*, 32–37.

35. Koche, D. K., Shirsat, R. P., Syed, I., Mohd. Nafees, Zingare, A. K., & Donode, K. A. (2008). Ethnomedicinal survey of Nagzira wild Life Sanctuary, District Gondia (M.S.) India- Part II. *Ethnobotanical Leaflets 12*, 532–537.

36. Kottaimuthu, R. (2008). Ethnobotany of the Valaiyans of Karandamalai, Dindigul district, Tamil Nadu, India. *Ethnobot Leaflets 12*, 195–203.

37. Kumar, R. P. (2014). Ethno Medicinal Plants used for oral health care in India. *Intern. J. Herbal Medicine. 2*, 81–87.

38. Lewis, M. E. (1990). Plants and Dental health. *J. Preventive Dentistry. 6*, 75–78.

39. Meena, K. L., & Yadav, B. L. (2010). Some ethnomedicinal plants of Rajasthan, *Indian J. Trad. Knowl. 9*, 191–202.

40. Mohana, V. R., Rajesh, A., Athiperumalsami, T., & Suthae, S. (2008). Ethnomedicinal plants of the Tirunelveli District, Tamil Nadu, India. *Ethnobot Leaflets 12*, 79095.

41. Mohanty, R. B. (2003). Oral and dental healthcare in folklores of Orissa: An ethnobotanical observation. *Ethnobotany. 15*, 125–126.

42. Muhammad, S., & Lawal, M. T. (2010). Oral hygiene and the use of plants. *Scientific Research and Essays. 5*, 1788–1795.

43. Munisamy, A., & Padmavathy, A. A. (2010). Ethno-medicinal plants in five Sacred Groves in Cuddalore district, Tamil Nadu, India. *Ethnobot. Leaflets. 14*, 774–80.

44. Murthy, E. N., Sudhakar, R. C., Reddy, K. N., & Raju, V. S. (2008). Ethnomedicinal observations from the Maha-Muthuram and Yamanpally tribal villages of Kari-mangar, East Forest Division of Andhra Pradesh, India. *Ethnobotanical Leaflets 12*, 513–19.

45. Natarajan, D., Balaguru, B., Nagamurugan, N., Soosairaj, S., & Natarajan, E. (2010). Ethno-medical-botanical survey in the Malliagainatham Village, Kandankathri taluk, Pudukottai district, Tamilnadu. *Indian J. Trad. Knowl. 9*, 768–774.

46. Ocasio, N. A., Solomowitz, B. H., & Sher, M. R., (1999). Natural remedies recommended for the management of oral health. *New York State Dental Journ. 65*, 22–24.

47. Pandi, K. P., Ayyanar, M., & Ignacimuthu, S. (2007). Medicinal Plants used by Mala-sar tribes of Coimbatore district, Tamil nadu. *Indian J. Trad. Knowl. 6*, 579–582.

48. Patil, M. V., & Patil, D. A. (2005). Ethno medicinal practice of Nasik district of Maharashtra. *Indian J. Trad. Knowl. 4*, 287–290.

49. Peterson, P. E., Bourgeois, D. Ogawa, H. Estupinan-Day, E., & Nidiaye, C. (2005). The global burden of oral diseases and risks to oral health. *Bulletin of the World Health Organization. 9*, 661–669.

50. Phondani, P. C., Maikhuri, R. K., Rawat, L. S., Farooquee, N. A., Kala, C. P., & Vish-vakarma, S. C. R. (2010). Ethnobotanical uses of plants among the Bhotiya tribal communities of Niti Valley in Central Himalaya, India. *Ethnobotany Research & Applications 8*, 233–244.

51. Pranjiv, S., Dudam, S., Anju, J., Moushumi, D., & Hirendra, N. S. (2009). Traditional health practices among the Tagin tribe of Arunachal Pradesh. *Indian J. Trad. Knowl. 8*, 127–130.

52. Prasanna, K. S., Pitamber, P. D., & Mihin, D. (2010). Indigenous medical practices of Bhotia tribal community in Indian Central Himalaya. *Indian J. Trad. Knowl. 9*, 140–144.

53. Pratap, A., Kumar, A., & Yadav. D. K. (2007). Herbal remedies for dental care system in Gaya district, Bihar. pp. 167–170. In: Singh, V. (Ed.). Indian folk medicine and other plant based products. Scientific Publishers, Jodhpur.

54. Praveen, K. S., Sethi, G. S., Sharma, S. K., & Sharma, T. K. (2006). Ethnomedicinal observations among the inhabitants of cold deserts of Himachal Pradesh. *Indian J. Trad. Knowl. 5*, 358–361.

55. Prusti, A. B., & Behera, K. K. (2007). Ethnobotanical exploration of Malkangiri district of Orissa, India. *Ethnobot Leaflets 11*, 122–140.

56. Punjani, B. L. (1998). Plants used as toothbrush by tribes of district Sabarkantha (North Gujarat), *Ethnobotany 10*, 133–135.

57. Rao, B. N. S., Rajasekhar, D., Raju, D. C., & Nagaraju, N. (1996). Ethnomedicinal notes on some plants of Tirumala Hills for dental disorders, *Ethnobotany 8*, 88–91.

58. Reddy, K. N., Reddy, C. S., & Raju, V. S. (2008). Ethnomedicinal observations among the Kondareddis of Khammam district, Andhra Pradesh, India. *Ethnobot Leaflets 12*, 916–26

59. Rethy, P., Singh, B., Kagyung, R., & Gajural, P. R. (2010). Ethnobotanical studies of Dehang-Debang biosphere reserve of Arunachal Pradesh with special reference to Membe tribe. *Indian J. Trad. Knowl. 9*, 61–67.

60. Revathi, P., & Parimezhagan, T. (2010). Traditional knowledge on medicinal plants used by the Irula tribe of Hasanur Hills, Erode district, Tamil Nadu, *Ethnobotanical Leaflets 14*, 136–60.

61. Rout, S. D., & Panda, S. K. (2010). Ethnomedicinal plant resources of Mayurbhaj District, Orrisa. *Indian J. Trad. Knowl. 9*, 68–72.

62. Semwal, D. P., Pardhasaradhi, P., Kala, C. P., & Sajwan, B. S. (2010). Medicinal plants used by local vaidhyas in Ukhimath block, Uttharakhand. *Indian J. Trad. Knowl. 9*, 480–485.

63. Shanmugan, S., Gayathri, N., Sakthivel, B., Ramar, S., & Rajendran, K. (2009). Plants used as Medicine by Paliyar Tribes of Shenbagathope in Virudhunagar District of Tamil Nadu. *Indian Ethnobotanical Leaflets 13*, 370–78.

64. Shubangi, P., & Patil, D. A. (2004). Observation on folkloric medicinal plants of Jalgaon District, Maharaastra. *Indian J.Trad. Knowl. 4*, 437–441.

65. Singh, H., Krishna, G., & Baske, P. K. (2013). Ethnomedicinal plants used for dental care in Sundargarh, Mayurbhanj, Angul and Balangir districts of Odisha, India. *Indian J. Nat. Prod. Resources. 4*, 419–424.

66. Sivaperumal, R., Ramya, S., Veera, R. A., Rajasekaran, C., & Jayakumarajaj, R. (2010). Ethnopharmacological studies on the medicinal plants used by tribal inhabitants of Kottur Hills, Dharmapuri, Tamilnadu, India. *Environ.We Int. J Sci, 5*, 57–64.

67. Szyszkowska, A., Koperm, J., Szczerba, J., Pulawska, M., & Zajdel, D. (2010). The use of medicinal plants in dental treatment. *Herba polonica. 56*, 97–106.

68. Udhayan, P. S., Sateesh, G., Thuskar, K. V., & Indra, B. (2005). Ethno medicine of the Chellipale community of Namakkal district, Tamil Nadu, *Indian J. Trad. Knowl.4*, 437–442.

69. Umapriya, T., Rajendran, A., Aravindhan, V., Binu Thomas. & Maharajan, M. (2010). Traditional medication of Namakal district, Tamil Nadu. *Global J. Pharmacol. 4*, 107–110.

70. Van Ooster, M. A., Mikx, F. H., & Rengi, H. H. (1987). Microbial and clinical measurement of periodontal pockets during sequential periods of non-treatment, mechanical debridement and metronidazole therapy. *J. Clinical Periodontol. 14*, 197–204.

71. Vanila, D. Ghanthikumar, S., & Manickam, V. S. (2008). Ethnomedicinal uses of plants in the plains area of the Tirunelveli District, Tamil Nadu, India. *Ethnobotanical Leaflets 12*, 1198–1205.

72. Veeramuthu, D., Muniappan, A., & Savarimuthu, I. (2006). Antimicrobial activity of some ethnomedicinal plants used by Paliyar tribe from Tamil Nadu, India, *BMC Complement Altern. Med. 6*, 35.

73. Yatsu, M. (1985). Miscellaneous records of medico-dental and Pharmacological history. Secret book on oral medicine published in 1762. *Shikai Tenbo. 66*, 1138–1139.

INDEX

A

Aagya, 64, 71, 72
Aalaav, 213
Aboriginal tribes, 61, 210, 211, 238
Abortifacient, 99
Abortion, 217, 220, 229, 245, 257
Abrus precatorius, 109, 212, 216, 239, 320, 359, 366
Acacia, 62, 64, 68, 78, 79, 81, 82, 109, 171, 187, 211, 216, 239, 321, 356–359, 366
Academic ethnobotany, 272
Academicians, 49, 252
Accountability, 59
Adiantum
    caudatum, 62, 110
    phillippense, 62
Administrative districts, 28
Aegle marmelos, 110, 187, 216, 321
African tribes, 281
Agarsita, 81
    Xanthium strumarium, 81, 149
Ageratum conyzoides, 108, 110, 171, 172, 184, 187, 216, 366
Agricultural
    crops, 210
    expansion, 42, 87
    recession, 41
    sustainability, 48
    technologies, 8
Agro
    chemicals, 278
    ecological, 58
    ecosystem, 41
Agroforestry, 35, 36, 44–48, 50, 101, 167
Agro-industries, 278
Agronomical, 45
Ailments, 9, 94, 98–108, 182, 183, 186, 234, 250, 255, 257, 259–261, 304, 344, 335

Akhuni, 64, 72, 74
Alamus andamanicus, 214
Alangium salvifolium, 322
Albizzia
    odoratissima, 165
    procera, 165
Alcoholic
    beverage, 57, 75–77, 79–82, 86, 88
    drinks, 75
Alcoholic ethnic foods, 71
Alkaloids, 94, 281, 322, 330, 358
Alleppey turmeric, 294
Allium, 63, 78, 111, 187, 253, 322
Allopathic, 12, 178, 186, 256
Alluvial plains, 97
Alnus nepalensis, 47, 48, 111
Aloysia gratissima, 283
Alpinia nigra, 108, 111
Aluminum vessels, 213
    buchu, 213
Ammonification, 40
Amomum dealbatum, 62
Amylase, 331
Anamirta cocculus, 171, 217
Ancestral spirits, 71, 75, 85
Ancient literature, 94, 95, 280
Ancistrocladus korupensis, 281
Andaman and Nicobar Islands, 1, 3–5, 6, 9, 10, 12, 17, 60, 61, 178, 183, 186, 203, 208, 210, 211, 213, 215, 234, 238, 298
Andhra Pradesh, 294, 295, 353
Andrographis paniculata, 113, 320, 321, 323
Andrographolide, 323
Anemia, 59, 136, 304
Angami, 6, 19, 20, 25, 26, 63, 74, 77, 84, 105, 108, 253, 260
Angiosperms, 100, 106, 261

Angkur, 81, 82
Animal
  feeds, 61
  husbandry, 9, 46, 181, 183
Animism, 6
Anishi, 64, 72, 74
Annesia fragrans, 102
Anodendron paniculatum, 211, 217, 235, 245
Anthropogenic, 36, 282
  pressure, 277
  training, 271
Anthropologists, 238
Anthropology, 271
Antibacterial, 305–307
Antibiotics, 184, 355
Anticancer/anticough/antifever, 102
Antidandruff effects, 306
Antidiabetic, 12, 102, 103, 115, 120, 125, 131, 139, 309, 318–322, 324, 326, 327, 331–333, 335, 337, 340, 342, 343, 345
  activity, 103, 318, 319, 324, 327, 331, 332, 340, 345
  plants, 2, 12, 318
Anti-diarrheal, 102
Antifertility, 99, 107, 261
Antifungal, 305
Anti-fungal properties, 251
Antihyperglycaemic, 330, 343
Antihyperglycemic
  action, 326
  activity, 324
Antihypertensive, 102
Anti-inflammatory, 100, 229, 304–307, 309
  agent, 304, 306
  properties, 100
Anti-jaundice plants, 98
Antimalarial
  compound, 279
  plants, 108
  therapies, 254
Antimutagen, 305
Antioxidant property, 181
Antiparasitic, 305

Antiperiodic, 219, 305
Antiseptic, 124, 128, 132, 136, 145, 259, 308, 356
Apatanis, 50
Aperient, 219, 305
Apong, 77, 80
Araceae, 243, 255, 322
Archaeological evidence, 180
Areca catechu L. (Betel palm), 5, 113, 188, 218, 323, 356
Arecaceae, 165, 168, 239, 240, 242, 323, 326
Arisaema leschenaulti, 62
Arnam Kethe, 71
Aroma, 67, 76, 85
Aromatic, 80, 299, 303, 356
  resin, 245
Arora, 61
Artabotrys speciosus, 214, 239
Artemisia annua L, 96
Arthritis, 104, 107, 110, 131, 138, 145, 197, 223, 257, 260, 308
Artocarpus chaplasha, 214
Artocarpus heterophyllus, 62, 78, 79, 114, 166, 167, 188, 324, 366
Artocarpus lakoocha, 214
Arunachal Pradesh, 4, 6, 15, 17, 19, 24, 25, 30, 31, 35, 36, 38, 42, 61–63, 71, 76, 82, 97, 100–104, 168, 170, 171, 183, 186, 249, 252, 253, 255, 256
Asparagus racemosus, 108, 114, 189, 324
Aspirin, 280, 309
Assam, 4, 15, 17–19, 24–26, 28, 29, 31, 55, 63, 64, 69, 73, 80–83, 85, 86, 93, 98–104, 106–108, 150, 168, 177, 181–183, 186, 207, 249, 252–255, 323
Asteraceae family, 183
Astringent, 133, 186, 216, 305, 344
Atherogenesis, 319
Atingba/Yu, 80
Australoid, 17, 18
Austro-Asiatic, 6, 15, 17, 18, 215
Ayurveda, 100, 180, 181, 186, 294, 304, 305, 318, 319, 358
Ayurvedic drug company, 280

B

Baccahris articulata, 283
Baccaurea ramiflora, 114, 214, 239
Baccharis crispa, 283
Baiga tribes, 323
Baisakhi, 31
Baked, 66, 241, 243, 307
Baked products, 307
Bakhor, 81
Balms, 307
Balphakrah Wildlife Sanctuary, 98
Bamboo, 20, 27, 30, 38–40, 43, 48, 62, 66–68, 70–75, 80–86, 165, 167, 173, 210, 215
   communities, 167
   containers, 30
   cups, 84
   productivity, 48, 167
   shoot, 64, 84
   thickets, 38
Bambusa spp, 62
   nutans, 64, 69
   spinosa, 186, 189
Bambusa tulda, 62, 115, 171, 189
Banana, 68, 69, 72, 73, 80, 82, 85, 86, 244, 307
Barak valley, 29, 97, 252
Barbadensis, 111, 187, 322
Barringtonia asiatica, 212, 218, 235, 239
Begonia roxburghii, 103, 115
Bejas/Bejins, 99
Bekang, 64, 72
Belphuar tree, 72
Berberis aristata DC, 115, 325
Beverages, 10, 63, 71, 75, 76, 80, 83, 173, 307
Beyul Demojong, 30
   hidden valley of rice, 30
Bhoot jolokia, 85
Bhutan, 17, 30
Bhutias, 30, 170
   wood crafts, 170, 171
Big momos, 86
Biguanides, 319

Bio-amelioration, 48
Biodiversity, 5, 7, 39, 43, 56–59, 61, 93, 97, 106, 108, 164, 210, 244, 249–252, 257, 260, 262, 280
Bioinformatics revolution, 10
Biological
   compounds., 178
   diversity, 8, 38, 56, 97, 103, 179, 284, 309
   invasions, 38
   traits, 18
Biomass, 40, 46, 48
Biomes, 97, 252
Biomolecules, 273
Biophytum sensitivum, 325
Bioprospecting, 7, 8, 10, 11, 270, 273, 275, 278–281, 285, 286
Bioresources, 186, 281, 282, 285
Biscuits, 307
Bisdemethoxycurcumin, 299
Bixa orellana, 169, 189
Blood purifier, 113, 129, 136, 305
Blood thinning medications, 309
Blood Urea Nitrogen (BUN), 326
Bodo tribes, 19
Body ache, 110, 122, 257
Boiled, 66, 166, 331, 367
Boiling process/boils, 112, 114, 115, 124, 131, 141, 148, 149, 217, 220, 223, 226, 229, 230, 232, 257, 299, 305
Boric acid, 308
Botanical
   families, 76, 238
   name, 261, 318
Botanical Survey of India, 214
Botanical training, 271
Botanist, 283
Botano-chemicals, 164
Brahmaputra, 3, 4, 29, 97, 98, 99, 252
Brewing, 75
British Pharmacopoeia (BP), 15, 17,, 185
Broad implementation, 44
Brucia javanica L., 325
Buddhist monasteries, 171
Burns, 118, 122, 132, 226, 257

C

Curcuma
  aeruginosa, 297, 298, 303
  angustifolia, 281, 297, 298
  aromatica, 297, 298, 300–302
  auriculata, 327
  collina, 168
  decipiens, 297, 298
  erectus, 168
  flagellum, 168
  floribundus, 168
  guruba, 168
  inermis, 168
  kwangsiensis, 298
  latifolius, 168
  leptospadix, 168
  longa, 11, 169, 296, 297, 299,
    300–302, 331
  malabarica, 298
  montana, 297, 298
  ochrorhiza, 298
  pierreana, 298
  pseudomontana, 297, 298
  tenuis, 168
  zedoaria, 297, 298, 300, 301, 303
Caatinga vegetation, 282
Caesalpinia bonduc, 108, 219
Caesalpinia bonducella (L.) Fleming
    Bonduc nut (Cesalpinaceae), 326
Calamoideae, 168
Calamus tenuis, 103
Calculus formation, 355
Callicarpa arborea, 103, 117
Canarium euphyllum, 219, 235, 245
Cane strips, 215
Canes, 20, 168, 173
Canna indica L, 326
Capparis jacobinae, 282
Car Nicobar Island, 234
Caraway seeds, 304
Carbohydrates, 214, 299, 359
Cardamom, 47, 358
Cardiac glycosides, 280
Cardiovascular diseases, 11

Carica papaya, 118, 190, 211, 240, 245,
    326, 361, 366
Caries, 354–356, 359, 369
Carminative, 117, 305
Carthamus tinctorius L, 169
Cassia
    auriculata, 308, 321, 327
    podocarpa, 281
Castanopsis indica, 172
Caucasoid, 18
Cedrela odorata L, 282
Cedrus deodora, 108, 366
Celastrus stylosa, 5
Celosia argentea L, 119, 328
Cephalostachyum capitatum, 62
Cereals, 37, 46, 67, 307
Chakma tribe, 106, 261
Chamdo region of Tibet, 27
Cheese, 306, 359
Chemical drugs, 184
Chemoprospecting, 278
Chewing stems, 238
Child birth, 98, 144, 218, 225, 257
Chilies, 66, 67, 72, 73, 85, 86
Chinampa cultivation, 42
Chinese medicinal system, 304
Cho-Jun, 64, 68, 69, 71
Choko/Jonga-mod, 81
Cholagogue, 305
Cholera, 98, 119, 128, 131, 138, 143,
    217, 219, 257
Chromosomal aberrations, 181
Chronic
    cough, 304
    diseases, 8
    hyperglycemia, 11, 319
Chutneys, 306
Cinchona officinalis, 95
Cissus quadrangularis, 120, 186, 191
Citation richness (CR), 276, 277, 278
Citrullus vulgaris, 76, 328
Civilization, 96, 100, 180, 215, 256, 271
Clan, 26, 28
Classic, 41, 42
Clerodendron
    odoratum, 169

colebrookianum, 102
infortunatum, 108, 191
Climate fluctuation, 56
Clinical
   persons, 270, 279
   practice, 250
Codified, 355, 358, 359
Coffee based agroforestry, 47
Colonial rule, 210
Coloring agent, 11
Coloring butter, 306
Colquhounia coccinea, 256
Commiphora mukul, 304, 366
Compact mass, 299
Complexion, 304, 307
Conceptual reorientation, 272
Concerted multidisciplinary, 88
Condiments, 62, 67
Consensus, 270, 275, 276, 284, 286
Conservation, 31, 43, 45–47, 56–58, 88,
   95, 96, 103, 166, 178, 185, 212, 250,
   254–258, 270, 273, 275, 277, 278,
   280, 282, 285, 286
   priority index (CPI), 270, 277,
     282–285
Constipation, 107, 119, 132, 135,
   138–140, 143, 148, 150, 190, 192,
   194, 196, 197, 200, 229, 230, 257
Construction materials, 40, 61
Convention on Biological Diversity
   (CBD), 279, 280
Conventional crops, 88
Cooked beans, 72, 73
Coptis teeta, 108, 122
Coral bedded sea, 245
Cordial, 305
Cortex, 298, 299
Cortical
   meristeles, 299
   vascular bundles, 299
Cosmetics, 11, 270, 278, 286, 301, 307
   uses, 307
Cottage cheese, 86
Cough, 107, 109, 110, 112–116, 120,
   121, 124, 127–136, 138, 139–142,
   145–149, 182, 187, 189, 194–198,

219, 221–223, 226, 230, 231, 233,
   257, 261, 306
Cow therapy, 181
Crafts and furniture, 20
Crateva magna, 330
Creatinine, 336
Crocodile hunting, 244
Crop
   diversity, 18
   improvement, 296, 298, 301
Croton
   caudatus, 123, 169, 191
   joufra, 78, 81
   rhamnifolius, 282
   tiglium, 171
Crude extracts, 96, 106
Cucumis sativus, 64, 108, 192
Cuisines, 244
Culinary methods, 55, 56, 60, 66, 68, 84
   food products, 66
Cultic dish, 305
Cultural Agreement Index (CAI), 277,
   285
Cultural
   continuity, 58
   diversity, 18, 59, 60, 103, 252
   elements, 57
   importance index, 277, 284
   practices, 57, 88, 97
   significance, 270, 275
   value, 61, 63
Cumbersome processes, 244
Curanga amara, 108, 123
Curative properties, 94, 96, 102
Curcuma, 11, 64, 69, 71, 123, 124, 169,
   192, 194, 196, 222, 294–302, 308, 330
   longa L., 192, 294, 295, 308
Curcumin, 294, 299, 300, 305, 306, 308,
   309
Curcuminoids, 11, 299, 301, 302, 306,
   308, 309
Cured rhizome, 298
Curry
   paste, 307
   powders, 306
Cuscuta reflexa, 103, 124, 222

Customary laws, 254
Cycads, 104, 254
Cycas rumphii, 212, 214, 240
Cyclosorus extensus, 78, 171, 172

D

Daemonorops jenkinsianus, 168
Dairy products, 307
Darjeeling Himalayas, 104, 260, 320, 322, 324–330, 333–344
Darlong community, 261
Dasain, 31
Data acquisition, 60
Data
    compilations, 272
    information, 258
Dead tissue decomposition, 41
Debang Biosphere Reserve, 63, 101
Decentralization, 42
Decision-makers, 59
Decoction, 320–325, 328–330, 333, 334, 336, 338, 340–344, 359–362, 365, 366, 368
Deep ravines, 29
Defensive protection, 250, 251
Deforestation, 36, 38, 186
Degree of attention (DA), 277, 278
Demarcation, 17
Demethoxycurcumin, 299
Demineralize, 355
Dental
    care, 354, 355, 369
    pathologies, 359
    problems, 2, 12, 354, 355, 358
    therapeutic applications, 368
Deori
    ethnic group, 76
    tribe, 254
Derris scandens, 172
Despotic chiefs, 15, 25
Detergent, 305
Deterrent, 71, 261
Detrimental effects, 36
Dexamethasone administered rats, 322
Dhemaji district, 29, 104, 182, 255

Diabetes mellitus (DM), 11, 181, 318–321, 325, 327, 338, 343, 345
Diabetic treatment, 318, 320, 323, 327
Dialects, 17, 24, 31, 61
Dibang valley, 25
Dietary, 56, 60, 86, 102, 238, 244, 354
    taboos, 56
Digestive properties, 186, 294
Digitalis purpurea, 280
Digitoxin, 280
Digoxin, 280
Dillenia, 68, 103, 108, 125, 167, 192
Dilution, 87
Diminution, 334
Diocorea alata, 62
Dioscorea
    bulbifera, 125, 214, 223, 240
    glabra, 212, 214, 240
    vexans, 214
Diospyros andamanica, 214, 240
Diphenylalkanoids, 299
Diphenylheptanoids, 299
Diplazium esculentum, 103
Dipterocarpaceae, 39, 357, 361
    Shorea robusta, 357
Direct compression tablets, 307
Disintensification, 42
Dissemination, 185
Diuretic, 131, 220, 223, 227, 305, 325
Diverse
    ethnicity, 17
    stakeholders, 10
Diversitiesethnic, 86
Diversity, 1, 15, 62, 63, 207, 239
    food plants, 55, 60, 238
Documentation, 2, 10, 11, 12, 48, 60, 87, 94, 95, 96, 98, 105, 167, 179, 249, 250, 251, 255, 262, 272, 369
Domestication, 178, 180
Donax canaeformis, 214, 223
Draft animals, 9
Dravidian, 17
Dried bamboo, 73
Drug
    development, 262, 276, 279
    discovery, 95, 270

Dual heath care, 256
Duggirala turmeric, 294
Dugong dugon, 245
Dugout canoe making, 211
Dupka community, 105
Dye
   dyeing wool, 307
   producing plants, 164
   yielding plants, 169, 173, 256
Dyslipidemia, 337
Dysoxylum procerum, 62

E

Earthen
   containers, 75
   pitcher, 81
East Khasi hills, 100
East Siang district, 104, 255
Eastern Himalayas, 4, 61, 97, 102, 105, 252, 258
Eco-friendly methods, 44
Ecological tools, 283
Economic
   activities, 171, 258
   constraints, 44
   potential, 62
   social compulsion, 26
Eco-sustainable model, 36, 48, 50
Ecotourism, 56, 88
Edible flowers, 63
Edible plants, 60– 62, 104, 165, 212, 238, 250, 253, 255, 262, 271
Efficacy, 12, 103, 185, 250, 320, 345, 355
Electronic storage, 10
Eleusine corocana, 76
Emblica officinalis, 47, 62, 127, 140, 165, 166, 308, 332
Emmenagogue, 219, 225, 305
Empirical evidence, 58
Encroachment, 87
Endangered
   orchids, 47
   plant species, 5, 184
Endemic plants, 5

Endemism, 62
Endodermoid ring, 298, 299
Endogamous groups, 17
Endogamy, 15
Endogenous institutions, 59
Environmental
   management, 95
   stress, 88
Ephedrine, 280
Ephemeral fever, 183
Epilepsy, 98, 120, 149, 225, 232
Ergometrine, 280
Eromba, 67, 68, 70
Eryngium foetidum, 244
Ethanolic extract (turmeric), 305, 324, 330, 332, 336, 337, 340, 342
Ethnic
   beverages, 75
   communities, 6–9, 15, 25, 27, 28, 30, 72, 84, 102, 106, 164, 179, 285, 318, 355
   cuisine, 67, 69
   culture, 31, 96
   diversity, 2, 5, 6, 8, 12, 18, 30, 31, 86
   foods, 55–61, 66, 67, 84, 86–88, 181, 208, 238
     plants, 61
     systems, 55, 88
     diversity, 61
   languages, 31
   linguistic, 8
   multiplicity, 15, 93
   people, 60, 95, 103, 208, 262, 320, 369
   plants, 88
   racial groups, 17
   richness, 18
   tapestry, 18
   traditional knowledge, 11
   tribes, 5, 63, 67, 98, 99, 107, 108, 165, 208, 250, 253, 322–329, 331, 332–336, 338–344, 355
Ethnicity, 26, 28, 36, 57, 58, 167, 210

Ethno, 7, 11, 12, 26, 36, 49, 101, 107,
    166, 178, 182, 183, 256, 257, 259,
    261, 275, 278, 281, 282
Ethno documentation, 12
Ethnoagriculture, 2, 7, 35, 36, 41, 49, 50
Ethnobiological studies, 274
Ethnobiologists, 282
Ethnobotanical
    appraisal, 254
    claims, 270
    data, 272, 274, 275, 284
    data techniques, 274
    exploration, 164, 208
    information, 10, 96, 103, 105, 238,
    270
    knowledge, 2, 6, 10, 249, 250, 262,
    282, 284, 318
    phytoresources, 285
    profile, 234
    research, 10, 252, 253, 255, 270–275,
    277, 281–286
    studies, 60, 97, 99, 102–104, 250,
    260, 284
Ethnobotanicity index (EI), 285
Ethnobotanists, 10, 12, 270, 272, 277,
    279, 283, 284
Ethnobotany, 2, 8, 10, 12, 60, 61, 88, 95,
    98, 101, 105, 108, 164, 165, 171, 179,
    238, 245, 253, 262, 269–273, 277,
    281–286, 293–295, 310, 355
Ethnodirected approaches, 281
Ethnoecology, 36, 50, 270, 285
Ethnofood, 2, 245
Ethnographic component, 369
Ethnography, 368
Ethnomedical
    experts, 12
    treatment, 12, 368, 369
Ethnomedicinal
    diversity, 94
    knowledge, 106, 260
    plants, 2, 94, 98, 100–102, 105,
    106–108, 151, 165, 182, 234, 245,
    250, 252, 258–261, 275, 278, 345
    practices, 102
    survey, 257

    treatment, 12, 257
    utility, 100
Ethnomedicine, 97, 99, 164, 165, 279,
    283, 368
Ethnopedology, 48, 167
Ethnopharmacological, 255
Ethnopharmacology, 253, 368
Ethnosciences, 178
Ethnoveterinary, 2, 7, 9, 11, 178, 179,
    181, 182, 183, 184, 185, 186, 203
    medicine, 179, 181, 183, 184, 185
    medicinal plants, 183
Ethnoveterinary practices (EVP), 9, 178,
    181, 182, 183
Ethnozoology, 179
Eupatorium nodiflorum, 102, 128
Euptelia, 5
European Patent Office (EPO), 251
Exploitation, 11, 40, 60, 186, 281

F

Facial
    hair, 307
    proximity, 24
Factor of informant consensus (FIC),
    275, 284
Fallow period, 38–41
Family influence, 256
Famine food, 58, 62
Fenugreek, 343
Fermentation, 57, 67, 72, 73, 77, 76,
    80–84, 86, 87
    process, 72, 73
    technologies, 57
Fermented
    bamboo shoots, 67, 73, 74
    beans, 72
    ethnic foods, 71, 84
    foods, 57, 67, 76, 86
    millet, 30
Fertile plains, 26
Fertility restoration capacity, 36
Festive occasions, 254
Fiber yielding
    plants, 164

properties, 256
Ficus, 73, 129, 167, 193, 194, 211, 214, 224, 236, 240, 241, 254, 332, 333, 356, 357, 361, 362, 366
  benghalensis L.: Banyan tree (Moraceae), 332
Fidelity level (FL), 275, 276, 284
Filtration, 80, 82, 83, 87
Fishing technology, 245
Fistula, 118, 190, 259, 304, 327
Flavonoids, 94, 96, 179, 299, 322, 330
Flavonol compound, 299
Flavoring
  agent, 303
  purpose, 307
Flemingea strobilifera, 108
Flora, 2, 4, 10, 31, 95, 97, 105, 168, 212, 250, 256, 277, 282, 285, 355
Floral diversity, 40, 93, 101
Faunal diversity, 17
Floristic diversity, 8, 318
Flossing, 356
Flotsam, 214
Folk
  knowledge, 178, 270
  medical systems, 11
  medicine, 99, 234, 254, 257, 298, 303, 305, 325, 327
Folklore claim, 333
Folkloric treatment, 104
Folkloristic significance, 95
Food additives, 278
Food and Agricultural Organization(FAO), 38, 44, 57
Food
  applications, 306
  colorant, 294, 301
  culture, 84, 245
  flavoring, 293
  plants, 7, 8, 10, 12, 55–57, 60–63, 87, 88, 212, 238, 255
  practices, 58
  systems, 7, 8, 56–60, 84, 87, 88, 178, 211
Fungus-infested balls, 83
Future prospects, 270, 286

G

Galo tribe, 71, 76, 82
Garcinia
  cowa, 129, 194, 214, 241
  kola, 281
  xanthochymus, 169
Garo Hills, 28, 98, 259
Garos, 28, 253
Gastrointestinal, 106, 115, 126, 131, 146
  ailments, 106
Gelatin capsules, 307
Gelatinized lumps, 298
Gelatins, 307
Genetic
  disorder, 319
  potential, 47
  resources, 57, 278
Germplasm, 42
Ginger based agroforestry system, 47
Gingival, 354, 355, 356, 369
Gingivitis, 354, 355, 359
Ginsenodies, 96
Glaphylopteriosis erubescens, 73
Global
  consumers, 172
  ecosystem, 5
  level, 164
  perspective, 286
Globalization, 8, 56, 59, 87
Glucose absorption, 326
Glutinous rice, 76, 80, 82
Gnetum gnemon, 64, 65, 68, 70
Gohpur, 99, 182
Gompas, 30
Grain maturity stage, 43
Grazing, 40
Great Andamanese, 6, 171, 208, 210–212, 238–243, 245
Gymnema sylvestre, 308, 320, 323, 330, 333
Gymnocladus assamicus, 184
Gynocardia odorata, 130, 171, 334, 362

H

Hajong community, 103

Haldi, 294
Halitosis, 354, 356
Hangla, 80
   Alocasia sp., 80, 111, 322
Hanmoi, 64, 68
Hanserong anempo, 64, 68
Hanthor (ethnic food), 64, 68
Haridra, 294, 296
Harpoon lines, 171, 211
Ha-un (Andaman pig), 186
Hawaizaar (ethnic food), 64, 72
Health
   care
      needs, 258
      system, 96, 256
   practice, 178
   practitioners, 106, 254
Heart burn, 304
Heartwood, 340
Hedeoma multiflora, 283
Hedgerow cropping, 47
Hedychium coronarium Koenig, 4, 130
Helicteres isora, 334
Hemorrhages, 98
Hemostatic, 122, 123, 135, 141, 305
Hepatic cells, 335
Hepatoprotective, 99, 106, 280, 305
Herbal
   formulations, 345
   medicinal remedies, 252
   medicine, 43, 101, 184, 261, 262, 270
   mixtures, 306
   plants, 12, 255, 318, 319
   practices, 186
   remedies, 256, 345
Herbalists, 320
Herbarium curator, 283
Herbomineral formulation, 308
Heterogeneity, 19, 67
Hexokinase, 343
Hibiscus, 64, 65, 68, 70, 130, 171, 194,
   225, 241, 244, 245, 334, 356
   sabdariffa, 64, 65, 68, 70, 130, 194,
   244
High
   blood pressure control, 257

demographic growth, 38
   intensity sweetener, 281
   yield crops, 8
Hilly tracts, 7, 26, 186
Him duk/Sang aduk, 68
Himadri, 2, 3
Himalayan bear, 172
Himalayas flowers, 326
Him-et, 64, 69
Hmar tribal, 6, 18, 19, 21, 27, 28, 64,
   73, 107
Holud/haldi, 294
Homalanthus nutans, 280
Homemade jaggery, 69
Homeostasis, 319
Homogeneity, 276
Hor, 81
Horis, 215
Human
   civilization, 95
   immunodeficiency virus (HIV), 280,
   305, 306
Humankind, 293
Hunter-gatherer, 7, 214
Hypoglycemic effect, 321, 322, 325,
   329, 334, 338, 342
Hypolipidemic, 305, 323, 329, 340
Hyponidd, 308
Hypotensive drug, 309
Hypothetical growth model, 41

I

Ibuprofen, 309
Ichnocarpus frutescens, 108, 225
Immature fruits, 244
Impatiens, 4, 108
   balsamina, 108
Imperata cylindrica, 40, 131, 335
Importance value index, 275, 277
Incantations, 75
Indian Council of Agricultural Research
   (ICAR), 48
Indian
   government, 251
   linguistic groups, 17

Pharmacopoeia, 185
population, 18
scenario, 286
Indices (quantitative/statistical), 270, 272, 275, 277, 284, 286
Indigenous
beverages, 75
community, 258
dugouts, 215
knowledge, 57, 63, 88, 95, 105, 107, 108, 172, 179, 181, 256, 258, 260
people, 57–61, 66, 95, 238, 255, 279, 282
protocols, 76
tribal, 6, 210
Indigestion, 107, 109–112, 117, 120, 127, 131, 137, 138, 141, 146, 149, 187, 191, 197, 198, 257
Indigo, 169, 307
Indigofera tinctoria, 169, 367
Indo-Burma, 61, 102, 164, 166, 172, 252, 257, 259
Indo-European, 11, 17, 18
language speakers, 17
Indogangetic plains, 2
Indo-Myanmarese Range, 3
Induced diabetic rats, 321, 324, 326, 327, 332, 334, 337, 340–342
Industrialization, 96
Inflamed joints, 305
Influenza, 124, 135, 150, 233, 257
Informants, 257, 270, 274, 276
Inhabitants, 19, 25, 26, 29, 81, 97, 213, 215, 234, 244, 343
Inhospitable terrians, 256
Insulin
deficiency, 319
gene, 11
secretion, 11, 319
Insulin-sensitizing activity, 334
Intellectual property, 88
Interviews, 254, 274
Intoxicants, 185
Investigators, 97
Ipomoea batatas, 131, 172, 194, 335

Irregular menstruation, 135, 140, 254, 257

J

Jadoh, 64, 69, 70, 85
Jaintia
Hills, 28, 62, 98
tribes, 258
Jantias, 29
Jarawas, 6, 208, 210, 213, 214, 238
Jaundice, 98, 104, 107, 111, 113–115, 117–121, 127, 133, 137, 139, 140, 148, 218, 219, 229, 233, 255, 257, 259–261, 304, 305
Jeopardizing, 59
Jhoom
cycles, 39, 41
system, 44, 45
Jhooming, 36, 38–40, 45
Jhum
cultivation, 7, 27
ecosystems, 8
system, 41
Jonai sub-division, 182
Jonga, 81
Jou, 81
Judima, 77, 82
Julocroton argenteus, 283
Jungle-clad ridges, 29
Justicia comata, 169

K

Kabui, 19, 21, 27, 253
Kacha Naga, 27
Kalanchoe pinnata, 336
Kameng district, 25
Kamrup district, 254
Kangchendzonga, 30
Karbi
ethnic group, 63, 76
tribe, 19, 68, 70, 71, 73
Karbi-Anglong district, 19, 29
Karbis, 19, 68–71, 81, 85, 252
Karnataka, 207, 294, 295, 297, 298, 353
Kerala, 294, 295, 297, 298

Khaimungan, 25
Khangchendzonga Biosphere Reserve, 100, 182
Khariff season, 210
Khasis, 17, 19, 28–30, 76, 99, 186
Kiad, 82
  khawiang, 82
Kidney stone, 102, 259
Kinema, 64, 72, 73
Kitchen garden plants, 62
Kokrajhar districts, 29
Kolakhar, 64, 69, 85
Kolaviron, 281
Kom tribe, 182
Komba, 244
Ksharasoothra, 304
Kuki-Chin-Mizo, 26
Kum dye, 170
Kurkum, 294

L

Lactuca gracilis, 103
Lagenaria leucantha, 186, 194
Lake Texcoco, 41
Lalramnghinglova, 62, 102, 125, 164, 182, 187– 200, 259
Lamiaceae, 255, 338, 341, 362, 367
Land management units, 44, 45
Land use systems, 36, 44, 45, 48
Langpong, 73
Leaf trace bundles, 299
Leech therapy, 304
Legitimacy, 59
Lekok, 186
Lepcha dances, 30
Lepchas, 30, 100, 105, 170
Lepidocaryoideae, 168
Leprosy, 98, 113, 119, 138, 220, 304, 305, 344
Leucorrhea, 254
Life-saving drugs, 273
Limboo, 22, 105
Lipid reduction, 306
Lippia turbinata, 283
Litchumsu, 84

Literacy rate, 28
Litter fall, 40, 48
Livestock
  health management, 203
  owners, 179
Local conservation priority index (LCPI), 270, 277, 278, 282, 285, 286
Local
  development, 88
  economy, 46
  inhabitants, 282
  Level Conservation of Phytoresources Employing, 282
  liquor, 82
  name, 99, 261
Locality, 87, 276, 277, 282, 283
Lohit district of Arunachal Pradesh, 25, 103
Lungseiji, 64, 69
Lushai Hills, 97, 252

M

Machilus gamblei, 169
Macrophages, 181
Magnolia, 5, 241
Maiba/Maibi, 107, 256
Maibra joubishi, 82
Makar Sankranti, 31
Malaxis acuminata, 5
Malevolent spirits, 212
Malnutrition, 8
Mangifera
  andamanica, 214, 241
  comptospermum, 211, 241
  indica, 62, 134, 195, 211, 242, 336, 356, 357, 362
Mannihot esculenta, 172
Manthu, 68
Marine products, 244
Marsdenia tinctoria, 169
Masala mixtures, 307
Materialistic life, 87
Matha joubishi, 82
Maththi, 244
Matriarchal law of inheritance, 29

Maturant, 305
Mautam, 62
Mechanical soil, 45
Medicinal
   folklore, 280
   parts, 261
   plants, 7, 8, 10, 12, 43, 47, 63,
      97–108, 182–186, 250, 254–262,
      318–320
      cultivation, 47
   preparations, 102, 185, 308
   purposes, 93–95, 101, 294, 318, 323
   uses, 98, 107, 234, 257, 259, 294,
      305, 310
   values, 87, 185, 186
Medicine, 10, 57, 63, 94–96, 98, 100,
   103, 104, 107, 178–185, 208, 215,
   234, 250, 251, 255–257, 259, 261,
   275, 294, 298, 303–305, 318, 369
   naturopathy, 104, 259
Meghalaya, 3, 4, 6, 15, 17, 19, 24, 28,
   30, 32, 38, 40, 48, 61–63, 69, 73, 74,
   82, 84–86, 98–100, 107, 165, 166,
   168, 171, 186, 249, 252, 253, 258, 259
Meitei
   community, 72–74, 107, 257, 320,
      321, 327, 329, 343
   tribe, 80, 325, 339
Meliosma simplifolia, 254
Melocana bambosoides, 62
Melocanna baccifera, 62
Melting pot, 18, 86
Menstruation problems, 104, 255
Mental yoga, 180
Metabolic diseases, 11
Methai community, 26
Methanol extract, 327, 333
Methodological tools, 284
Methods of preparation, 7, 56, 104, 259
Michelia oblonga, 48
Microbial
   growth, 86
   strains, 355
Microscopical characters, 294
Mikir hills, 3, 4, 26, 253
Millingtonia hortensis, 103, 227

Minthostachys mollis, 283
Mishing
   people, 80
   tribe, 104, 255
Mizo Tribe, 28
Mizoram, 4, 15, 17, 19, 24, 32, 35, 37,
   38, 45, 47, 49, 62, 72, 99–101, 163,
   165, 173, 182, 250, 252, 253, 259
Mod pitha, 76, 83
Modern medications, 256
Molar basis, 281
Molded mass, 76
Molecular interactions, 345
Molecules of medicinal importance, 8
Mollusk, 213
Momordica charantia, 136, 196, 227,
   308, 337, 367
Mompa tribe, 25
Mongoloid, 17, 18, 31, 211, 215, 234
Mongoloid
   aborigines, 215
   racial stock, 18
Monitor lizard, 213, 214
Mon-Khmer family, 29
Monoculture, 8, 44, 45
Monoterpenes, 299
Morinda angustifolia, 169
Moringa oleifera, 136, 196, 244, 337,
   363
Mouth ulcers, 114, 147, 366–369
Mucus production, 41
Multipronged stick, 170
Muruku, 244
Musa, 62–64, 69, 72, 76, 85, 137, 184,
   196, 211, 242, 244, 338
   balbisiana, 64
   paradiasica, 62
Mustard, 67, 68, 86

N

Naga Hills, 25, 252, 253
Nagaland, 4, 6, 15, 17, 19, 24–26, 32,
   38, 46, 82, 84, 85, 98, 101, 102,
   105–108, 164, 168, 186, 250, 252,
   253, 259, 260

Nagbeli, 325
National Bureau of Plant Genetic
　Resources (NBPGR), 4
Natural
　communities, 39
　compounds, 94
　ecosystems, 47
　habitats, 56, 87
　products, 94, 172, 270, 280, 281,
　　286, 318
Natural resource management., 44, 57
Naturalness rank, 277
Negrito, 17, 210, 211, 213, 214, 234
Negrito stock, 210
Nematicidal activities, 106
Nempo, 69
Nepalese, 30
Nephropathy, 11, 319
Neuropathy, 11, 319
Nicobarese, 6, 17, 183, 208, 215, 234
Nicotiana tabacum, 137, 186, 196
Nidzurku Hills, 26
Nitrogen cycle, 41
N-mineralization, 40
Nogin Apong, 80
　e'pob, 78, 80
Non Insulin Dependent Diabetes
　Mellitus (NIDDM), 319, 344
Non-alcoholic foods, 71
Non-codified, 355, 359
Non-fermented ethnic foods, 67
Non-timber forest produce (NTFP), 164
Non-tuberous species, 295
North East India, 1, 3, 4–6, 8–10, 17–19,
　25, 31, 33, 35, 36, 48, 49, 55, 94,
　97–99, 101–106, 108, 109, 151, 163,
　164, 167, 169, 182, 249, 251, 262,
　327, 328, 341
Northeast region, 252
Nutraceuticals, 8, 58, 255, 270, 286
Nutrient cycling, 48, 164, 167
Nutritional
　contents, 58, 63
　importance, 281
　profiles, 87
Nypa fruticans, 211, 228, 237, 242

O

Ocimum gratissimum, 71, 108, 138, 196
Ointment, 305, 308
Onge shelters, 212
Onges, 6, 208, 210, 212, 239–243, 245
Onlawangkhrai, 85
Opo, 82
Opoh, 80
Opop, 83
Oral
　administration, 326, 329, 330, 332,
　　342
　compositions, 308
　dental hygiene, 12
　hygiene, 354, 355, 369
Orchidaceae, 39
Oroxylum indicum, 102, 139, 196, 228,
　242, 338
Osomar nempo chori, 69
Oxalis griffithii, 103
Oxygenating agents, 355

P

Psidium
　odaratissimus, 244
　tectorius, 244
Paddy cultivation, 43
Paite, 6, 23, 27
Pakora, 244
Palatability, 67
Panax pseudoginseng, 99, 139, 339
Pancreatic beta cells, 321, 322
Pandanus, 5, 66, 211, 212, 215, 228,
　237, 242, 305
　leram, 244
　andamanensium, 211, 242
Papaver somniferum, 95, 139
Paralysis, 98, 111, 127, 144, 220
Paravachasca valley, 283
Parenchyma, 274, 298, 301
Parkia roxburghii, 48, 140, 339
Participatory rural appraisal (PRA), 183,
　274
Pasania pachyphylla, 169, 170
Passiflora caerulea, 283

Pastoralists, 9
  yak pastoralists, 170
Peppercorn hairs, 210
Peppery taste, 306
Pericarp, 335
Perpur, 83
Petioles, 230, 238
Phagocytosis, 181
Phanek, 169
Phap, 81
Pharmaceutical products, 8, 94, 185,
  270, 277–279, 286, 307
Pharmacokinetic properties, 319
Pharmacological evidence, 333
Pharmacologists, 270, 279
Pharmacopoeias, 355
Phenylpropene derivatives, 299
Phlogacanthus thyrsiformis, 108, 257
Pholo, 68, 85
Pholobisir, 68, 85
Phosphoglucoisomerase, 343
Phytochemical screening, 186
Phytochemistry, 12, 278, 294, 295, 310
Phytochemists, 11, 270, 279
Phytomedicines, 279
Phytoresources, 270, 273, 275, 278, 281,
  285
    quantitative ethnobotany, 278
    quantitative ethnobotany,
      bioprospecting, 278
    conservation, 281
Piazu, 84
Pickles, 164, 165, 244, 298, 306
Pilchards, 212
Pinanga manii, 99, 214, 242, 244
Pinus kesiya, 48
Piperr longum, 108
Pisciculture, 43
Pith, 211, 242, 298, 331
Plant and bird communities recovery, 39
Plant
    bark decoction, 323
    knowledge, 272
    populations, 258
    specimens, 271
    uptake, 40

Plantago major, 141, 184, 197, 363
Plastic mesh, 84
Plectocomia bractealis, 168
Pochury tribe, 25, 26
Polyalthia jenkinsii, 212, 237
Polygonum, 68, 142, 171, 172, 197
    hydropiper L., 142, 171, 172
Polyherbal drug, 321, 322, 327
Pometia pinnata, 213, 214, 243
Pongamia pinnata, 142, 230, 243, 339,
  356, 363
Powders, 354, 358
Prawn aquaculture, 46
Preparation methods, 56, 61, 208, 238
Primitive angiosperms, 5
Principles of patrilineal descent, 26
Prostratin, 280
Protein, 11, 214, 299, 319
Protium serratum, 62
Prunus persica, 102, 142, 197
Psidium guajava L, 78, 142, 197, 243,
  340
Pteridophyte, 106, 261, 283
Pteridophytic flora, 101
Pterocarpus marsupium, 308, 331, 340,
  363
Pushpangadan model, 280
Pyrnium pubinerve, 72

Q

Quality use value (QUV), 285
Quantitative
    approaches, 10, 272
    ethnobotany, 12, 278, 281, 286
    indices, 270, 272, 275, 282, 284–286
    technique, 270, 273, 275
Quenching, 238
Quercus spp, 170
    dealbata, 170
    wallichiana, 170
Quinine, 279

R

Radical, 87
Raja mircha, 85

Raphidophora sp, 68
Rapid rural appraisal(RRA), 274
Rasasastra, 304
Rawolfia serpentina, 95
Reang
   communities, 106, 261
   tribe, 105
Reangs, 86, 98, 106
Reciprocity, 57
Relative cultural importance, 275
Relative density (RD), 277, 278
Relative frequency of citation (RFC), 277, 284
Rengma tribe, 26
Researchers, 282, 285
Reserpine, 280, 309
Respiratory disorders, 106
Retinopathy, 11, 319
Retrieval databases, 10
Rheumatoid arthritis, 306
Rhizome, 109–113, 122, 123, 126, 130–132, 135–137, 140, 143, 148, 150, 183, 187, 189–192, 195, 198, 200, 216, 221, 222, 226, 233, 293, 294, 298–300, 305–307, 322, 330–332, 335, 336, 339, 344, 361, 365
Rhododendron, 4, 105, 143, 170, 171, 197
Rhus javanica, 62, 197
Rhynchotecum ellipticum, 68
Rice, 64, 67, 70, 76, 85
Rice beer preparation, 81, 254
Ritual
   ceremonies, 294
   occasions, 68
Roasted, 62, 66, 239, 240, 326
Root
   decomposition, 40
   powder, 298, 322
Root canal treatment, 354
Rubia
   cordifolia, 144, 198, 256, 364
   sikkimensis, 256
Rubus rugossus, 108
Rural
   development, 58

populations, 104, 255, 345

S

Sabroom, 106, 261
Saccharifying agent, 79
Saccharum spontaneum, 103
Safflower, 307
Sakthi worship, 296
Salem turmeric, 295
Sangtam, 23, 25, 108, 253, 260
Sanjivani, 181
Santirbazar subdivision, 261
Sapientum var. *simiarum*, 211
Sarchoclamys pulcherrima, 254
Saya a-an, 70, 71, 85
Schinopsis brasiliensis, 282, 283
Scientific
   discipline, 271
   education, 59
   evaluation, 181
   publications, 180
Scorpion sting, 117, 129, 182, 191, 219
Seafoods, 244
Sema, 6, 19, 23, 25, 26, 105, 253, 260
Semangs, 210
Sensitivity rank, 277
Sentinelese, 208, 210, 214, 215, 238–243
Sesame, 66–71
Sesamum orientale, 68, 69, 145
Sesbania sesban L, 341
Sesquiterpenes, 299
Shephoumaramth Nagas, 99
Shifting agricultural cycle, 46
Shifting agriculture, 36
Shifting cultivation, 36–39, 41, 43–45, 49, 50, 57, 61, 178
Shompen, 208, 215
Shorea robusta, 170, 357, 364
Short fallow rotation, 40
Shrubs, 44, 45, 47, 283
Siiyeh, 79, 83
Sikkim, 4, 15, 17, 24, 29–32, 47, 62, 64, 72, 84, 86, 98, 100, 103, 165, 168,

171, 182, 186, 250, 252, 253, 260, 320, 322, 324–330, 333–344
Myel Lyang, 29
Sikkimese society, 30
Sing river, 63
Sino-Tibetan language family, 6, 25
Skeleto-muscular disorders, 182
Skin diseases, 104, 107, 257, 260
Slash and burn
    agriculture, 36, 39, 56
    agroecosystem, 46
    system, 38
Small pox, 116, 221, 230, 233, 257, 304
Smoke shield, 308
Smoked, 66
Snuhi, 304
Socio cultural
Soibum, 64, 73, 74
Soil
    erosion, 38, 44, 45
    fertility, 40, 43, 45, 46, 167
        depletion, 40
    hydro-physical behavior, 48
    organic carbon (SOC), 47, 48
    perception, 48, 167
Soil quality index (SQI), 48, 167
Solanaceae, 255, 341, 344, 361, 362, 368
Solanum myriacanthum, 108
Solanum viarum, 78, 103, 364
Soluble turmeric, 307
Sovereign rights, 280
Spatial arrangement, 44, 45
Spilanthes acmella, 108, 146, 172, 364
Spinacia oleracea L, 341
Spiranthes oleracea, 171
Spiritual life, 87, 258
Sprains, 144, 217, 257, 304
Starch grains, 298, 299
Starter cakes, 76, 79–81, 86
Statistical
    analysis, 270, 272
    indices, 272, 286
    measurements, 283
Stellaria reticulata, 5
Stemona tuberosa, 108

Steroids, 94, 322
Stimulant, 120, 218, 220, 225, 230, 303, 305
Stir fried, 67
Stomach problems, 114, 140, 304
Stomachic, 219, 228, 305
Streptozotocin, 324, 327, 337, 342
Strobilanthes
    cusia, 170
    flaccidifolia, 170
Stupefying, 171
Subabul, 47
Sub-Himalayan Terai, 63
Submerged alcoholic fermentation, 76
Succession, 39, 40
Sujen, 83, 254
Sulphonylureas, 319
Suppresses thrombosis, 306
Surachi, 81
Sustainable
    development, 164
    food-production systems, 36
    utilization, 273, 282
Swertia chirata, 108, 147, 198, 199
Symbiotic relationship, 37
Synergistic effect, 94, 97
Systemic interactions, 42
Syzygium cumini, 106, 147, 199, 320, 321, 324, 336, 337, 342, 365, 368

T

Taboos, 211, 234, 257
Tai-Kadai languages, 6
Tai-Khamyangs, 102, 252
Tamang, 23, 80, 105
Taxa, 5, 9, 62, 98, 107, 168, 276, 282, 283
Taxonomist, 283
Taxus baccata, 99, 148
Techniques, 8, 272, 274, 275, 283, 284
Technological development, 59
Tectona grandis, 170, 365
Telangana, 207, 293–295, 317, 353
Teohar, 31
Teotihuacan era, 42

Tephrosia candida, 171
Terminali bellirica, 170
Terminali
    catappa, 211, 214, 243
    chebula, 148, 199, 324, 368
Terpenoids, 94, 299, 322, 358
Tethyys Himalaya, 3
Tetracentron, 5
Thalictrum foliolosum, 148, 183, 199
Thanka painting, 30
Thap aphi, 81
Thatch grasslands, 38
Thaumatin, 281
Thaumatococcus danielli, 281
The Tropical Botanic Garden and
    Research Institute (TBGRI), 280
Therapeutic
    drugs, 318
    efficiency, 354
    potentiality, 331
    potentials, 75
    skills, 180
    value, 8
    weight loss, 306
Therapeutics aids, 179
Thingtam/Mautam, 62
Thirumoorthy hills, 322, 328
Thukpa, 86
Tibet, 3, 5, 19, 24, 30
    Tibeto-Burman, 17, 29
Tonic, 112, 115, 123, 127, 146, 188, 190,
    195, 216, 219–222, 228, 280, 305
Tooth paste/powders, 369
Toothache, 107, 109, 114, 123, 128–132,
    136, 138, 145, 149, 228, 230, 257
Tooth
    brushes, 356
    pastes, 358
Total
    state population, 24
    tribal population, 26–29
    use value, 275
Totemism, 6
Traditional
    cattle, 178
    communities, 7, 9, 105

customs, 254
drugs, 318
eco-technologies, 46
foods, 8, 57, 58, 59, 60, 63, 87
healers, 101, 102, 104, 178, 183, 256,
    258, 260, 262, 279, 345
herbal drugs, 177
knowledge, 6–11, 20, 31, 36, 56–61,
    75, 86, 88, 95–104, 107, 172, 182,
    186, 245, 250, 251, 258, 259, 261,
    271, 274, 280, 282, 284, 285
    Digital Library (TKDL), 251
languages, 250
medicinal
    practices, 61, 186
    safety, 250
medicine, 108, 178, 184, 250, 258,
    260, 279, 304, 318, 345
practices, 19, 41, 60, 95, 100, 105,
    178, 253, 260, 271
shamans, 71
uses, 104, 254, 303
vegetables, 244
Trial and error method, 97, 271
Tribal
    communities, 5, 9, 10, 15, 18, 19, 25,
    27–29, 31, 63, 75, 87, 97, 208, 252,
    255, 285
    diversity, 60, 211
    medicine, 100, 151, 260
    nutrition, 61
    segment, 18
    societies, 42, 46, 256
Tribals, 5, 6, 61, 62, 75, 85, 178,
    211–213, 234, 253, 320, 337, 354
Tripura, 4, 15, 17, 18, 24, 27, 32, 39,
    86, 100, 101, 105, 106, 168, 250, 252,
    253, 260, 261
Trixis divaricata, 283
Trochus, 213
Tropical forests, 101
Tuaithur, 64, 73
Tubers, 62, 66, 211, 213, 214
Tubocurarine, 279, 280
Tungrymbai, 64, 73, 74

Turbo, giant clams, 213
Turmeric, 2, 11, 12, 69, 70, 71, 73, 190, 210, 293–296, 298, 299, 301–310, 330, 331
  leaves, 307
  paste, 307
  uses, 294, 295, 301, 304
Turtles eggs, 213
Typhoid, 98, 120, 138, 145

U

Up-thor, 73
Up-vai, 71
Urbanization, 31
Urea, 336
Use value (UV), 270, 275, 276, 284
Utilitarian ethnobotany, 11

V

Vaiphui, 27
Valuable heritage, 252
Vanaspati, 306
Vascular bundles, 298–301
Vegetable dyes, 20
Vegetation, 2–5, 39–41, 44, 45, 272, 273, 282, 283
Vekur pitha, 83
Veterinary
  fees, 179
  plants, 12
  science, 180, 181
Vinblastine, 280
Vitamins, 94, 122, 214, 299
Vitex negudo, 108

W

Warfarin, 309
Watershed programs, 45
Watery-milky juice, 245
Wedding rituals, 305
Weed
  biomass, 38, 46

infestation, 40
West Khasi hills, 100
Wild
  boars, 213, 244
  food plants, 61
  fruits, 238
Wildlife Institute of India (WII), 39
Wokha Hills, 26
Wooden
  mortar, 68, 69, 73, 84
  skewer, 66
Woodfordia fruticosa, 256
World Health Organization (WHO), 11, 95, 178, 184, 318–320

X

Xaj Pani, 83
Xochimilco-Chalco area, 42

Y

Yellow
  cakes, 307
  dye, 169, 303, 307
Yogurts, 307

Z

Zanthoxylum nitidum, 171
Zea mays, 149, 172, 200
Zingeberous plant, 83
  oko, 83
Zingiber
  cassumunar, 102, 150
  officinale, 78, 102, 150, 200, 233, 308, 344, 365
  squarossum, 238
  zerumbet, 102, 233
Zingiberaceae, 4, 11, 100, 101, 255, 294, 295, 330, 336, 365
Zingiberaceous plants, 98, 101
Ziro valley, 42, 43, 255
Ziziphus joazeiro, 282, 283
Zutho, 77, 84